# Scientific Aspects of Steroids

# Scientific Aspects of Steroids

Edited by **Janet Hoffman**

FOSTER
ACADEMICS

New Jersey

Published by Foster Academics,
61 Van Reypen Street,
Jersey City, NJ 07306, USA
www.fosteracademics.com

**Scientific Aspects of Steroids**
Edited by Janet Hoffman

International Standard Book Number: 978-1-63242-361-0 (Hardback)

Printed in the United States of America.

# Contents

# Preface

This book presents various scientific and technical aspects of steroids. It provides an explanation of the basic science of steroids and is aimed at catering to the professionals engaged in health services. It should be kept in mind that medical science evolves at a rapid pace and a few important concepts, like the understanding of steroids and their therapeutic use, may readily transform with emergence of new concepts. Steroids can be either synthetic fat-soluble or naturally occurring organic compounds. They are present in fungi, plants and animals. They mediate a varied set of biological responses. Among these, cholesterol is the most common steroid in the body. It is an important part of cell membranes and also the starting point for the synthesis of other steroids. The aim of this book is to provide valuable information to the readers and enrich their knowledge about this interesting medical topic of steroids.

The information contained in this book is the result of intensive hard work done by researchers in this field. All due efforts have been made to make this book serve as a complete guiding source for students and researchers. The topics in this book have been comprehensively explained to help readers understand the growing trends in the field.

I would like to thank the entire group of writers who made sincere efforts in this book and my family who supported me in my efforts of working on this book. I take this opportunity to thank all those who have been a guiding force throughout my life.

**Editor**

# Part 1

# Physiology of Steroid Hormones

# Hormonal and Neural Mechanisms Regulating Hormone Steroids Secretion

Roberto Domínguez[1], Angélica Flores[1] and Sara E. Cruz-Morales[2]
[1]Facultad de Estudios Superiores Zaragoza,
[2]Facultad de Estudios Superiores Iztacala
Universidad Nacional Autónoma de México
México

## 1. Introduction

Hormonal and neural signals participate in regulating the synthesis and release of steroid hormones from the adrenals, ovaries and testicles. Hormonal signals arise from the hypothalamus, pituitary, thyroid, thymus, adipose tissue, as well as from the adrenals, ovaries and testicles. Neural signals originating in the hypothalamus and other regions of the central and peripheral nervous system modulate the responses to the hormonal signals sent to the adrenals, ovaries and testicles.

In female, the involvement of the adrenal and ovarian innervations in regulating the synthesis and release of steroid hormones have shown that right and left organs have different abilities to carry out these functions (Gerendai et al., 2000; Domínguez et al., 2003). The asymmetric capacity to release steroid hormones is related to differences in the origin and type of innervations received by right and left organs (Tóth et al., 2007; Gerendai et al., 2009). In addition, the way neuroendocrine signals participate in regulating steroid hormones secretion is different for each hormone, and the release of ovarian hormones is regulated according to the day of the estrus cycle.

Scientific reviews on the biochemical steps that take place during the capture and processing of cholesterol and synthesis of steroid hormones, as well as in the regulation of the enzymes activities have been published in the last decade (Auchus & Miller, 2000; Straus & Hsue, 2000; Stocco, 2008; Boon et al., 2010; Chung et al., 2011). In such regard, the present chapter presents only a summary of those aspects we think are relevant to analyze the neuroendocrine regulation of steroid hormones secretion.

## 2. Steroid hormones

Steroid hormones are classified according to the number of carbon (C) atoms in the molecule deriving from the pregnane (C-21), androstane (C-19) or estrane (C-18) nucleus. C-21 hormones include progesterone, cortisol, corticosterone and aldosterone; C-19 testosterone, androstenedione (A4) and dihydrotestosterone; and C-18 estradiol, estrone and estriol. Based on its functional actions, steroid hormones are classified into five principal classes: estrogens (estradiol, estrone, estriol), progestins (progesterone), androgens (testosterone, A4, dihydrotestosterone), glucocorticoid (cortisol, corticosterone), and mineralocorticoids (aldosterone, deoxicorticosterone).

All steroid hormones derive from cholesterol in a process that includes:

- *de novo* synthesis of cholesterol from acetate, the cholesterol release from cholesterol esters stored in lipid cytoplasmic droplets, and the capture and processing of blood cholesterol
- the transport of cholesterol to the mitochondria;
- the conversion of cholesterol to pregnenolone;
- the transport of pregnenolone to the smooth endoplasmic reticulum;
- modifications of the pregnenolone molecule and the synthesis of active hormones;
- the transport of active hormones to the cell membrane and the release of hormones to the blood stream;
- the biosynthesis of new hormones in the peripheral tissues through enzymes acting on steroid hormones as precursors;
- the activation or inactivation of steroid hormones by organs or tissues; the catabolism and elimination of catabolites by urine, bilis or feces;
- the esterification of the steroid hormone molecules and its elimination through the urine, bilis or feces.

## 3. Capture and processing of cholesterol

Cells synthesizing steroid hormones (steroidogenic cells) use several pathways that ensure the constant supply of cholesterol for steroid hormone synthesis, including:

1. De novo synthesis from acetate in the endoplasmic reticulum;
2. The mobilization of cholesterol esters stored in lipid droplets through cholesterol-ester hydrolase;
3. The uptake of blood lipoproteins carrying cholesterol (low-density (LDL) and high-density lipoproteins (HDL).

The incorporation of lipoproteins into the cells is mediated by a receptor-endocytic mechanism that delivers the lipoproteins to the lysosomes where apolipoproteins are degraded. High density lipoproteins (HDL) are incorporated by the scavenger receptor class B, type I (SR-BI)-mediated selective uptake. Depending on the cell, the synthesis of lipoprotein receptors is stimulated by the adreno-corticotropin-hormone (ACTH) and luteinizing hormone (LH). The source of cholesterol for steroidogenesis varies according to the animal studied (Azhar et al., 2003; Hu et al., 2011). SR-BI synthesis in adrenal cells is stimulated by ACTH and inhibited by glucocorticoids (Mavridou et al., 2010).

The membrane-bound transcription factor sterol regulatory element binding protein (SREBP) is the main regulator for cholesterol synthesis and cellular uptake. In mammalian cells, protein Insig, an endoplasmic- reticulum membrane protein, controls the activity of SREBP and the sterol-dependent degradation of the biosynthetic enzyme HMG-CoA reductase (Espenshade & Hughes 2007).

The cholesterol side chain cleavage reaction is the first step, and also the rate-limiting process in steroid hormone synthesis. The reaction takes place on the inner mitochondrial membranes and is catalyzed by the cholesterol-side-chain cleavage enzyme, cytochrome P-450scc; Cyp11a1 (Straus & Hsue, 2000). The translocator protein (TSPO) and the steroidogenic acute regulatory (StAR) protein mediate this transfer. TSPO is a high-affinity cholesterol-binding mitochondrial protein and StAR is a hormone-induced mitochondria protein that initiates the transfer of cholesterol into the mitochondria (Hu et al., 2010). In *vitro* studies show that treating Leydig cells with testosterone decreases the expression of SR-BI, TSPO, StAR and cytochrome P-450scc (Kostic et al., 2011). In the adrenals, ACTH induces StAR synthesis by stimulating the synthesis of cyclic adenosin mono phosphate (cAMP), while the early steps in steroidogenic synthesis are mediated by post-transcriptional and post-translational changes in the StAR protein (Spiga et al., 2011). In the gonads, gonadotropic hormones transcriptionally control StAR gene expression via a cAMP second messenger (Sugawara et al., 1997). A characteristic feature of steroidogenic cells is the presence of numerous cytoplasmic lipid droplets containing cholesterol esters. Cholesterol esters in these droplets are synthesized by acyl coenzymeA-cholesterol acyltransferase, an endoplasmic reticulum-enzyme. The esters synthesized by cholesterol acyltransferase accumulate within the endoplasmic reticulum membranes and bud off as lipid droplets. Cholesterol esters in lipid droplets are hydrolyzed by a soluble sterol ester hydrolase. Gonadotropins stimulate the activation of cAMP-dependent-protein kinase that activates this enzyme by phosphorylating specific serine residues, thus promoting binding of the sterol esterase to lipid droplets and the hydrolysis of cholesterol esters.

Cholesterol is converted into pregnenolone, and the rate of pregnenolone synthesis is determined by:

1. The rate of cholesterol delivery to the mitochondria;
2. The access of the inner mitochondrial membranes to cholesterol;
3. The available quantity of cholesterol side chain cleavage enzyme and, secondarily its flavoprotein and iron sulfur protein electron transport chain;
4. The catalytic activity of P-450scc.

Acute alterations in steroidogenesis generally result from changes in the delivery of cholesterol to P-450scc, whereas long-term alterations involve changes in the quantity of enzyme proteins, as well as cholesterol delivery (Straus & Hsue, 2000).

## 4. Enzymes participating in the synthesis of steroid hormones

The synthesis of the numerous enzymes participating in steroid hormones synthesis is under the stimulatory effects of hormones secreted by the pituitary ACTH, LH and follicle stimulating hormone (FSH). Other pituitary hormones, such as growth hormone (GH) and prolactin (PRL), also play a role regulating the synthesis of some of these enzymes.

Based on the progression of changes occurring to the cholesterol molecule, four enzymes seem to be crucial for hormone synthesis: cytochrome P-450scc, 3β-hydroxysteroid dehydrogenase/Δ5-4-isomerases (3β-HSDs), 17 α-Hydroxylase/17,2O-desmolase, and aromatase cytochrome P450

### 4.1 Cytochrome P-450scc

The cytochrome P-450scc side chain cleavage is an enzyme present in the inner mitochondrial membranes. The enzyme is involved in three catalytic cycles on the cholesterol molecule: the introduction of hydroxyl groups at positions C-22 and C-20, and the subsequent scission of the side chain between these carbons. ACTH and LH stimulate cytochrome P-450scc synthesis in a mechanism that depends on cAMP synthesis as a second messenger (Auchus & Miller, 2000; Straus & Hsue, 2000).

### 4.2 3β-Hydroxysteroid dehydrogenase/Δ5-4-isomerases

3β-Hydroxysteroid dehydrogenase/Δ5-4-isomerases (3β-HSDs) are located at the microsomal fraction, and are expressed in the adrenal cortex and in steroidogenic cells of the gonads. The expression of 3β-HSDs is enhanced by ACTH and LH. These isomerases catalyze the formation of Δ4-3-ketosteroids from A5-3β-hydroxysteroids, an obligate step in the biosynthesis of progestins, androgens, estrogens, mineralocorticoids and glucocorticoids. 3β-HSDs catalyze the dehydrogenation of the 3B-equatorial hydroxyl group and the subsequent isomerization of the olefinic bond to yield the $A_4$ 3-ketone structure; converting pregnenolone into progesterone, l7α-hydroxypregnenolone into 17α-hydroxyprogesterone, and dehydroepiandrosterone into A4.

Protein kinase A signaling activators (forskolin, dibutyrylcAMP) increase the synthesis of dehydroepiandrosterone and A4, as well as the levels of 3β-HSD and P-450c17 mRNA transcripts. Activation of the protein kinase C pathway by phorbol ester treatment also elevates 3β-HSD mRNA levels and lowers P-450cl17 mRNA levels (Auchus & Miller. 2000).

### 4.3 17 α-Hydroxylase/17,2O-Desmolase

The 17 α-Hydroxylase/17,2O-Desmolase (P-45Oc7f or CYP17A1 ITl) is a cytochrome P450 enzyme with 17 α-hydroxylase and 17,20-lyase activities that catalyzes two reactions: the hydroxylation of pregnenolone and progesterone at carbon 17, and the conversion of pregnenolone into C-19 steroids. P-450c17 is a key enzyme in the steroidogenic pathway producing all steroid hormones (progestins, mineralocorticoids, glucocorticoids, androgens, and estrogens). The theca cells of the follicle and the theca lutein cells of the corpus luteum, as well as the ovarian stroma, the adrenal gland, and Leydig cells express P-450c17. (Auchus & Miller, 2000; Straus & Hsue, 2000).

### 4.4 Aromatase cytochrome P-450c17

Aromatase cytochrome P-450 c17 is an enzyme found in the endoplasmic reticulum membrane that acts on aromatizable androgen. Aromatase P 450 catalyses the biosynthesis of all estrogens from androgens by transforming the A-ring of steroids to an aromatic state through the oxidation and elimination of the C19 methyl group (Ghosh et al., 2009; Straus & Hsueh, 2000). Aromatase expression is present in fetal and immature ovaries, and in rodents, aromatase expression/activity is restricted to the gonads and the brain. In humans, aromatase activity is expressed by the adrenal medulla (Belgorosky et al., 2008), adipose tissue, breast, skin, and bone (Czajka-Oraniec & Simpson, 2010).

FSH is the main factor inducing aromatase activity in mural granulosa cells located on the outer edge of healthy large antral follicles and luteal cells. Aromatase is not expressed in cumulus granulosa cells. The stimulatory effects of FSH are modulated in an inhibitory way by glucocorticoids, prolactin, progestins, inhibin, triiodothyronine and thyroxine (T3-T4) (Chen et al., 2010). Transforming growth factor-β (TGF-β) enhances FSH effects (Stocco, 2008).

Bone morphogenetic protein 15 (BMP-15) and growth differentiating factor 9 (GDF9) produced by the oocytes also stimulate aromatase expression and the stimulatory effects of the tumor necrosis factor- α (TNF- α), epidermal growth factor (EGF), transferrin, nitric oxide (NO), and superoxide dismutase (Stocco 2008). Leptin has stimulatory or inhibitory effects on aromatase expression depending on the animal studied (Sirotkin & Grossman, 2007).

Acting as an autocrine signal, estradiol enhances the stimulatory effects of FSH on aromatase activity in granulosa cells, and its effects are mediated by the activation of estrogen receptor β (Wang et al., 2010).

Androgens enhance FSH effects on aromatase expression by increasing cAMP levels. Aromatizable androgens synthesized by theca-internal cells are the substrate for estrogen synthesis. The stimulating actions of FSH on aromatase are potentiated by insulin-like growth factor-1 (IGF-1), because IGF-I stimulates the capacity of granulosa cells to respond to FSH (Stocco 2008).

FSH stimulates the synthesis of cAMP, which in turn acts as an intracellular messenger mediating FSH stimulation of aromatase expression, leading to the activation of the cAMP-dependent protein kinase A (PKA) which is cAMP-dependent (Stocco, 2008). FSH stimulates the mRNA for LH receptor synthesis, explaining why LH is the main aromatase inductor before ovulation (Boon et al., 2010).

## 5. Hormonal signals

The regulation of steroid hormones synthesis is mediated by hormones secreted by the pituitary, thyroid, adipose tissue, neuropeptides, adrenals, ovaries and testicles.

### 5.1 Pituitary hormones

The pituitary secretes several hormones that stimulate the release of steroid hormones. In this process, two key hormones are the ACTH and LH, and their release is pulsating. Higher cortisol, progesterone, testosterone, and estradiol levels in serum are observed minutes after each ACTH or LH pulse. By acting on the expression of several genes, ACTH and LH stimulate the synthesis of enzymes participating in the conversion of cholesterol to steroid hormones, a process that can take hours or even days. The rapid increase in steroid hormone concentrations after the injection of ACTH or LH cannot be explained by the synthesis of enzymes participating in steroid hormones synthesis and release. Based on several studies, it has been proposed that the rapid increase in steroid hormones levels is mediated by a c-AMP action resulting in StAR synthesis, one of the proteins carrying the cholesterol to the mitochondria, the first step in steroid hormones synthesis (Auchus & Miller, 2000).

The first step in the acute response to hormonal stimulation for steroid biosynthesis is the delivery of cholesterol from the outer to the inner mitochondrial membrane; a process that depends on *de novo* StAR protein synthesis and phosphorylation. LH and ACTH stimulate the synthesis of StAR by increasing cAMP levels and its phosphorylation rate (Luo et al., 2010).

LH plays a dual role in regulating P-450 enzymes participating in the synthesis of steroid hormones. Following the initial stimulation synthesis of the enzyme, LH exerts a down regulation on the synthesis of granulosa-specific CYP19A1 and theca-specific CYP17A1 transcripts and lowers the abundance of HSD3B1 transcripts (Nimz et al., 2010).

In female rabbits, hyperprolactinemia inhibits the peripheral and ovarian venous progesterone and 20 alpha-hydroxypregn-4-en-3-one (20 alpha-OHP) levels increase stimulated by human chorionic gonadotropin (hCG), without causing changes in the estradiol, androstenedione and testosterone levels (Lin et al., 1987).

### 5.2 Adipose tissue hormones

The adipose tissue secretes several adipose-derived polypeptidic hormones. Together, adipose-derived polypeptidic hormones receive the name of adipokines. Adipokines act locally and distally through autocrine, paracrine and endocrine effects (Ronti et al., 2006), and participate in the regulation of appetite and metabolic processes. Experimental studies show that some adipokines play a role regulating steroid hormones secretion by different organs.

### 5.2.1 Leptin

Leptin is a hormone secreted by the adipose tissue, and its participation in the regulation of steroid hormones is controversial. *In vitro* studies show that the participation of leptin in the regulation of steroid hormones release depends on the species studied. In avian ovarian cells leptin stimulates the release of progesterone and estradiol, blocks testosterone secretion, and does not affect arginine-vasotocin secretion (Sirotkin & Grossmann 2007). In granulosa cells from rats, high leptin concentrations inhibits the stimulatory effects of insulin-like growth factor I (IGF-I) on FSH-stimulated estradiol secretion, but does not affect progesterone secretion (Zachow and Magoffin, 1997; Duggal et al., 2002; Ricci et al., 2006). In cultured granulosa cells leptin also suppresses the stimulating effect of the transforming growth factor β (TGF-β) on FSH-dependent estrone and estradiol secretion, as well as in aromatase mRNA expression and aromatase activity (Zachow et al., 1999).

Leptin inhibits insulin-induced estradiol secretion by granulosa cells and decreases the insulin-induced increases of progesterone production in bovine granulosa cells (Spicer & Francisco, 1997). Co-stimulated by FSH and dexamethasone, leptin blocks steroid hormone synthesis by the ovaries and the synthesis of pregnenolone, progesterone, and 20alpha-hydroxy-4-pregnen-3-one. Leptin also reduces the expression of adrenodoxin, an enzyme in the P50scc electron transport system (Barkan et al., 1999), and inhibits the synthesis of insulin-stimulated progesterone production from human luteinized granulosa cells (Brannian et al., 1999). The synthesis of functional leptin receptors depends on pituitary hormones, since hypophysectomized rat theca cells do not have such receptors (Zachow et al., 1999).

Studies in human granulosa cells suggest that *in vitro* the effects of leptin on the secretion of estradiol and progesterone depend on the doses used; with low doses of leptin having a stimulatory effect and high doses an inhibitory effect (Karamouti et al., 2009). Leptin and leptin fragments enhance the secretory activity of aldosterone and corticosterone by the adrenal cortex of rats (Malendowicz et al., 2003; Markowska et al., 2004). However, later studies by Malendowicz et al., (2007) reported that leptin inhibits steroid-hormone secretion from the adrenal cortex by lowering the response to stress of the hypothalamic-pituitary-adrenal (HPA) axis and by increasing the release of catecholamines from the adrenal medulla. Because leptin Ob-receptor is expressed in the adrenal gland, it seems that leptin modulates adrenal hormones secretion by acting as a circulating hormone (Malendowicz et al., 2007). Leptin blocks the ovarian steroid synthesis co-stimulated by FSH and dexamethasone. *In vitro* studies show that leptin inhibited the secretion of pregnenolone, progesterone, and 20alpha-hydroxy-4-pregnen-3-one, as well as the secretion of progesterone induced by the co-stimulation by forskolin and dexametasene; without modifying the forskolin induction of cAMP (Barkan et al., 1999).

### 5.2.2 Adiponectin

Adiponectin is an adipocyte hormone participating in lipid metabolism and glucose homeostasis. Adiponectine receptors and its mRNA are expressed in the ovaries and testicles. Pituitary gonadotropins have low effects on adiponectin mRNA testicular levels. Metabolic signals, such as glucocorticoids, thyroxine, and peroxisome proliferator-activated receptor-gamma modulate the expression of adiponectin mRNA. *In vitro* studies show that recombinant adiponectin inhibits basal and human chorio-gonadotropin-stimulated testosterone secretion by adult rat testicles (Caminos et al., 2008).

## 5.3 Gut hormones

The gut secretes several polypeptidic hormones that participate in regulating the brain-gut relationship with different organs in the digestive system. Experimental studies show that some gut hormones also play a role regulating the secretion of steroid hormone.

### 5.3.1 Secretin and gastric inhibitory polypeptide

Secretin and gastric inhibitory polypeptide (GIP), together with glucagon, parathyroid hormone (PTH), vasoactive intestinal peptide (VIP) and pituitary adenylate cyclase-activating polypeptide, belong to the VIP-secretin-glucagon super family.

Secreted by the duodenum, secretin is a hormone that selectively depresses the glucocorticoid response to ACTH of dispersed zona fasciculata-reticularis cells. By inhibiting the cascade of AC/protein kinase A, glucagon, and glucagon-like peptide-1 secretin depresses the response of cells in the zona fasciculata-reticularis to ACTH. PTH and PTH-related protein stimulate aldosterone and glucocorticoid secretion of dispersed zone glomerulosa and zone fasciculata-reticularis cells (Nussdorfer, 2000).

The intra-peritoneal injection of GIP increases corticosterone plasma concentrations in a dose-dependent manner, without affecting aldosterone levels. GIP did not affect aldosterone and cyclic-AMP release by dispersed zone glomerulosa cells, but increased basal corticosterone secretion and cyclic-AMP release by dispersed inner adrenocortical cells. In rats, GIP stimulates the basal secretion of glucocorticoids by acting through specific receptors coupled with the adenylatecyclase/PKA-dependent signaling pathway (Mazzocchi et al 1999).

### 5.3.2 Obestatin

Produced in the stomach and other tissues, obestatin is one of the metabolic hormones that has effects on systems other than the digestive system. In *in vitro* porcine granulosa cells, obestatin increases the secretion of progesterone, without modifying testosterone or estradiol secretion (Mészárosová et al., 2008). Thus, it is possible that obestatin stimulates StAR phosphorylation without affecting the activity of the enzymes participating in androgen synthesis.

## 5.4 Neuropeptides

The term neuropeptide refers to polypeptidic molecules synthesized and released by neurons that can act neurotransmitters and/or hormones. Common neuropeptides include orexins (A & B) and galanin.

### 5.4.1 Orexins

Orexin-A and orexin-B (hypocretin-1 and -2) are two neuropeptides produced by neurones located in the lateral hypothalamus. Orexins A and B bind to two different receptors that are coupled to G proteins. Both neuropeptides raise basal corticosterone secretion by dispersed cells obtained from the rat's fasciculate-reticular zone, and do not affect either maximally

ACTH stimulated corticosterone production by cells of the fasciculate-reticular zone or the basal and agonist-stimulated aldosterone secretion of dispersed cells from the glomerulosa zone. The ACTH-receptor antagonist corticotropin-inhibiting peptide blocks the secretion of corticosterone induced by ACTH to cells from the fasciculate-reticular zone, but does not modify orexins effects. Both orexins enhance cyclic-AMP release by cells in the fasciculate-reticular zone. The selective inhibitor capacity of protein-kinase A (PKA) H-89 decreased corticosterone responses to both ACTH and orexins. A subcutaneous injection of orexin A and B evokes a clear-cut increase in the plasma concentration of corticosterone, but not of aldosterone. The effect of orexin-A on corticosterone release is higher than the effect of orexin-B. Based on these results the authors suggest that orexins exert a selective and direct glucocorticoid secretagogue action on the adrenals of the rat, acting through a receptor-mediated activation of the adenylate cyclase/PKA-dependent signaling pathway (Malendowicz et al., 1999).

Stimulating orexin receptors results in higher ACTH secretion by the pituitary and has a direct stimulatory effect on adrenocortical cells (Malendowicz et al., 1999; Spinazzi et al., 2006; Kagerer & Jöhren 2010).

### 5.4.2 Galanin

Galanin is a 29- or 30- amino acid long neuropeptide expressed in the brain, spinal cord, and gut that acts via three subtypes of G protein-coupled receptors. Galanin increases the basal secretion of cortisol from dispersed inner adrenocortical cells, without affecting the effects of ACTH (Belloni et al., 2007). Galanin stimulates the release of corticotrophin releasing hormone (CRH) and ACTH, enhances glucocorticoid secretion by the adrenal cortex, and directly stimulates corticosterone secretion from the adrenals through GAL-R1 and GAL-R2 receptors and the release of noradrenaline from the adrenal medulla. Other results suggest that galanin increases corticosterone release via an indirect paracrine mechanism involving the local release of catecholamines, which in turn activates beta-adrenoceptors located on adrenocortical cells (Tortorella et al., 2007).

### 5.4.3 Vasoactive intestinal peptide and neuropeptide Y

The VIP and neuropeptide Y (NPY) are the most abundant transmitter-peptides in the adrenal gland (Whitworth et al., 2003). These peptides act as neurotransmitters and exert endocrine, paracrine or autocrine effects in numerous cell types, particularly in the adrenals and ovaries. *In vitro*, the adrenal responsiveness to VIP depends on the model used: in rats, VIP stimulates aldosterone production by the adrenal capsular tissue (Cunningham & Holzwarth, 1988) and by intact perfused adrenal glands (Hinson et al., 1992), but not by dispersed zona glomerulosa cells (Enyedi et al., 1983; Hinson et al., 1992). There is evidence that VIP acts on chromaffin cells present beneath the adrenal capsule, stimulating the release of catecholamines, which in turn stimulate aldosterone secretion (Whitworth et al., 2003). It seems that the mechanisms used by NPY in the adrenals are the same as those used by VIP (Renshaw et al., 2000).

### 5.4.4 Pituitary Adenylate Cyclase-Activating Polypeptide (PACAP)

The pituitary adenylate-cyclase activating polypeptide (PACAP) and its receptors are present in the central nervous system (CNS), the testicles, adrenals, and ovaries. LH increases PACAP mRNA levels in pre-ovulatory follicles, and stimulates estrogen and progesterone secretion by granulosa cells stimulated with hCG (Lee et al. 1999). In the adrenals, PACAP stimulates VIP synthesis, which in turn stimulates hormones release (Ait-Ali et al., 2010).

## 5.5 Adrenal hormones
The adrenals secrete steroid hormones, catecholamines and peptidergic hormones. Evidence suggests that almost all the adrenal hormones play a role on their own regulatory process.

### 5.5.1 Endothelins
Endothelins (ETs) are a family of vasoactive peptides secreted by vascular endothelium. ETs play autocrine/paracrine regulatory functions, acting via two subtypes of receptors, ET-A and ET-B. The endocrine cells in the glomerulosa cells of the adrenal cortex express both ET-A and ET-B. The cells of the zone fasciculata/reticularis mainly express ET-B. ETs stimulate the secretion of mineralocorticoids by glomerulosa cells. Its effects on glucocorticoid secretion are lower (Nussdorfer et al., 1997). The effects of ETs on steroidogenic cells are mediated through the activation of various signaling mechanisms, including the stimulation of phospholipase C, phospholipase A2 and adenyl cyclase activity, as well as calcium influx through plasma channels (Delarue et al., 2004).

### 5.5.2 Noradrenaline
Noradrenaline (NA) is a cathecolamine secreted by neurons in the adrenal medulla and by chromaffin cells present in the adrenal cortex. In luteal bovine cells NA stimulates progesterone secretion through the beta 1- and beta 2-adrenoceptors. NA also increases cytochrome P-450scc and 3 beta-HSD activity. Prostaglandin F (PGF) inhibits the luteotropic effect of NA on the luteal tissue (Miszkiel&, Kotwica, 2001).

### 5.5.3 Dopamine
Human granulosa cells (GCs) express 4 out of 5 dopamine (DA) receptors (D1 and D5 coupled and linked to cAMP increase, D2 and D4; Gi/Gq coupled and linked to IP3/DAG. *In vitro*, the stimulation of human granulosa cells with hCG did not increase mRNA or protein levels of DA receptors. D1 and D2 receptors are also present in the ovaries of rats (Rey-Ares et al., 2007).

## 5.6 Thyroid hormones
The thyroid mainly secretes triyodo tyrosine (T3), tiroxine (T4) and calcitonin. T3 and T4 play several roles in regulating all the mammalian organs and systems.
Rats with hypothyroidism present high progesterone and low testosterone levels, without apparent changes in basal estradiol levels (Hatsuta et al., 2004). Acute experiments with murine Leydig cells, T3 induced StAR expression and progesterone production (Manna et al., 1999). In contrast, chronically stimulating mice Leydig tumor cells with T3 inhibits StAR expression and progesterone production, mainly by decreasing the delivery of cholesterol to the inner mitochondrial membrane (Manna et al., 2001). In cultivated Leydig cells, T3 treatment increased testosterone and estradiol secretions in a dose dependent manner (Maran et al., 2000).

## 5.7 Protein kinases and cAMP

Protein kinases (PKs) are a group of enzymes that modify other enzymes by adding phosphate groups (phosphorylation), which changes the enzyme's activity.

PKs participate in regulating the release of steroid hormones. Ovarian cells produce a number of PKs whose expression depends on the type of cell, their state and the action of hormones and other PKs (Sirotkin et al., 2011). In mammalian ovarian cells, PK-A stimulates the release of progesterone and estradiol (Makarevich et al., 2004); while others affirm that PKA inhibits progesterone, testosterone and estradiol release by mammalian ovarian follicular cells (Dupont et al., 2008). In chickens, PK-A either stimulates or suppresses the release of progesterone, testosterone and estradiol (Sirotkin & Grossmann, 2006, 2007b). In corpus luteum, PK-A promotes the release of progesterone by large luteal cells, while PK-C inhibits the release of progesterone and maintains luteal prostaglandin 2 alpha release (Diaz et al., 2002; Niswender, 2002). According to Makarevich (2004) PK-A type II is more important for the control of ovarian steroidogenesis than PK-A type I.

Rabbit ovaries treated *in vitro* with dbcAMP secrete less progesterone and testosterone, but basal estradiol release remained unchanged. Adding FSH, IGF-I, and ghrelin reduced progesterone release, and adding only ghrelin increased the release of testosterone without modifying estradiol output. Previous treatment with dbcAMP inverted the inhibitory to stimulatory action of FSH, IGF-I and ghrelin on progesterone release (Chrenek et al., 2010).

## 5.8 Ovarian signals

Like the adrenal glands, the ovaries secrete steroid and polypeptidic hormones that regulate / modulate the synthesis and release of ovarian hormones.

Estradiol regulates the synthesis of androgens by the follicular theca interna in an inhibitory way. Estrogens and androgens inhibit progesterone secretion by the human corpus luteum. The effects of testosterone and androstenedione are mediated by their conversion to estrogens (Tropea et al., 2010). Androgens stimulate cytochrome P450 aromatase mRNA concentrations in granulosa cells. The effects depend on the androgen studied, suggesting that the expression of the aromatase gene has differential regulation in the developing follicle (Hamel et al., 2005). GnRH-like peptides in the testicle and ovary play an inhibitory regulation on steroidogenesis (Franchimont, 1983).

# 6. Neuroendocrine signals

At present there is no doubt that in addition to pituitary and non-pituiraty hormone control, ovarian functions, hormone synthesis and ovulation, as well as adrenal cortex secretions, and perhaps the secretion of hormones by the testicles and even spermatogenesis, are under direct local neural modulation.

Kawakami et al. (1979, 1981) obtained the first unequivocal results indicating that the regulation of ovarian functions is accomplished by hormonal signals that are modulated by neural signals. Applying electric stimulation to the ventromedial hypothalamus and the medio-basal prechiasmathic area in hypophysectomized and adrenalectomized rats provoked the release of progesterone and estradiol without modifying ovarian blood flow.

The synthesis and secretion of steroids from the adrenal cortex and ovaries are also under direct modulation by local neurons. Without making synaptic contact, many noradrenergic nerve endings are in close proximity to zona-glomerulosa cells. NA acts as a direct modulator of local steroid secretion. Catecholamines and adenosine triphosphate (ATP) diffuse into zone glomerulosa cells and modulate the synthesis of aldosterone in a paracrine way. The enzymes that may terminate the effect of ATP are present in the nerve endings, suggesting that ATP and its metabolites influence the production of aldosterone. Thus, catecholamines and ATP play a paracrine non-synaptic modulator role of in the regulation of adrenocortical steroid secretion (Szalay et al., 1998).

Stimulation of beta-adrenoreceptors, VIP receptors or the forskolin-induced activation of cAMP formation of 2-day-old rat ovaries increases the steady state levels of the mRNAs encoding P-450aromatase and FSH receptors. Based on these results it was suggested that ovarian nerves, acting via neurotransmitters coupled to the cAMP generating system, contribute to the differentiation process by which newly formed primary follicles acquire FSH receptors and responsiveness to FSH. Follicles that grow in more densely innervated ovarian regions may have a selective advantage over those not exposed to neurotransmitter-activated, cAMP-dependent signals; and thus may become more rapidly subjected to gonadotropin control (Mayerhofer et al., 1997).

The intra-cerebro-ventricular injection (icv-i) of isoproterenol (beta-adrenergic agonist) to rats in diestrus 2 lowers progesterone levels in the ovarian vein blood. However, no apparent effects are observed when both superior ovarian nerves (SON) are sectioned before the icv-i treatment. Blocking the beta-adrenergic receptors with propranolol icv-i increased progesterone levels, an effect that was not observed when both SONs were sectioned (De Bortoli et al., 1998, 2002). According to De Bortoli et al. (2000), the neural signals arriving to the ovary through the SON antagonize the ovarian LH regulation of progesterone and androstenedione.

## 7. Ovarian and adrenal innervations

The adrenal gland and the ovaries receive innervation from several nerve fibers of extrinsic and intrinsic origin. Most of the extrinsic innervations in the adrenal derive from the sympathetic nervous system, including cholinergic fibers containing nitric oxide synthase (Holgert et al., 1995), thyrosine hydroxylase- and neuropeptide Y-positive postganglionic sympathetic fibers (Holgert et al., 1998; Kondo, 1985). Encephalin was exclusively found in choline-acethyl-transferase positive fibers among adrenaline chromaffin cells (Holgert et al., 1995). Intrinsic innervation originates from two different types of medullary ganglion cells: Type I and Type II cells. Type I cells are NPY-positive noradrenergic, while type II ganglion cells synthesize VIP and nitric oxide synthase (Holgertet al., 1998; Ulrich-Lai et. al., 2006).

The adrenals have efferent fibers connecting to the dorsal motor nucleus of the vagus nerve, while other fibers of vagal origin reach the gland via the celiac or suprarenal ganglion (Berthoud and Powley, 1993; Coupland et al., 1989). In the rat, the motor and sensory vagal innervations of the adrenal gland originate from bilaterally situated cell bodies that have slight ipsi-lateral predominance (Coupland et al., 1989). Nerve fibers that go to and from the adrenal gland also possess afferent viscero-sensory fibers. According to Tóth et al. (2007), the steroid feedback mechanism affects the cerebral structures that send descending input to the sympathetic preganglionic neurons innervating the adrenal gland.

The bilateral sectioning of the thoracic splanchnic nerve resulted in lower corticosterone plasma levels measured in the afternoon seven days after treatment, without apparent changes in ACTH levels; results that suggest that the splanchnic adrenal innervation modulates the response to ACTH. The effects are related to functional changes in the adrenal medulla and do not depend on the sensitive of the afferent fibers (Ulrich-Lai et al., 2006).

The ovaries receive motor innervations from the sympathetic and the parasympathetic system via the vagus nerve, and possess afferent fibers travelling sympathetic and vagal routes (Burden et al 1983; Klein and Burden, 1988, Gerendai et al., 2000, 2009). The vagus nerve connects the ovaries with the area postrema, the nucleus of the solitary tract, the dorsal vagal complex, the parapyramidal nucleus, A1, A5, and A7 -cell groups, the caudal raphe nuclei, the hypothalamic paraventricular nucleus, the lateral hypothalamus, the Barrington's nucleus, the locus coeruleus, the periaqueductal gray, and the dorsal hypothalamus. All of these areas form a neural circuit that directly participates in the neural communication between the CNS and the ovaries (Gerendai et al., 2000; Tóth et al., 2007).

As in the adrenals, the ovaries have micro-ganglia with tyrosine hidroxilase positive neurons (D'Albora & Barcia, 1996; Dees et al., 1995; D'Albora et al., 2002), and along some capillaries there are neurons resting on the basal (D'Albora & Barcia, 1996).

## 8. Methodologies used to analyze the participation of neural signals

The participation of the peripheral nervous system in the regulation of adrenal, ovarian and testicular functions is studied using two main experimental approaches: *in vitro* and *in vivo* methods. Studies *in vitro* allow for the understanding of the isolated participation of one, two or even three neurotransmitters in the regulation of hormones secretion by one type of cell, or even an organ tissue. Studies *in vitro* have certain advantages, such as the possibility of analyzing the cellular mechanisms regulated by neurotransmitters, identifying the receptors participating in the regulation, and the molecular changes that occur. *In vitro* methods also have disadvantages, since in many studies the amount of neurotransmitters added to the culture medium is much higher than the normal concentration measured in the organ. Another problem of *in vitro* studies is the loss of the interplay occurring between different kinds of cells.

*In vivo* methods include the analysis of nerve stimulation and/or sectioning, the extirpation of one or both organs, the denervation of the *in situ* organ, as well as the local or systemic injection of neurotransmitters or blocking agents. The information obtained from *in vivo* studies gives an idea about the animal's response to such manipulations (changes in hormone levels; metabolic modifications, etc.). In general, the cellular mechanisms participating in the modifications resulting from such manipulations are not clearly evident.

### 8.1 *In vitro* methods

Taken together, the results of *in vitro* and *in vivo* studies give an idea about the participation of neurotransmitters in regulating steroid hormone secretion. Studies on the participation of different systems regulating the secretion of steroid hormones analyze the effects of directly injecting neurotransmitters or substances known to block its receptors. Incubating steroid-hormones producing cells, with or without specific neurotransmitters, or in neurotransmitters "cocktails", is the main methodology used for studying the participation of neural signals regulating the secretion of steroid hormones.

Serotonin inhibits testosterone, dihydrotestosterone, and androstane-3alpha, 17beta-diol production from testicles of peripubertal and adult hamsters maintained in long or short photoperiods. Serotonin also inhibits the stimulation induced by hCG, cAMP and testosterone production, by its union to 5-HT1A and 5-HT2A receptors subtypes. The testicular activity of the serotoninergic system is mediated by the corticotrophin releasing hormone (CRH) and by the noradrenergic system. CRH has an inhibitory modulation of testosterone, dihydro-testosterone, and androstane-3alpha, 17beta-diol secretion, while epinephrine and norepinephrine have a stimulatory effect through alpha1/beta1-adrenergic receptors (Frungeri et al., 2002).

Stress induced by sleep deprivation results in lower testosterone levels in serum and lower testicular StAR protein expression, while serotonin and corticosterone serum levels are elevated (Wu et al., 2011). These results suggest that serotonin regulation of steroid hormones release depends on the cells where such sterols originate.

Acting through β-1 and β-2 receptors, NA stimulates progesterone secretion from luteal slices of heifers, and increases cytochrome P-450scc and 3 beta-HSD activity (Miszkiel & Kotwica, 2001). Nitric oxide (NO) inhibits the activity of cytochrome P450 aromatase and the secretion of estradiol by granulosa cells in culture (Ishimaru et al., 2001). In vitro studies show that in the rat, the participation of neurotransmitters regulating the secretion of ovarian progesterone varies throughout the day of the estrous cycle. In diestrus-1, NPY, NA, and VIP inhibit progesterone secretion by the ovaries, while on diestrus-2 these neurotransmitters stimulate progesterone secretion. In diestrus 1 and 2, NA+VIP or NA+NPY had a synergic effect on progesterone secretion, since measured concentrations were higher than VIP or NPY treatment alone (Aguado, 2002). In the rat, ovarian denervation reduces the synthesis and secretion of progesterone by inhibiting 3-betaHSD activity (Burden & Lawrence, 1977). Sectioning the plexus nerve and the SON of pigs led to lower LH, progesterone, androstenedione (A4), testosterone, estrone and estradiol-17beta plasma levels. In addition, a significant increase in the immune-expression of cholesterol side-chain cleavage cytochrome P450 occurs in follicles, as well as a decrease in 3-betaHSD activity, and in LH, progesterone, androstenedione (A4), testosterone, estrone and estrogen plasma levels (Jana et al., 2007).

Using an ex vivo celiac ganglion (CG)-SON-ovary (CG-SON-O) system, Aguado's research group has contributed to the understanding of the participation of the SON, the plexus ovarian nerve and the vagus nerve in regulating the secretion of ovarian hormones. In in vitro studies, the release of ovarian hormones is modulated by the stimulation/inhibition of neurons present in the CG.

According to Morán et al., (2005), the CG form a bilateral structure with the superior mesenteric ganglia in the rat, receiving the name of celiac-superior mesenteric ganglion (CSMG) which is composed of noradrenergic neurons called principal neurons, small intensely fluorescent cells, and peptidergic interneurons.

In in vitro studies, adding NPY, VIP or substance P (SP) to the ovaries obtained from rats in diestrus 1 resulted in lower release of progesterone, while the same treatment to ovaries obtained from rats in diestrus 2 increased it. Adding these three neuropeptides to the CG from rats in diestrus 2 resulted in higher progesterone secretion (Garraza et al., 2004). These results suggest that the way neural signals participate in the regulation of steroid secretions depends on the day of the estrous cycle and the type of cells receiving the signal.

Adding NA to the CG obtained from rats on diestrus 1 resulted in ovarian dopaminergic and noradrenergic activity increases, while adding NA to the CG system from rats on diestrus 2 only increased noradrenergic activity. Such changes in dopaminergic and noradrenergic ovarian activities resulted in lower release of androstenedione in systems obtained from rats on diestrus 1, and higher release of androstenedione in systems obtained from rats on diestrus 2 (Bronzi et al., 2011).

The results presented above suggest that the adrenergic activation of the CG plays a role in regulating ovarian androgen secretion, and that this role varies along the estrous cycle. Therefore, steroidogenesis appears to be controlled by a balance between the stimulatory effects of hormones secreted by the pituitary, the inhibitory effects of other hormones, and the modulating participation of the ovarian innervations.

Pituitary hormones and innervations, including sympathetic and sensory nerves, also regulate the adrenal cortex secretion of hormones. The nerves innervating the adrenal cortex include heterogeneous populations containing various different neuropeptides (Kondo, 1985). The sympathetic innervation is composed of cholinergic preganglionic fibers and catecholaminergic postganglionic fibers that are positive for tyrosine hydroxylase (TH) and NPY (Kondo, 1985; Holgert et al., 1998). Sensory innervations consist of primary afferent fibers that are positive for calcitonin gene–related peptide (CGRP) and SP (Kuramoto et al. 1987). Intrinsic innervations on the adrenal cortex arise from two types of medullar ganglion cells: Type I cells are noradrenergic and NPY-positive, whereas Type II cells produce neuronal nitric oxide synthase and VIP (Holgert et al., 1998). Preganglionic sympathetic and primary afferent fibers are carried in the thoracic splanchnic nerve (Ulrich-Lai & Engeland 2000).

## 9. Experimental methods *in vivo*

Figure 1 shows the innervations received by the ovaries and adrenals originating in the CMSG and the centers originating in the vagus nerve (Vagus centers). The CMSG and the

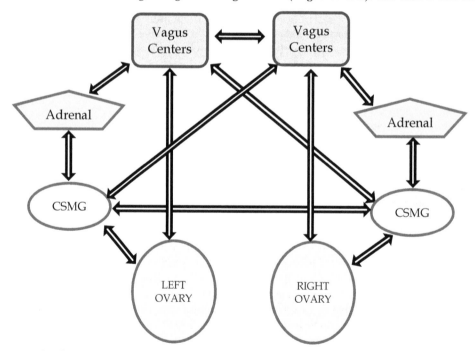

Fig. 1. The diagram shows the neural pathways connecting the adrenals and ovaries with the celiac-superior mesenteric ganglia (CSMG). The interconnections between the right and left CSMG, as well as the innervations to the vagus nerves are also represented.

vagus centers seem to be the place where information from other regions of the CNS converges. Both centers send and receive neural information that modulates the reactivity of the endocrine cells to hormonal signals from the ovaries and adrenals. The existence of neural communication between the right and left CMSG implies the existence of neural communication between the ovaries. The modulation exerted by the neural signals over the ovaries and the adrenals varies during the estrous cycle (ovaries) and along the day (adrenals and ovaries). Such modulation is asymmetric, and the asymmetry varies during the estrous cycle and the hour of the day.

Extirpating one ovary or one adrenal result in acute neural stimulation of the *in situ* ovary and/or adrenal, that modifies the response of endocrine cells to the hormonal signals. Sectioning one nerve also results in an acute neural stimulation of the denervated organ, though such stimulation is more restricted. For the ovaries and adrenals, the partially denervated organ still has neural pathways regulating its functions and, in theory, the innervated organ received only one different neural signal.

To study the role played by the ovarian innervations in regulating progesterone, testosterone and estradiol levels in serum we have used five experimental models. The experimental models were performed on cyclic rats and our studies analyzed the influence of the day of the estrous cycle on treatment results.

1.  The effects of dorsal and ventral surgery to reach the ovaries and their innervation.
2.  The effects of bilateral ovariectomy or adrenalectomy
3.  The effects of unilateral ovariectomy
4.  The effects of unilateral or bilateral section of the SON
5.  The effects of unilateral adrenalectomy.

## 9.1 The effects of dorsal and ventral surgical approaches

The unilateral perforation of the dorsal or ventral abdominal wall results in different changes in progesterone, testosterone and estradiol serum levels. Irrespective of the day of the estrous cycle surgery was performed, rats with a ventral sectioning of the abdominal wall showed higher progesterone and testosterone levels in serum than control rats and rats with dorsal sectioning of the abdominal wall (Figure 2). The increase in hormone release could be explained by an increase in StAR protein phosphorylation and/or synthesis stimulated by the neurotransmitters released by the neural terminals arriving to the ovaries and adrenals. Changes in ACTH, LH and FSH serum levels induced by sectioning the abdominal wall cannot be ruled out. Since estradiol levels were not modified, we presume that P-450 aromatase activity is not influenced by the neural information arising from the abdominal wall.

Uchida et al. (2005) showed the existence of asymmetry in the neural reflexes arising from the abdominal skin that arrive to the ovaries and affect the ovarian blood flow and the activity of the SON. Stimulating the left abdomen produced a much stronger effect on the activity of the left ovarian sympathetic nerve than stimulating the right abdomen. The magnitude of the changes in hormone levels induced by ventral or dorsal surgery depend on both, the dorsal or ventral side (left or right) of the surgery and the day of the estrous cycle when surgery is performed. These results suggest the existence of a multi-synaptic neural pathway between the abdominal wall, the adrenals and the ovaries, a pathway that is mediated through the innervations of the adrenals and ovaries (Flores et al., 2008).

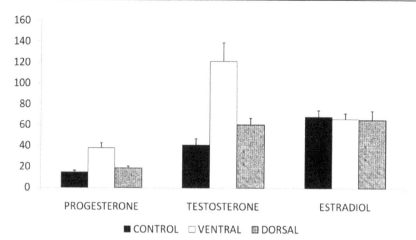

Fig. 2. Comparative effects of ventral or dorsal sectioning the abdominal wall on progesterone, testosterone, and estradiol serum levels. Based in data published by Flores et al., (2008) * $p<0.05$ vs. control (MANOVA followed by Tukey's test)

### 9.2 The effects of bilateral ovariectomy or adrenalectomy performed using a dorsal or ventral approach

Compared to animals with a ventral abdominal wall surgery, the effects of ventral bilateral ovariectomy one hour after surgery include lower testosterone and estradiol levels; while ventral bilateral adrenalectomy resulted in lower the progesterone levels (Figure 3). Similar effects were observed when surgeries were performed using the dorsal approach.

The effects of bilateral ovariectomy depend on the day of the cycle when surgery is performed (Flores et al., 2008). For instance, ventral bilateral ovariectomy on diestrus 1 resulted in lower progesterone levels than in animals with ventral wall surgery. These effects were not observed when the treatment was performed on diestrus 2, proestrus or estrus. In turn, dorsal bilateral ovariectomy on proestrus or estrus resulted in higher progesterone levels in serum than in rats with ventral abdominal wall surgery. The effects of bilateral adrenalectomy on progesterone were not impacted by the day of the cycle when surgery was performed or by the surgical approach (Flores et al., 2008). These results suggest that the neural information arriving to the adrenals and ovaries play different roles in regulating progesterone secretion by both organs.

Compared to ventral approach wall surgery treatment, animals with ventral bilateral ovariectomy had lower testosterone serum levels on each day of the estrous cycle. Similarly, ventral bilateral adrenalectomy performed on estrus resulted in lower hormone levels. Testosterone levels were not modified when the adrenals were removed on diestrus 1, diestrus 2 or proestrus. Compared to animals with dorsal wall surgery treatment, testosterone serum levels were lower in rats with dorsal bilateral ovariectomy performed on diestrus 2 or proestrus and higher when treatment was performed on estrus (Flores et al., 2008).

Compared to ventral or dorsal abdominal wall surgery treatment, ventral or dorsal bilateral ovariectomy performed on proestrus resulted in lower estradiol serum levels. Ventral bilateral adrenalectomy performed on diestrus 1 or 2 resulted in higher hormone levels, and lower when surgery was performed using a dorsal approach; and an inverse result occurred when the animals were treated on estrus (Flores et al., 2008).

Bilateral ovariectomy and adrenalectomy modify progesterone, testosterone and estradiol serum levels depending on the day of the cycle and the surgical approach. Analyzing the effects of dorsal or ventral bilateral ovariectomy or adrenalectomy on progesterone, testosterone and estradiol levels, suggest that the stimulatory/inhibitory signals arising from the dorsal or ventral abdominal wall modifies the sensitivity of the theca interna and granulosa cells to the hormonal signals regulating their functions.

The results obtained from rats with bilateral ovariectomy or adrenalectomy suggests that the ovaries mainly produce testosterone and estradiol, while the adrenals are the main producer of progesterone. The effects of bilateral adrenalectomy performed on different days of the estrous cycle on testosterone and estradiol serum levels (Flores et al., 2008) suggest that endocrine signals arising from the adrenals (corticosterone and progesterone) play a role regulating ovarian steroids release. It is possible that at the CSMG level, bilateral adrenalectomy modified the functions of the neurons originating in the SON and the nerve of the ovarian plexus that innervate the ovaries.

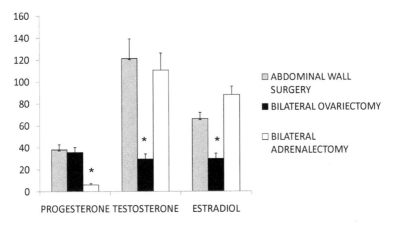

Fig. 3. Comparative effects of ventral bilateral ovariectomy or ventral adrenalectomy on progesterone, testosterone and estradiol serum levels. Based on data published by Flores et al., (2008) * $p < 0.05$ vs. abdominal wall surgery (MANOVA followed by Tukey's test)

### 9.3 The effects of unilateral ovariectomy

The acute effects of hemiovariectomy on progesterone, testosterone, estradiol, and LH concentrations in serum depends on the surgical approach and the day of the cycle when surgery is performed (Barco et al., 2003; Flores et al., 2005, 2006, 2011; Cruz et al., 2006).

Figure 4 shows the comparative effects of ventral unilateral mechanical stimulation of the SON and unilateral ventral ovariectomy, performed on each day of the estrous cycle, on progesterone, testosterone and estradiol serum levels analyzed one hour after treatment. The ventral mechanical stimulation of the left or right SON of rats in estrus resulted in higher progesterone levels. While extirpating the left ovary eliminated the progesterone levels increase, extirpating the right ovary did not. Regardless of the day of the estrus cycle

Progesterone                                 Testosterone

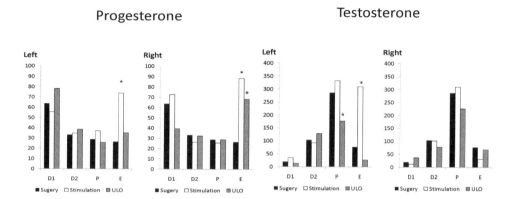

Estradiol

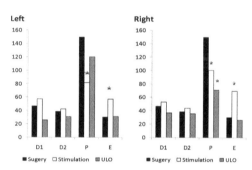

Fig. 4. Comparative effects of ventral unilateral mechanical stimulation of the SON and ventral unilateral ovariectomy performed each day of the estrous cycle on: progesterone (ng/mL), testosterone and estradiol (pg/mL) one hour after surgery. * p<0.05 vs. surgery. ■ Ventral surgery; □ mechanical stimulation of the SON; ▨ unilateral ovariectomy (ULO)

rats were treated on, stimulating the left SON resulted in higher testosterone levels, while stimulating the right SON did not have an apparent effect on testosterone. Higher testosterone levels in serum resulting from the stimulation of the left SON were eliminated when the right ovary was subsequently removed. In rats on estrus, stimulating the left or right SON increased estradiol levels, and ventral ovariectomy eliminated it.

These results suggest that mechanically stimulating the SON on estrus day stimulates the transport of cholesterol to the mitochondria, and the performance of the enzymes participating in the synthesis of progesterone and estradiol in both ovaries. Effects on testosterone levels were observed only when the left ovary was manipulated, suggesting an asymmetric participation of the ovarian innervation in regulating testosterone, and that such asymmetry depends on the day of the estrous cycle.

In other studies, the acute and non-acute effects of dorsal unilateral ovariectomy on progesterone, testosterone and estradiol serum levels vary according to the time elapsed between surgery and autopsy (Morales et al., 2011).

## 9.4 The effects of unilateral or bilateral ovarian denervation

The ovaries receive innervations arriving through the SON, the ovarian plexus nerve, and the vagus nerve. Since each nerve carries different neural information, we postulate that the unilateral or bilateral sectioning of each nerve will produce different effects on the secretion of steroid hormones by the ovaries.

The SON and the ovarian plexus nerve carry catecholaminergic fibers that innervate endocrine ovarian cells. These fibers are distributed in the peri-follicular theca layer and are closely related to the theca internal cells. According to Burden (1978) and Aguado (2002), most neurons originating in the SON fibers are located in the CSMG. Aside from the catecholaminergic innervation, the SON provides VIP (Garraza et al., 2004) and NO (Casais et al., 2007) innervations to the ovaries. 24 and 72 hrs after unilateral or bilateral sectioning of the SON of pre-pubertal rats, NA levels in the denervated ovary were lower than in untouched (control) or laparotomized animals (Chávez et al., 1994).

Aguado & Ojeda (1984) observed that after sectioning both SON on proestrus the secretion of progesterone and estradiol from both ovaries dropped immediately (four minutes). Progesterone secretion was recovered 15 minutes later, but estradiol levels kept low. Sectioning the SON on estrus did not modify hormone secretion. The effects of denervation depended on the hour of the day when surgery was performed. According to the authors, their results support the idea that the CNS controls directly the hormone release by the ovaries.

In gilts, sectioning the plexus and the SON during the middle luteal phase of the estrous cycle lowered the number of dopamine-beta-hydroxylase- and/or neuropeptide tyrosine-immunereactive nerve terminals. The treatment also lowered the levels of progesterone, androstenedione, and testosterone in the fluid and the wall of follicles. Neurectomy increased the immune expression of cholesterol side-chain cleavage cytochrome P450, lowered the expression of 33-hydroxysteroid dehydrogenase, and lowered the plasma levels of LH, progesterone, androstenedione, testosterone, estrone and estradiol-17beta. The results suggest that ovarian innervations play a role regulating the steroidogenic activity of the ovary (Jana et al., 2007).

Figure 5 shows the comparative effects of ventral unilateral mechanical stimulation of the SON on ovarian hormone secretion. From the graph, it is apparent that progesterone and testosterone levels in serum were modified by mechanically manipulating the SON, while changes in estradiol serum levels are not significant.

As with unilateral ovariectomy, the acute effects of ventral unilateral sectioning of the SON on progesterone, testosterone and estradiol serum levels presents asymmetry and vary according the day of the cycle when surgery was performed (Flores et al., 2011).

Ovarian denervation performed by unilaterally sectioning the vagus nerve, by a ventral approach, has different effects on normal cyclic rats and ULO rats. Sectioning the left vagus nerve resulted in lower ovulation rates than in sham operated animals; while sectioning the right vagus nerve did not modify ovulation rates. Sectioning the right or left vagus nerves to right-ULO rats (left ovary in-situ) reduced compensatory ovarian hypertrophy. Sectioning the left vagus nerve to ULO rats induced different effects depending on which ovary remained in-situ. Left-side vagotomy performed to right ULO rats (left ovary in-situ) resulted in higher ovulation rates, compensatory ovarian hypertrophy, and number of ova shed; while the same procedure to left ULO rats (right ovary in-situ) resulted in a decrease of the same parameters.

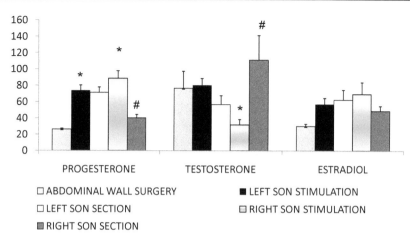

* p<0.05 vs. abdominal wall surgery; # p<0.05 vs. ipsilateral stimulation (MANOVA followed by Tukey's test)

Fig. 5. Comparative effects of ventral abdominal wall surgery, unilateral stimulation or sectioning of the superior ovarian nerve on progesterone (ng/mL, testosterone and estradiol serum levels (pg/mL).

Sectioning the right or left vagus nerves to right-ULO rats (left ovary in-situ) reduces compensatory ovarian hypertrophy, while the effects of sectioning the left vagus nerve depended on which ovary remained in-situ. Left-side vagotomy performed to right ULO rats (left ovary in-situ) resulted in higher ovulation rates, higher compensatory ovarian hypertrophy, and higher number of ova shed; while the same procedure to left ULO rats (right ovary in-situ) resulted in lower levels of the same parameters (Chávez et al.1987, 1989).

Sensorial innervations also play a role in regulating ovarian functions. Sensorial denervation induced by injecting capsaicin subcutaneously or into the ovarian bursa lowered spontaneous ovulation and secretion of progesterone and estradiol. Capsaicin treatment to ULO rats affected ovulation and the secretion of ovarian steroids, and these effects depended on which ovary remained in situ and the day of the cycle when treatment was performed (Trujillo et al., 2001, 2004).

### 9.5 The effects of unilateral adrenalectomy

Figure 6 shows the acute effects (one hour after surgery) of unilateral adrenalectomy, conducted on each day of the estrous cycle, on progesterone, testosterone and estradiol serum levels. The results show that the lack of one adrenal modified in different ways the concentration of the three hormones. The results suggest that the acute diminution and recovery of adrenal hormones affects the transportation of cholesterol to the ovaries in different ways, and the hormone secretion by the in situ ovary is only affected in diestrus 1, when unilateral adrenalectomy resulted in lower progesterone levels.

The effects of unilateral ovariectomy on testosterone and estradiol serum levels are asymmetric, mostly when surgery was performed on diestrus 2 (testosterone) or proestrus (testosterone and estradiol). The results suggest that the activity of enzymes participating in the synthesis of testosterone and estradiol are regulated by the levels of adrenal hormones and are not related to the synthesis of progesterone, since progesterone levels were not modify when the surgery was performed on diestrus 2 or proestrus.

# Progesterone

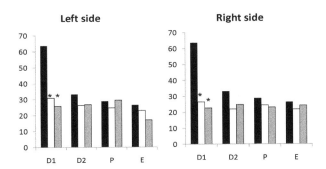

# Testosterone

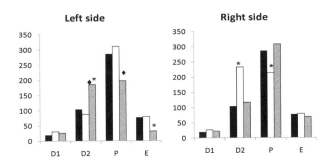

# Estradiol

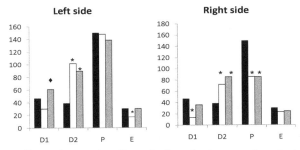

Fig. 6. Comparative effects of ventral unilateral adrenalectomy and ventral unilateral adrenalectomy followed by sectioning the SON ipsilateral to the extirpated adrenal, performed on each day of the estrous cycle on: progesterone (ng/mL), testosterone and estradiol (pg/mL) one hour after surgery. *p<0.05 vs. surgery. ■ Ventral surgery; □ unilateral adrenalectomy; ▨ unilateral ovariectomy followed by the SON section.

Some of the effects of unilateral adrenalectomy seem to be related to the SON ovarian innervation since the unilateral section of the SON modified some of the changes in testosterone and estradiol serum levels induced by unilateral adrenalectomy. Thus, the extirpation of one adrenal could modify the activity of the neurons in the CSMG originating SON fibers.

## 10. Ovarian and adrenal asymmetries

The supra-spinal innervations of the adrenals and ovaries show left side predominance, and some neurons exclusively innervate a given organ (Gerendai et al., 2009). Each adrenal gland is innervated both by side-specific neurons and by neurons that project to both organs (Tóth et al., 2007). The left and right ovaries have different abilities to spontaneously release oocytes. Such differences appear to be related to the ovarian innervations, and the left ovary appears to be more competent to spontaneously release oocytes (Domínguez et al., 1989).

According to Klein and Burden (1988), the number of neural fibers received by the right ovary is higher than in the left; while Toth et al., (2007) showed that the left ovary sends more neural information to the CNS than the right ovary. The right and left ovaries show different ovulatory responses to surgical denervation, and these responses vary according to the day of the estrous cycle when surgery is performed (Chávez et al., 1987, 1989; Chávez & Domínguez, 1994). These results suggest that the endocrine performances by the ovaries and adrenals present asymmetries, which are related to the innervations received by the organs.

## 11. Conclusions

Taken together the results obtained by different experimental approaches show that the synthesis and release of hormone by the adrenals and ovaries are under multiple controls. The hormonal signals arise from different sources, including the adrenals and ovaries. The adrenal and ovarian innervations modulate the effects of the hormonal signals, possibly by differences in the frequency and amplitude release of different neurotransmitters.

Because the mechanisms regulating the release of steroid hormones changes during the estrous cycle and throughout the day, it is possible that circadian signals arising from the suprachiasmatic nucleus exert a fine modulation of adrenal and ovarian cells to hormone and neural signals (Buijs et al.,2006).

Currently we do not have a clear hypothesis to explain why the organs secreting steroid hormones are asymmetric, or why such asymmetry varies during the estrous cycle and the hour of the day. Questions arising in the intent to present a hypothesis include:

1.   Is the expression of hormones and/or neurotransmitters receptors secreted by endocrine cells under the control of proteins synthesized under the directions of the clock genes present in the cells?

2.   Do the release characteristics (frequency and amplitude) of neurotransmitters by the axons arriving to the endocrine cells vary during the day, and do they present differences between one organ and the other?

3.   What are the functions of the micro-ganglia in the adrenals, testicles and ovaries?

## 12. Acknowledgments

We thank MSc Álvaro Domínguez-González for assistance in the English revision. DGAPA-UNAM Grants IN 200405, IN209508 and IN218911-3 supported the studies whose results are presented herein.

## 13. References

Aguado, L. I. (2002). Role of the central and peripheral nervous system in the ovarian function. *Microscopy Research and Technique,* Vol. 59, No.1 (December 2002), pp. 462-473, ISSN 1097-0029.

Aguado, L. I. & Ojeda, S. R. (1984) Ovarian adrenergic nerves play a role in maintaining preovulatory steroid secretion. *Endocrinology,* Vol. 114, No 5, (May 1984), pp. 1944-1946, ISSN 0013-7227.

Auchus, R. J. & Miller, W. L. (2000). The principles, pathways and enzymes of human steroidogenesis. *In Endocrinology Fourth Edition* Edited by LJ De Groot and JL Jameson. Vol 3, Chap. 115, pp. 1616-1631. ISBN 0-7216-7840-8 (set). WB Saunders Co.

Azhar, S., Leers-Sucheta, S, & Reaven, E. (2003). Cholesterol uptake in adrenal and gonadal tissues: the SR-BI and 'selective' pathway connection. *Frontiers in Bioscience,* Vol. 8, (September 2003) pp. 8,s998-1029, ISSN 1093-4715.

Barco, A. I., Flores, A., Chavira, R., Damian-Matsumura, P., Dominguez, R. & Cruz, M. E. (2003). Asymmetric effects of acute hemiovariectomy on steroid hormone secretion by the in situ ovary. *Endocrine,* Vol. 21, No.3 (August 2003), pp. 209-215, ISSN: 1559-0100.

Barkan, D., Jia, H., Dantes, A., Vardimon, L., Amsterdam, A. & Rubinstein M. (1999). Leptin modulates the glucocorticoid-induced ovarian steroidogenesis. *Endocrinology,* Vol. 140, No. 4, (April 1999), pp. 1731-1738, ISSN 1945-7170.

Barreiro, M. L. & Tena-Sempere, M. (2004). Ghrelin and reproduction: a novel signal linking energy status and fertility? *Molecular and Cellular Endocrinology,* Vol. 226, No.1-2, (October 2004), pp. 1-9, ISSN 0303-7207.

Belgorosky, A., Baquedano, MS., Guercio, G. & Rivarola ,M. A. (2008). Adrenarche: postnatal adrenal zonation and hormonal and metabolic regulation. *Hormone Research,* Vol. 70, No.5, (September 2008), pp. 257-67, ISSN 0301-0163.

Belloni, A.S., Malendowicz, L. K., Rucinski, M., Guidolin, D. & Nussdorfer, G. G. (2007). Galanin stimulates cortisol secretion from human adrenocortical cells through the activation of galanin receptor subtype 1 coupled to the adenylate cyclase-dependent signaling cascade. *International Journal of Molecular Medicine,* Vol.20, No.6, (December 2007), pp. 859-864, ISSN 1107-3756.

Berthoud HR, Powley TL. (1993). Characterization of vagal innervation to the rat celiac, suprarenal and mesenteric ganglia. J Journal of the autonomic nervous system.Vol. 42, No. 2 (February), pp.153-169. ISSN 1872-7484

Boon, W. C., Chow, J. D. & Simpson, E. R. (2010). The multiple roles of estrogens and the enzyme aromatase. In *Neuroendocrinology: The Normal Neuroendocrine System,* Edited by Luciano Martini, George Chrousos, Fernand Labrie, Karel Pacak, Donald Pfaff, Progress in Brain Research. Vol.181, pp. 209-232, ISBN 13: 978-0-444-53617-4 Elsevier.

Brannian, J.D., Zhao, Y., & McElroy, M. (1999). Leptin inhibits gonadotrophin-stimulated granulosa cell progesterone production by antagonizing insulin action. *Human Reproduction*, Vol.14, No. 2 (June 1999), pp.1445-1448, ISSN 1460-2350.

Bronzi, D., Orozco, A.V., Delgado, S.M., Casais, M. & Rastrilla, A.M.,& Sosa, Z.Y. (2011.) Modulation of the noradrenergic activity index by neural stimulus, and its participation in ovarian androstenedione release during the luteal phase. *Fertility & Sterility*, Vol. 95, No.4, ( December 2010), pp. 1211-1216, ISSN 0015-0282.

Burden, H.W., Lawrence, I.E. Jr. (1977). The effects of denervation on the localization of delta5-3beta-hydroxysteroid dehydrogenase activity in the rat ovary during pregnancy. *Acta Anat (Basel)*. Vol. 97, No. 3 (March), pp. 286-290. ISSN 0001-5180.

Burden, H.W., Leonard,M,, Smith, C,P., Lawrence, I. E. Jr. (1983). The sensory innervation of the ovary: a horseradish peroxidase study in the rat. *The Anatomical Record*. Vol.207, No. 4 (December), pp. 623-627. 0003-276X.

Buijs, R.M., Scheer, F.A., Kreier, F., Yi, C., Bos, N., Goncharuk, V.D. & Kalsbeek A. (2006) Organization of circadian functions: interaction with the body. *Progress in Brain Research*, Vol. 153 , No., (2006), pp. 341-360. Hypothalamic Integration of Energy Metabolism, Proceedings of the 24th International Summer School of Brain Research, held at the Royal Netherlands Academy of Arts and Sciences Amsterdam, The Netherlands 29 August-01 September 2005. Edited by: A. Kalsbeek, E. Fliers, M.A. Hofman, D.F. Swaab, E.J.W. van Someren and R.M. Buijs ISBN 978-0-444-52261-0.

Caminos, J. E., Nogueiras, R., Gaytán, F., Pineda, R., González, C.R., Barreiro, M.L., Castaño, J.P., Malagón, M.M., Pinilla, L., Toppari, J., Diéguez, C. & Tena-Sempere, M. (2008). Novel expression and direct effects of adiponectin in the rat testis. *Endocrinology*, Vol. 149, No. 7, (July 2008), pp. 3390-3402, ISSN 1945-7170.

Casais, M., Delgado, S.M., Vallcaneras, S., Sosa Z., & Rastrilla, A.M. (2007). Nitric oxide in prepubertal rat ovary contribution of the ganglionic nitric oxide synthase system via superior ovarian nerve. *Neuroendocrinology letters*, Vol. 28, No. 1, (February), pp. 39-44, ISSN 0172-780X.

Chávez, R., Cruz, M.E. & Domínguez, R. (1987). Differences in the ovulation rate of the right or left ovary in unilaterally ovariectomized rats: effect of ipsi- and contralateral vagus nerves on the remaining ovary. *Journal of Endocrinology*, Vol.113, (June 1987), pp. 397-401, ISSN 0022-0795.

Chávez, R., Morales, L., Gonzalez, M. E. & Domínguez, R. (1994). Ovarian norepinephrine content in prepubertal rats with superior ovarian nerve section. Temporally studies. *Medical Science Research* 1994, Vol.22, (n.d.), pp.789-790, ISSN .

Chávez, R., Sánchez, S., Ulloa-Aguirre, A. & Domínguez, R. (1989). Effects on estrous cyclicity and ovulation of unilateral section of the vagus nerve performed on different days of the estrous cycle in the rat. *Journal of Endocrinology* ,Vol.123 , No.3, (December 1989), pp. 441-444,ISSN 0022-0795.

Chen, M. C., Wang S.W., Kan S.F., Tsai S.C., Wu Y.C. & Wang P. S. (2010) Stimulatory effects of propylthiouracil on pregnenolone production through upregulation of steroidogenic acute regulatory protein expression in rat granulosa cells. *Toxicological Sciences*, Vol.118, No.2, (October 2010), pp. 667-74 , ISSN 1096-0929.

Chrenek, P., Grossmann, R. & Sirotkin, A. V. (2010). The cAMP analogue, dbcAMP affects release of steroid hormones by cultured rabbit ovarian cells and their response to

FSH, IGF-I and ghrelin. *European Journal of Pharmacology*, Vol. 640, No.1-3, (August 2010), pp. 202-205, ISSN 0014-2999.

Chung. S., Son, G.H., & Kim, K. (2011). Circadian rhythm of adrenal glucocorticoid: its regulation and clinical implications. *Biochimica et biophysica acta,*Vol.1812, No. 5, (May), pp. 581-591. ISSN 0006-3002.

Coupland, R. E., Parker, T. L., Kesse, W. K. & Mohamed, A. A. (1989). The innervation of the adrenal gland. III. Vagal innervation. *Journal of Anatomy*, Vol.163 , (April 1989), pp. 173-181, ISSN 1469-7580.

Cruz, M. E., Flores, A., Palafox, M. T., Meléndez, G., Rodríguez, J. O., Chavira, R. & Domínguez R. (2006). The role of the muscarinic system in regulating estradiol secretion varies during the estrous cycle: the hemiovariectomized rat model. *Reproductive Biology and Endocrinology*, (August 2010), pp. 4-43, ISSN 1945-7170.

Cunningham, L. A. & Holzwarth, M. A. (1988). Vasoactive intestinal peptide stimulates adrenal aldosterone and corticosterone secretion. *Endocrinology*. Vol. 122, No. 5, (May 1988), pp. 2090-2097, ISSN 0013-7227.

Czajka-Oraniec, I. & Simpson, E. R. (2010). Aromatase research and its clinical significance. *Endokrynolia Polska*, Vol.61 , No.1, (February 2010), pp. 126-34, ISSN 0423-104X.

D'Albora, H. & Barcia, J. J. (1996). Intrinsic neuronal cell bodies in the rat ovary. *Neurosciense Letters*, Vol.205, No.1, (1996), pp. 61-67, ISSN 0304-3940.

D'Albora, H., Anesetti, G., Lombide, P., Dees, W.L. & Ojeda, S.R.(2002). Intrinsic neurons in the mammalian ovary. *Microscopy Research Technology*. Vol.59, No. 6 (December 15), pp. 484-489.ISSN 1097-0029.

De Bortoli, M.A., Garraza, M.H., &Aguado, L. I. (1998). Adrenergic intracerebroventricular stimulation affects progesterone concentration in the ovarian vein of the rat: participation of the superior ovarian nerve. *Journal of Endocrinology*, Vol. 159, No.9, (October 1998), pp. 61-68, ISSN 0022-0795.

De Bortoli, M. A, Garraza, M. H., & Aguado, Ll. (2000). Epinephrine intracerebroventricular stimulation modifies the LH effect on ovarian progesterone and androstenedione release. *Journal of Steroid Biochemistry & Molecular Biology*, Vol. 74, No.1-2, (September 2000), pp.19-24 , ISSN 0960-0760.

De Bortoli, M. A., Garraza, M. H., &Aguado, L. I. (2002). Involvement of beta-adrenoceptors in a central regulation of the ovarian progesterone release in rats. *Neuroendocrinology Letters* Vol.23 , No.3, (February 2002), pp. 27-31, ISSN 0172–780X.

Dees WL, Hiney JK, Schultea TD, Mayerhofer A, Danilchik M, Dissen GA, Ojeda SR. (1995). The primate ovary contains a population of catecholaminergic neuron-like cells expressing nerve growth factor receptors. *Endocrinology*, Vol. 136, No.12, (December 1995, pp. 5760-5768, ISSN 0013-7227.

Delarue, C., Conlon, J. M., Remy-Jouet, I., Fournier, A., & Vaudry, H. (2004). Endothelins as local activators of adrenocortical cells. *Journal of Molecular Endocrinology*, Vol.32, No.1, (February 2004), pp. 1-7, ISSN 0952-5041.

Diaz, F.J., Anderson, L.E., Wu, Y. L., Rabot, A., Tsai, S. J. & Wiltbank, M. C.(2002). Regulation of progesterone and prostaglandin F2alpha production in the CL. *Molecular Cell Endocrinology*, Vol. 191, No. 1 (May 2002), pp. 65-80.ISSN 1872-8057.

Domínguez, R., Cruz, M. E. & Chávez, R. (1989). Differences in the ovulatory ability between the right and left ovary are related to ovarian innervation. *In: Growth*

*Factors and the Ovary*. Editor Anne M.Hirshfield.. Chap. 39. pp.321-325. Plenum Press, New York

Domínguez, R., Morales, L. & Cruz, M.E. (2003). Ovarian asymmetry. *Annual Review of Biological Sciences*. Vol.5, No. Pp. 95-104

Duggal, P.S., Ryan, N.K., Van der Hoek, K.H., Ritter, L.J., Armstrong, D.T., Magoffin, D.A., & Norman R.J. (2002) Effects of leptin administration and feed restriction on thecal leucocytes in the preovulatory rat ovary and the effects of leptin on meiotic maturation, granulosa cell proliferation, steroid hormone and PGE2 release in cultured rat ovarian follicles. *Reproduction*, Vol. 123, No.6, (June 2002), pp. 891-898, ISSN 1470-1626.

Dupont, J., Chabrolle, C., Ramé, C., Tosca, L., & Coyral-Castel, S. (2008). Role of the peroxisome proliferator-activated receptors, adenosine monophosphate-activated kinase, and adiponectin in the ovary. *PPAR Research*, Vol. 2008, p. 176275 , ISSN 1687-4765.

Enyedi, P., Szabó, B. & Spät, A. (1983) Failure of vasoactive intestinal peptide to stimulate aldosterone production. *Acta Physiologica Hungarica*. Vol. 61, No. 1-2, (n.d.)pp. 77-79.ISSN 0231-424X

Espenshade, P. J, & Hughes, A.L. (2007). Regulation of sterol synthesis in eukaryotes. *Annual Review of Genetics*, Vol.41, (July 2007), pp. 401-427, ISSN: 0066-4197.

Flores, A., Gallegos, A. I., Velasco, J., Mendoza, F. D., Montiel, C., Everardo, P. M., Cruz, M. E., Domínguez, R. (2008). The acute effects of bilateral ovariectomy or adrenalectomy on progesterone, testosterone and estradiol serum levels depend on the surgical approach and the day of the estrous cycle when they are performed. *Reproductive Biology and Endocrinology*, Vol. 6. (October 2011), p. 48, ISSN 1945-7170.

Flores, A., Meléndez, G., Palafox, M. T., Rodríguez, J., Barco, A. I., Chavira, R., Domínguez, R. & Cruz, M. E. (2005). The participation of the cholinergic system in regulating progesterone secretion through the ovarian-adrenal crosstalk varies along the estrous cycle. *Endocrine*, Vol. 28, No.2, (July 2005), pp. : 145-151, ISSN 1559-0100.

Flores, A., Rodríguez, J. O., Palafox, M. T., Meléndez, G., Barco, A. I., Chavira, R., Cruz, M. E. & Domínguez, R. (2006). The acute asymmetric effects of hemiovariectomy on testosterone secretion vary along the estrous cycle. The participation of the cholinergic system. *Reproductive Biology and Endocrinology*, Vol. 4, (March 2006), p. 11, ISSN 1945-7170.

Flores, A., Velasco, J., Gallego,s A. I., Mendoza, F. D., Everardo, P. M., Cruz, M. E. & Domínguez, R. (2011). Acute effects of unilateral sectioning the superior ovarian nerve of rats with unilateral ovariectomy on ovarian hormones (progesterone, testosterone and estradiol) levels vary during the estrous cycle. *Reproductive Biology and Endocrinology*, Vol. 9, No.34, (March 2011), pp. , ISSN 1945-7170.

Franchimont, P. (1983). Regulation of gonadal androgen secretion. *Hormone Research*, Vol.18, No. 1-3, pp.7-17, ISSN 1423-0046.

Frungieri, M. B., Zitta, K., Pignataro, O. P., Gonzalez-Calvar, S. I. & Calandra, R. S. (2002). Interactions between testicular serotoninergic, catecholaminergic, and corticotropin-releasing hormone e systems modulating cAMP and testosterone production in the golden hamster. *Neuroendocrinology*. Vol.17, No.1, (July 2002), pp. 35-46, ISSN 0028-3835.

Garraza, M. H., Aguado, L. I., & De Bortoli, M. A. (2004) In vitro effect of neuropeptides on ovary or celiac ganglion affects the release of progesterone from ovaries in the rat. *Medical Science Monitor,* Vol.10, No.12, (December 2004), pp.440-446, ISSN 1634-3750.

Gerendai, .I, Tóth, I.E., Boldogköi, Z., Medveczky, I., & Halász B. (2000) CNS structures presumably involved in vagal control of ovarian function. Journal of Autonomic Nervous System. Vol. 80, No. 1-2, (April 12), pp. 40-45.ISSN 0165-1838

Gerendai, I., Tóth, I.E., Boldogkoi, Z. & Halász, B. (2009). Recent findings on the organization of central nervous system structures involved in the innervation of endocrine glands and other organs; observations obtained by the transneuronal viral double-labeling technique. *Endocrine,* Vol.36, No.2, (October 2009), pp. 179-188, ISSN 1559-0100.

Ghosh, D., Griswold J, Erman M. & Pangborn W. (2009). Structural basis for androgen specificity and oestrogen synthesis in human aromatase. *Nature,* Vol.457 , No.7226, ( January 2009), pp. 219-223 , ISSN 0028-0836.

Hamel, M., Vanselow, J., Nicola, E.S. & Price CA. (2005). Androstenedione increases cytochrome P450 aromatase messenger ribonucleic acid transcripts in nonluteinizing bovine granulosa cells. *Molecular Reproduction and Development.* Vol. 70, No. 2, (February 2005), pp.175-183. ISSN 1098-2795

Hinson, J.P., Kapas, S., Orford, C.D. & Vinson, G.P. (1992). Vasoactive intestinal peptide stimulation of aldosterone secretion by the rat adrenal cortex may be mediated by the local release of catecholamines. *The Journal of Endocrinology.* Vol. 133, No.2 (May 1992), pp.253-238,ISSN 1479-6805

Holgert, H., Aman, K., Cozzari, C., Hartman, B.K., Brimijoin, S., Emson, P., Goldstein, M. & Hökfelt, T. (1995). The cholinergic innervation of the adrenal gland and its relation to enkephalin and nitric oxide synthase. *Neuroreport,* Vol.15 , No.6, (December 1995), pp. 2576–2580, ISSN 09594965.

Holgert, H., Dagerlind, A., & Hökfelt, T. (1998). Immunohistochemical characterization of the peptidergic innervation of the rat adrenal gland. *Hormone Metabolic Research,* Vol.30 , No.6-7, (Julio 1998), pp. 315–322, ISSN 0018-5043.

Hu, J., Zhang ,Z., Shen, W. J. Azhar, S. (2010). Cellular cholesterol delivery, intracellular processing and utilization for biosynthesis of steroid hormones. *Nutrition & metabolism (Lond).* Vol. 7, (June 1), p. 47, ISSN 1743-7075.

Ishimaru, R. S., Leung, K., Hong L., & LaPolt, P. S. (2001). Inhibitory effects of nitric oxide on estrogen production and cAMP levels in rat granulosa cell cultures. *Journal of Endocrinology,* Vol. 168, No.8, (February 2001), pp. 249-255, ISSN 0022-0795.

Jana, B., Dzienis, A., Wojtkiewicz, J., Kaczmarek, M., & Majewski, M. (2007). Surgical denervation of porcine ovaries during the middle luteal phase of the oestrous cycle changes their morphology and steroidogenic activity. *Acta Veterinaria Hungarica,* Vol.55, No.5, (March 2007), pp. 107-122 , ISSN 1588-2705.

Kagerer, S. M. & Jöhren O. (2010). Interactions of orexins/hypocretins with adrenocortical functions. *Acta Physiologica (Oxford, England),* Vol.198 , No.3, (March 2010), pp. 361-371, ISSN 1748-1716.

Karamouti, M, Kollia, P, Kallitsaris, A, Vamvakopoulos, N, Kollios, G, & Messinis, IE. (2009). Modulating effect of leptin on basal and follicle stimulating hormone stimulated steroidogenesis in cultured human lutein granulosa cells. *Journal of Endocrinological Investigation*, Vol.32, No.5, (May 2009), pp. 415-419, ISSN 0022-0795.

Kawakami, M., Kubo K., Uemura, T. & Nagase, M.(1979). Evidence for the existence of extra-hypophyseal neural mechanisms controlling ovarian steroid secretion. *Journal of Steroid Biochemistry*, Vol.11, No.1C, (July 1979), pp. 1001-1005, ISSN 0022-4731.

Kawakami, M., Kubo, K., Uemura, T., Nagase, M. &., Hayashy, R.(1981). Involvement of ovarian innervation on steroid secretion. *Endocrinology*, Vol. 109, No.1, (July 1981), pp. 136-145, ISSN 1945-7170.

Klein, C. M. & Burden, H. W. (1988). Anatomical localization of afferent and postganglionic sympathetic neurons innervating the rat ovary. *Neuroscience Letters*, Vol.85 , No.2, (February 1988), pp. 217-222 , ISSN 0304-3940.

Kondo, H. (1985). Immunohistochemical analysis of the localizationof neuropeptides in the adrenal gland. *Archivum Histologicum Japonicum*, Vol. 48, No.5, (December 1985), pp. 453-481, ISSN 0004-0681.

Kostic, T. S., Stojkov, N. J., Bjelic, M. M., Mihajlovic, A. I., Janjic, M. M. & Andric, S. A. (2011) Pharmacological doses of testosterone up-regulated androgen receptor (AR) and 3-beta-hydroxysteroid dehydrogenase/delta-5-delta-4 isomerase (3{beta}HSD) and impaired Leydig cells steroidogenesis in adult rat. *Toxicological Sciences*, Vol.120, No.2, (April 2011), pp. 397-407, ISSN 10966080.

Kuramoto, H., Kondo, H., & Fujita, T. (1987). Calcitonin gene-related peptide (CGRP)-like immunoreactivity in scattered chromaffin cells and nerve fibers in the adrenal gland of rats. *Cell & Tissue Research*, Vol. 247, No.2, (February 1987), pp. 309-315, ISSN 1432-0878.

Lee, J., Park, H.J., Choi, H.S., Kwon, H.B., Arimura, A., Lee, B,J,, Choi, W.S. & Chun S.Y. (1999). Gonadotropin stimulation of pituitary adenylate cyclase-activating polypeptide (PACAP) messenger ribonucleic acid in the rat ovary and the role of PACAP as a follicle survival factor. *Endocrinology*. Vol. 140, No. 2 (February 1999), pp.818-826, ISSN 0013-7227.

Lin, K.C., Okamura, H. & Mori T. (1997). Inhibition of human chorionic gonadotropin-induced ovulation and steroidogenesis by short-term hyperprolactinemia in female rabbits. *Endocrinologia Japonica*, Vol. 34, No. 5, (October 1997), pp. 675-683, ISNN0013-7219

Luo, W., Gumen, A., Haughian, J. M. & Wiltbank, M. . (2011). The role of luteinizing hormone in regulating gene expression during selection of a dominant follicle in cattle. *Biology of Reproduction*, Vol.84, No.2, (February 2011), pp. 369-78, ISSN 1529-7268.

Makarevich, A.V., Sirotkin, A.V., & Genieser, H.G. (2004). Action of protein kinase A regulators on secretory activity of porcine granulosa cells in vitro. *Animal Reproduction Science*, Vol.81 , No.1-2, (March 2004), pp. 125-36, ISSN 0378-4320.

Malendowicz, L. K. Rucinsk, M., Belloni, A.S, Ziolkowska, A. & Nussdorfer, G. G. (2007). Leptin and the regulation of the hypothalamic-pituitary-adrenal axis. *International Reviews of Cytology*, Vol. 263, (August 2007), pp. 63-102, ISSN 0074-7696.

Malendowicz, L.K., Tortorella, C., & Nussdorfer, G. G. (1999). Orexins stimulate corticosterone secretion of rat adrenocortical cells, through the activation of the adenylate cyclase-dependent signaling cascade. *The Journal of Steroid Biochemistry & Molecular Biology*, Vol. 70, No.4-6, (Sep-October 1999), pp. 185-188, ISSN 0960-0760.

Malendowicz, L. K., Neri, G., Markowska, A., Hochol, A., Nussdorfer, G. G. & Majchrzak, M. (2003). Effects of leptin and leptin fragments on steroid secretion of freshly dispersed rat adrenocortical cells. The Journal of Steroid Biochemistry & Molecular Biology, Vol. 87, No. 4-5, (December 2003), pp. 265-2688, ISSN 0960-0760.

Manna, P.R., Kero J., Tena-Sempere, M., Pakarinen, P., Stocco, D.M., & Huhtaniemi, I.T. (2001). Assessment of mechanisms of thyroid hormone action in mouse Leydig cells: regulation of the steroidogenic acute regulatory protein, steroidogenesis, and luteinizing hormone receptor function. Endocrinology, Vol. 142, No.1, (January 2001), pp. 319-31, ISSN 1945-7170.

Manna, P.R., Tena-Sempere, M., Huhtaniemi, I.T. (1999). Molecular mechanisms of thyroid hormone-stimulated steroidogenesis: involvement of steroidogenic acute regulatory (StAR) protein. Journal of Biological Chemistry. Vol. 274, No.,9 (February 26), pp. 5909-5918, ISSN 1083-351X.

Maran, R.R., Arunakaran, J. & Aruldhas, M.M. (2000). T3 directly stimulates basal and modulates LH induced testosterone and oestradiol production by rat Leydig cells in vitro. Endocrinologia Japonica. Vol. 47, No. 4 (August 2000), pp.417-428, ISNN0013-7219.

Markowska, A., Neri, G., Hochol,A., Nowak, M., Nussdorfer ,G.G., & Malendowicz, L.K. (2004). Effects of leptin and leptin fragments on steroid secretion and proliferative activity of regenerating rat adrenal cortex. International Journal of Molecular Medicine Vol. 13, No.1, (January 2004), pp. 139-141, ISSN 1107-3756.

Mavridou, S., Venihaki, M., Rassouli, O., Tsatsani,s C., & Kardassis D. (2010). Feedback inhibition of human scavenger receptor class B type I gene expression by glucocorticoid in adrenal and ovarian cells. Endocrinology, Vol. 151, No.7, (July 2010), pp. 3214-24, ISSN 1945-7170.

Mayerhofer, A., Dissen, G. A., Costa, M. E., & Ojeda, S. R. (1997). A role for neurotransmitters in early follicular development: induction of functional follicle-stimulating hormone receptors in newly formed follicles of the rat ovary. Endocrinology, Vol.138, No.9, (August 1997), pp. 3320-3329, ISSN 1945-7170.

Mazzocchi, G., Rebuffat, P., Meneghelli, V., Malendowicz, L.K., Tortorella, C., Gottard,o G., & Nussdorfer, G. G. (1999). Gastric inhibitory polypeptide stimulates glucocorticoid secretion in rats, acting through specific receptors coupled with the adenylate cyclase-dependent signaling pathway. Peptides, Vol.20 , ( 1999), pp. 589-594 , ISSN 0196-9781.

Mészárosová, M., Sirotkin, A.V., Grossmann, R., Darlak, K., & Valenzuela, F. (2008). The effect of obestatin on porcine ovarian granulosa cells. Animal Reproduction Science, Vol. 108, No. 1-2, (October 2008), pp. 196-207, ISSN 0378-4320.

Miszkiel, G., & Kotwica, J. (2001). Mechanism of action of noradrenaline on secretion of progesterone and oxytocin by the bovine corpus luteum in vitro. Acta Veterinaria Hungarica, Vol.49, No.1, pp. 39-51, ISSN 1588-2705.

Morales-Ledesma, L., Ramírez, D.A., Vieyra, E., Trujillo, A., Chavira, R., Cárdenas, M. & Domínguez R. (2011). Effects of acute unilateral ovariectomy to pre-pubertal rats on steroid hormones secretion and compensatory ovarian responses. Reproductive Biology and Endocrinology. Vol. 9, (March 30 2011), p. 41, ISSN 1477-7827.

Morán, C., Franco, A., Morán, J,L,, Handal, A,, Morales, L, & Domínguez R. (2005). Neural activity between ovaries and the prevertebral celiac-superior mesenteric ganglia varies during the estrous cycle of the rat. *Endocrine* Vol. 26, No. 2 (March 2005), pp. 147-156, ISSN: 1559-0100.

Nimz, M., Spitschak, M., Fürbass, R., & Vanselow, J. (2010). The pre-ovulatory luteinizing hormone surge is followed by down-regulation of CYP19A1, HSD3B1, and CYP17A1 and chromatin condensation of the corresponding promoters in bovine follicles. *Molecular Reproduction and Development*, Vol.77, No.12, (December 2010), pp. 1040-1048, ISSN 1098-2795.

Niswender, G.D. (2002). Molecular control of luteal secretion of progesterone. *Reproduction*. Vol. 123, No. 3 (March 2002), pp. 333-339, ISSN 1741-7899.

Nussdorfer, G.G., Bahçelioglu ,M., Neri, G. & Malendowicz, L.K. (2000). Secretin, glucagon, gastric inhibitory polypeptide, parathyroid hormone, and related peptides in the regulation of the hypothalamus- pituitary-adrenal axis. *Peptides*, Vol. 21, No.12, (February 2000), pp. 309-324, ISSN 0196-9781.

Ramírez, D. A., Vieyra, E., Morales, L. & Dominguez, R. (2008). The acute effects of unilateral ovariectomy to prepubertal rats on gonadotropin and hormone ovarian secretion are asymmetric. Program No. 81.3 Washington, DC: Society for Neuroscience; 2008, Online.

Renshaw, D., Thomson, L.M., Carroll, M., Kapas. S. & Hinson J.P. (2000). Actions of neuropeptide Y on the rat adrenal cortex. *Endocrinology*. Vol. 141, No. 1 (January 2000), pp. 169-173, ISSN 1945-7170.

Rey-Ares, V., Lazarov, N., Berg, D., Berg, U., Kunz, L. & Mayerhofer, A. (2007). Dopamine receptor repertoire of human granulosa cells. Reproductive Biology & Endocrinology. Vol.5 , (October 25), pp. 40, ISSN 1477-7827.

Ricci, A. G., Di Yorio, M. P. & Faletti, A. G. (2006). Inhibitory effect of leptin on the rat ovary during the ovulatory process. *Reproduction*, Vol. 132, No. 5, (November 2006), pp. 771-780, ISSN 1741-7899

Ronti, T., Lupattelli. G. & Mannarino, E. (2006). The endocrine function of adipose tissue: an update. *Clinical Endocrinology (Oxf)*. 2006 Vol. 64, No.4, (April), pp.355-365. ISSN 0300-0664.

Sirotkin, A.V., Makarevich, A.V. & Grosmann R. (2011). Protein kinases and ovarian functions. Journal of Cellular Physiology. Vol. 226, No. 1(September), pp. 37-45, INSS 1097-4652.

Sirotkin, A.V. & Grossmann, R. (2007a). The role of ghrelin and some intracellular mechanisms in controlling the secretory activity of chicken ovarian cells. Comparative Biochemistry and Physiology. Part A. *Molecular & Integrative Physiology*, Vol.147, No.1, (May 2007), pp. 239-246, ISSN 1531-4332.

Sirotkin, A.V., & Grossmann, R. (2007b). Leptin directly controls proliferation, apoptosis and secretory activity of cultured chicken ovarian cells. Comparative Biochemistry and Physiology. Part A. *Molecular & Integrative Physiology*. Vol. 148, No.2, (October 2007), pp.422-429, ISSN 1531-4332.

Sirotkin, A.V, Makarevich A.V, & Grosmann ,R. (2011). Protein kinases and ovarian functions. *Journal of Cellular and Comparative Physiology*, Vol.226, No.1, (January 2011), pp. 37-45, ISSN 0095-9898.

Spicer, L. J . & Francisco, C. C. (1997). The adipose obese gene product, leptin: evidence of a direct inhibitory role in ovarian function. *Endocrinology*, Vol. 138, No.8, (August 1997), pp. 3374-3379, ISSN 1945-7170.

Spiga, F, Liu, Y., Aguilera, G. & Lightman, S.L. (2011). Temporal effect of adrenocorticotrophic hormone on adrenal glucocorticoid steroidogenesis: involvement of the transducer of regulated cyclic AMP-response element-binding protein activity. *Journal of Neuroendocrinology*, Vol. 23, No.2, (February 2001), pp. 136-142, ISSN 0028-3835.

Spinazzi, R., Andreis, P.G., Rossi, G.P. & Nussdorfe,r G.G. (2006). Orexins in the regulation of the hypothalamic-pituitary-adrenal axis. *Pharmacological Reviews*, Vol.58 , No.1, ( March 2006), pp.46-57, ISSN 1521-0081.

Stocco, C. (2008). Aromatase expression in the ovary: hormonal and molecular regulation. *Steroid*, Vol.73 , No.5, (May 2008), pp.473-478 , ISSN 0039-128x.

Strauss, J. R- III & Hsueh, A. J. W. (2000). *Ovarian hormone synthesis*. In: *Endocrinology* Fourth Edition edited by LJ De Groot and JL Jameson vol 3, Chap. 148, pp 2043-2052. WB Saunders Co. ISBN 0-7216-7840-8 (set). Philadelphia, Pennsylvania

Sugawara, T., Kiriakidou, M., McAllister, J. M., Holt, J. A., Arakane, F. & Strauss, J. F. 3rd. (1997). Regulation of expression of the steroidogenic acute regulatory protein (StAR) gene: a central role for steroidogenic factor 1. *Steroids*, Vol.62, No.1, (January 1997), pp.5-9, ISSN 0039-128x.

Szalay, K. S, Orsó, E., Jurányi, Z., Vinson, G. . & Vizi, E. S. (1998). Local non-synaptic modulation of aldosterone production by catecholamines and ATP in rat: implications for a direct neuronal fine tuning. *Hormone Metabolic Research*, Vol.30, No.6-7, (June-July), pp. 323-328, ISSN 0018-5043.

Tortorella, C., Neri, G. & Nussdorfer, G.G. (2007). Galanin in the regulation of the hypothalamic-pituitary-adrenal axis (Review). *International Journal of Molecular Medicine*, Vol.19 , No.4, (April 2007), pp. 639-647, ISSN 1107-3756.

Tóth I.E., Wiesel O., Boldogkoi, Z., Bálint, K., Tapaszti, Z. & Gerendai, I. (2007). Predominance of supraspinal innervation of the left ovary. *Microscopic Research Technique*. Vol. 70, No.8, (August 2007), pp.710-718, ISSN 1097-0029.

Tóth, I.E., Wiesel, O., Boldogkoi, Z., Bálint, K., Tapaszti, Z. & Gerendai I. (2007). Predominance of supraspinal innervation of the left ovary. *Microscopy Research Technique*. Vol. 70, No. 8 (August 2007), pp.710-718 ISSN 1097-0029.

Tropea, A., Lanzone, A., Tiberi,F., Romani, F., Catino, S. & Apa, R. (2010). Estrogens and androgens affect human luteal cell function. *Fertility & Sterility*, Vol. 94, No. 6, (November 2010), pp. 2257-2263, ISSN 0015-0282.

Trujillo, A., Morales, L., Dominguez, R. & Vindrola, O. (2001). Effects of sensorial denervation on the ovarian functions in the adult rat. Program No. 734.14 Neuroscience Meeting Planner. San Diego, Ca; 2001.

Trujillo, A., Morales, L., Vargas, X., Alba, L. & Domínguez R. (2004). Effects of capsaicin treatment on the regulation of ovarian compensatory hypertrophy and compensatory ovulation. *Endocrine*, Vol. 25, No. 2, (November 2004), pp. 155-162, ISSN: 1559-0100.

Uchida, S., Kagitani F., Hotta, H., Hanada, T. & Aikawa, Y. (2005). Cutaneous mechanical stimulation regulates ovarian blood flow via activation of spinal and supraspinal reflex pathways in anesthetized rats. *The Japanese journal of Physiology*, Vol. 55, No.5, (October 2005), pp.265-277, ISSN 1881-1396.

Ulrich-Lai, Y. M. & Engeland, W. C. (2000). Hyperinnervation during adrenal regeneration influences the rate of functional recovery. *Neuroendocrinology*, Vol.71, No.2, (February 2000), pp.107-123 , ISSN 0028-3835.

Ulrich-Lai, Y. M., Arnhold, M. M. & Engeland, W. C. (2006). Adrenal splanchnic innervation contributes to the diurnal rhythm of plasma corticosterone in rats by modulating adrenal sensitivity to ACTH. *American Journal of Physiology Regulatory, Integrative and Comparative Physiology*, Vol.290, No.4, (April2006), pp. R1128-1135, ISSN 1522-1490.

Wang, H., Eriksson, H. & Sahlin, L. (2000) Estrogen receptors α and β in the female reproductive tract of the rat during the estrous cycle. *Biology of Reproduction*, Vol. 63, No.5, (November 1, 2000), pp. 1331–1340, ISSN 1529-7268.

Whitworth, E. J, Kosti, O., Renshaw, D., & Hinson, J.P. (2003). Adrenal neuropeptides: regulation and interaction with ACTH and other adrenal regulators. *Microscopy Research and Technique*,Vol.61 , No.3, (June 15), pp. 259-267, ISSN 1097-0029.

Wu, J.L., Wu, R.S., Yang, J.G., Huang, C.C., Chen, K.B., Fang, K.H. & Tsai H. D. (2011). Effects of sleep deprivation on serum testosterone concentrations in the rat. *Neuroscience Letters*, Vol. 494, No.2, (April 25, 2011 ), pp. 124-129, ISSN 1872-7972.

Zachow, R.J. & Magoffin, D. A. (1997). Direct intraovarian effects of leptin: impairment of the synergistic action of insulin-like growth factor-I on follicle-stimulating hormone-dependent estradiol-17 beta production by rat ovarian granulosa cells. *Endocrinology*, Vol. 138, No. 2, (February 1997), pp. 847-850, ISSN 0013-7227.

Zachow, R. J, Weitsman, S. R., & Magoffin, D. A. (1999). Leptin impairs the synergistic stimulation by transforming growth factor-beta of follicle-stimulating hormone-dependent aromatase activity and messenger ribonucleic acid expression in rat ovarian granulosa cells. *Biology of Reproduction*, Vol. 61, No. 4, (October 1999), pp. 1104-1109. ISSN: 0006-3363.

# 2

# Evolving Trends in Estrogen Receptor Biology

Raghava Varman Thampan
*MIMS Research Foundation, A Division of Malabar Institute*
*of Medical Sciences, Ltd. (MIMS), Calicut, Kerala,*
*India*

## 1. Introduction

Discussions on receptors involved in estrogen action(Stanišić et al,2010) have so far focused on the two major forms of "classical" estrogen receptors, the estrogen receptor α (ER α) and estrogen receptor β (ER β). Both are DNA binding as well as hormone binding forms, with distinct, well-characterized functional domains. The differences between the two have mainly been in their respective molecular masses and shapes and in the target genes with which they interacted.

I have been involved in research in estrogen action for 4 decades and more. Since the focus of my work was chiefly on non-conventional estrogen receptors and receptor associated proteins, often the progress made was felt by me as slow.Nevertheless,it is my sincere belief that what has been unveiled in this direction over the years have not gone unproductive. The two proteins that have been identified in this context, one a non DNA binding estrogen receptor and the other a transcription factor that dimerises with this receptor in the nucleus, have pointed towards the existence of a unique system of receptor in estrogen action. For the first time ever, it has become clear that there is a form of estrogen receptor whose primary functional role is in post transcriptional regulatory mechanisms that include splicing, nucleocytoplasmic transport of RNA and finally, the translation of mRNA. Also, deeper insights into the functional biology of the transcription factor have unfolded certain experimental data hitherto unknown in the literature on steroid hormone action. What is being discussed in this chapter deals exclusively with these two proteins, one a plasma membrane localized estrogen receptor which moves into the nucleus to involve itself in gene regulatory events and the other a transcription factor with a parallel functional role in mitochondrial steroidogenesis

## 2. The concept of steroid hormone receptor activation

The favorite theme of the 60's and early 70's in descriptions of steroid hormone action, particularly with reference to estrogen action, used to be that the receptor primarily existed in the cytosol. Upon hormone binding and the consequent "receptor activation" the receptor entered the nucleus and interacted with the genetic elements. This "two-step mechanism", independently proposed by the research groups led by Jensen and Gorski (Jensen & DeSombre, 1973; Shyamala & Gorski, 1969; Mohla et al, 1972) formed the basis for all subsequent discussions on intracellular movements of the receptor –steroid hormone complex. It was proposed that the cytosolic receptor existed as a high molecular weight form that sedimented at 8-9S in low salt linear sucrose gradients. Later studies have revealed that in this cytosolic form, the receptor with an average sedimentation value of 4S, remained in association with heat shock protein 90(hsp 90) when there was no hormone bound to it (Pratt, 1990; Pratt &Toft, 1997). Hormone binding to the receptor initiated dissociation of the receptor form Hsp-90, which formed a key event in steroid receptor activation (Pratt, 1990). One of the major structural changes noticed in the receptor during its activation was the transformation of the 4S receptor to a form that sedimented at 5S in sucrose gradients containing 0.3M KCl (Shyamala & Gorski, 1969).

The 4S-5S conversion was the target of several hypotheses that attempted to explain the molecular event. In the Hsp-90 model, it was clear that association of the receptor with Hsp-90 prevented the nuclear migration of the receptor the reason for which was not clear at that time. It was the first ever report on the sequencing of amino acids of the human estrogen receptor α (ER α) by Chambon's group at Strasburgh that paved the way for a number of active studies in this direction (Green & Chambon, 1987 a, b). The identification of the nuclear localization signal (NLS) in ERα (Kumar et al., 1986; Kumar et al., 1987) was one such landmark observation. Thampan's group subsequently extended the studies using ERα isolated from goat uterus and purified and characterized a 55kDa protein (p55) that apparently recognized the nuclear localization signal (NLS) on ERα and initiated the nuclear entry of the receptor (Nirmala & Thampan,1995 a,b). The studies reported by Thampan's group gave additional validity to the role of p55 in the nuclear entry of ERα.

## 3. The role of estradiol in the nuclear entry of ERα

Sai Padma et al (2000)and Sai Padma & Thampan(2000) observed that there were three nuclear proteins that contributed to the regulated entry of ERα into the nuclei. (a) the p55 that recognized the NLS on ERα(b)a 28kDa protein,p28 that bound to the NLS signal on ERα and thereby prevented the p55-ERα interaction;(c)a 73 kDa protein,p73 that bound to the hormone binding domain(HBD)on ERα.Under hormone free conditions,p28 remained bound to the ERα NLS,blocking the NLS recognition by p55.Estradiol binding to the HBD and the consequent conformational change in the HBD brought the HBD-bound p73 in close interaction with p28.This resulted in the dissociation of p28 from the NLS which was subsequently occupied by p55.The interaction culminated in the nuclear entry of ERα,also mediated by the cytoskeletal elements, actin and tubulin(14).

## 4. Search for the "receptor-activator" protein and the discovery of E-RAF

There was a line of thinking that originated from Notides'(Notides & Nielson,1974)and Yamamoto's (Yamamoto,1974)laboratories that in estrogen action there was a possibility for the involvement of a DNA binding X-protein in converting the non-DNA binding estrogen receptor to a DNA binding form. Based on these observations and consideration of a potential possibility that a non-hormone binding transcription factor could be involved in the "activation" process, Thampan and Clark (1981,1983) presented the first ever experimental evidence for the existence of an estrogen receptor activation factor (E-RAF) in the rat uterus. A parallel thinking that contributed to the design of experiments was the already available information that many transcription factors were moderately basic proteins and also that such proteins failed to bind to DEAE cellulose. It was this information that primarily led to the separation of E-RAF from the estrogen receptor that it dimerises with during DEAE-cellulose chromatography. Thampan and Clark (1981) reported that a 3S protein of the rat uterine cytosol, that appeared in the DEAE cellulose flow through fraction, promoted the DNA binding of a specific class of non-DNA binding estrogen receptor. Thampan (1987,1989) in his reports on the purification of E-RAF observed that E-RAF existed in two molecular forms, E-RAF II and I.

While both forms displayed identical molecular weight of 66kDa, their molecular shapes appeared to be different as displayed by the results of gel filtration chromatography and also in their dissimilar sedimentation behavior in linear sucrose density gradients. Functional assays were carried out in which the proteins were incubated with labeled DNA, which was subsequently exposed to S1 nuclease in order to digest the single stranded regions. The results showed that while E-RAF II destabilized DNA double helix and enhanced strand separation, the reverse property (stabilization of double helical structure) was found associated with E-RAF I. In vitro transcription assays involving isolated nuclear RNA polymerases also highlighted this differential behavior of the two molecular forms. While E-RAF II enhanced transcription, in a system containing nuclear RNA polymerase purified from goat uterine nuclei, E-RAF I inhibited transcription in a dose-dependent manner.

## 5. A vision into the molecular identity of the type I and type II nuclear estrogen binding sites

The report in which functional characterization of E-RAF was described (Thampan,1989), also presented a method for the assay for E-RAF in association with the nuclear RNA polymerases. Nuclear RNA polymerases were extracted from isolated rat uterine nuclei and subjected to partial purification through chromatography on DEAE Sephadex A-25 and elution with linear $(NH_4)_2SO_4$ gradient. Ovariectomized rats were used in this study. While control rats received injection of the vehicle alone, experimental animals were subjected to subcutaneous injections of 3µg estradiol-17β for a duration of one hour. The RNA polymerase fractions derived from both control and experimental nuclei and eluted from DEAE-Sephadex A-25 column were subjected to the nuclear exchange assay that was developed earlier by Clark and coworkers (Clark & Peck,1979;Clark et al.,1979). It was through this nuclear exchange assay that Clark's group had demonstrated the existence of type I and type II estrogen binding sites in rat uterine nuclei (Eriksson et al.,1978).

Following DEAE Sephadex-A25 chromatography of nuclear sonicates, the fractions collected were subjected to the estradiol exchange assay as well as RNA polymerase assay with calf thymus DNA as the template .RNA polymerase peaks representing I, II, IIIa and IIIb were clearly demonstrated in the DEAE-Sephadex A-25column fractions. Also demonstrated was the estrogen binding function associated with all four peaks of RNA polymerase activity. The 'receptor' activity associated with the RNA polymerase II was subjected to further analysis. Sucrose density gradient analysis displayed two peaks of activity, a small peak at 5S and a large peak at 3S.While the 5S peak was distinctly DNA binding, the 3S peak which represented the major share of receptor activity, remained non DNA binding. Subsequent studies (Thampan,1989) have demonstrated that the DNA binding function of the 5S peak was due to the presence of E-RAF and an estrogen receptor that dimerised with E-RAF while the non DNA binding 3S fraction was represented by a receptor that did not dimerise with E-RAF.The same studies have concluded, subsequently that the receptor of the 5S peak was the non activated estrogen receptor (naER),a glycoprotein and a tyrosine kinase sensitive to the presence of estradiol and primarily localized at the plasma membrane(Karthikeyan & Thampan,1994). The naER was the only estrogen receptor that could dimerise with E-RAF.The 3S peak on the other hand, represented the nuclear estrogen receptor II (nERII), a tyrosine kinase insensitive to the presence of estradiol. The nuclear estrogen receptor II failed to dimerise with E-RAF, the obvious reason being the changes induced in naER conformation during its transformation to nERII (Karthikeyan & Thampan,1995;Thampan et al.,1996). The naER to nERII transformation was accomplished by a 61kDa nuclear naER-transforming factor (naER-TF), originally reported by Jaya and Thampan (2000).

## 6. Factors regulating nuclear entry of E-RAF

Endoplasmic reticulum is the primary site of localization of intracellular E-RAF.A 55kDa anchor protein, ap55, that binds estradiol with high affinity retains E-RAF at the endoplasmic reticulum (Govind et al.,2003 a,b). Figure 1 displays the immunolocalisation of E-RAF in the endoplasmic reticulum of a goat uterine cell.

E-RAF remains anchored to ap55, through the mediation of a 66kDa nuclear transport protein, tp66. The tp66 recognizes the NLS in E-RAF.Within the E-RAF-tp66 complex, tp66 is anchored by ap55 in an estrogen dependent manner. Presence of saturating levels of estradiol maintains a specific conformation of ap55 that keeps tp66-E-RAF complex anchored to it. Lowering of estradiol concentration results in altered ap55 conformation that facilitates the release of tp66-E-RAF complex from ap55. The complex moves to the nucleus during which tp66 gets docked to a 38kDa nuclear pore-complex protein, npcp38. E-RAF enters the nucleus.

E-RAF is a high affinity progesterone and cholesterol binding protein (Thampan et al., 2000). Under both conditions E-RAF dissociates from the ap55-tp66 complex and migrates to the nucleus (possibly also to the mitochondria as cholesterol bound form). Premkumar et al(1999)presented information on the functional domains of E-RAF.Nuclear run on transcription studies were carried out in order to identify the genes influenced by E-RAF.For this, subtractive hybridization approach was attempted (Jacob,2006). Free E-RAF which can be transported to the nuclei by tp66, and progesterone bound E-RAF that gets transported to the nuclei on its own displayed totally distinct response patterns. It was a 55kDa nuclear pore complex protein (npcp55) that docked progesterone bound E-RAF at the pore complex. On the contrary, the free E-RAF-tp66 complex was docked to npcp-38. While free E-RAF was found to enhance the expression of splicing factor(s) genes, a major gene that was shown to be influenced by progesterone bound E-RAF was the collagenase(s) gene(s). The gene(s) if any, that are under the regulatory influence of cholesterol bound E-RAF remain to be known. Also the nuclear pore complex protein that docks cholesterol bound E-RAF is to be identified.

It appears that cholesterol is a natural regulator of E-RAF mediated gene expression (Thampan et al,2000). The presence of an inhibitor that prevented the dimerisation between E-RAF and naER in goat uterus was recognized early in E-RAF studies. The inhibition in the formation of E-RAF –naER heterodimer and the subsequent decline in the nuclear binding of the receptor was the assay target employed for the identification of this inhibitor. GC-MS analysis of the purified molecule showed its identity as unmetabolised cholesterol (Thampan et al,2000).

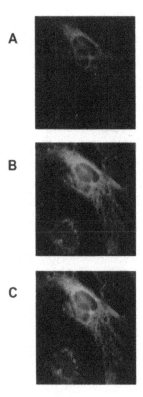

(A)The cells were fixed, permeabilised and exposed to rabbit anti-goat E-RAF IgG, followed by Cy3 labeled anti rabbit IgG.
(B)The cells were also stained with DiOC6 (3) to highlight the endoplasmic reticulum.
(C)The merged figures created by confocal microscopy clearly showed that endoplasmic reticulum is the primary site of localization of E-RAF.

Fig. 1. **Intracellular association of E-RAF with endoplasmic reticulum in goat endometrial cells in culture.** A primary culture of goat endometrial cells was exposed to estradiol-free medium for 48 hours following which the cells were examined under a Leica confocal microscope.

## 7. E-RAF in pregnant rat uterus: significance of the findings

Premkumar and Thampan (1995) examined the level of E-RAF in the uteri of pregnant rats during a full term of pregnancy. It was noticed that from day 1 of pregnancy the E-RAF titer in the uterus registered a steady increase. It reached an all time peak towards mid-pregnancy following which E-RAF level began to decline. The rate of decline was found to be very fast; two days before parturition the uterine E-RAF titer became virtually undetectable. It is known that progesterone is essential for maintaining the functional integrity of the pregnant uterus. The possibility, therefore, exists that the E-RAF titer is a reflection of the progesterone requirement of the pregnant uterus. The decline in E-RAF titer during the second half is again indicative of the need for progesterone withdrawal prior to parturition. The hypothetical presentation given in figure 2 takes into account the E-RAF titer in rat uterus during pregnancy.

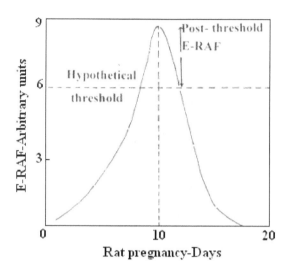

Fig. 2. **A generalized plan of E-RAF titer in rat uterus during pregnancy.** Uterine tissue was collected from a group of rats everyday during the 21-day pregnancy term. The tissue samples were homogenized in the coating buffer (10mM carbonate and 40mM bicarbonate buffer, pH 9.6), and the homogenates were centrifuged at 10,000Xg for 15 minutes. To the supernatant an equal volume of a suspension of DEAE cellulose in coating buffer was added. After 30 minutes of incubation in ice, the DEAE cellulose flow through fraction was collected. An aliquot of this fraction was used for E-RAF estimation through ELISA. The data takes into account the potential existence of an intracellular threshold level of E-RAF. It is being postulated that, beyond this threshold E-RAF enters the blood and gets transported to the specified site that, under conditions where E-RAF titer is low releases the hypothetical factor which, upon binding to its receptor on the uterine cell membrane, initiates the signal transduction events leading to enhanced E-RAF gene expression.
During the negative regulatory mechanism the enhanced level of E-RAF could inhibit the release of the stimulatory factor, thereby suppressing the signal transduction process leading to E-RAF gene activation.

If one assumes that there is an upper limit (threshold) in the uterine level of E-RAF, beyond which the E-RAF enters the blood, it is possible to reconstruct a molecular event. E-RAF is probably transported by the blood to an anatomical site (brain?), which is responsible for enhancing uterine E-RAF gene expression through distinct signal transduction mechanisms mediated by a specific macromolecular agent. Possibly, the presence of E-RAF in circulation could inhibit the release of this mediator, the eventual result being the decline in E-RAF synthesis, leading to the final disappearance of the proteins prior to parturition. Figure 3 illustrates the proposed mechanism of action of this hypothetical regulator of E-RAF gene expression in uterine cells.

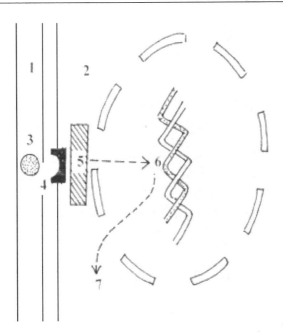

(1) Blood plasma (2) Target cell(3)E-RAF-GRA(E-RAF gene regulatory agent)(4)receptor for E-RAF-GRA(5)signal transduction events that succeed the receptor –GRA-interaction(6)E-RAF gene expression(7)synthesis of E-RAF in the cytoplasm.

Fig. 3. **A model that explains the role of an external factor, transported by the blood, on uterine E-RAF synthesis.** The factor recognizes its receptor on the target cell plasma membrane and induces signal transduction events which eventually terminate in enhanced expression of E-RAF gene.

The model indicates that the regulatory factor,E-RAF gene regulatory agent(E-RAF-GRA) transported by the blood, binds to its receptor on the plasma membrane of the uterine cell. This interaction initiates a cascade of signal transduction events, ultimately leading to the enhancement in E-RAF gene expression in the nucleus and synthesis in the cytoplasm. The decline in the circulating presence of the factor, as it may happen during the second half of pregnancy, will be reflected in the decline in uterine E-RAF gene expression. Preliminary report has already been made on the presence of E-RAF in the goat uterine mitochondria (Praseetha & Thampan,2009). Possibly one of the major functions of E-RAF is to transport cholesterol to the mitochondria where it will be converted enzymatically to pregnenolone and progesterone.

## 8. E-RAF and mammary cancer

E-RAF could play a role in the progression of mammary cancer. E-RAF II is a very active transcription factor and this molecular form of E-RAF represents more than 75%of total E-RAF population representing both E-RAFI and E-RAF II. If one assumes that the benign to malignant transformation of the mammary cancer is associated with enhanced expression of E-RAFII, that should be reflected in immunofluorescent detection of E-RAF in frozen biopsies of mammary tissue. Figure 4 presents the results of a recent study carried out in this direction where the tissue sections were exposed first to anti E-RAF IgG and subsequently to FITC labeled secondary antibody. There is a dominating presence of E-RAF in the cytoplasm and also in the nuclei (primarily stained with propidium iodide).

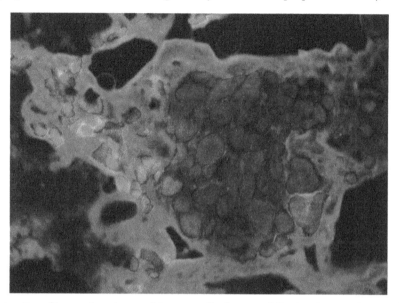

A cryostat section of human breast cancer biopsy was fixed, permeabilised and exposed overnight to rabbit anti goat E-RAF IgG at 4°C.Further exposure of the section to goat anti rabbit IgG labeled with FITC was conducted in the dark for 1 hr following which the nuclei were stained with propidium iodide. The sections were examined using a Leica fluorescence microscope. The green fluorescence indicates the cytoplasmic presence of E-RAF.The nuclei are stained red with propidium iodide. However the presence of E-RAF in the nuclei is marked by the transition of the red colour to light orange and even yellow.

Fig. 4. **Detection of E-RAF in human breast cancer biopsy.**

If what I discussed in the previous paragraph regarding the brain derived regulator of E-RAF gene expression is proven correct, it is possible to suggest that defects in this regulatory protein mechanism and its action could lead to uncontrolled expression of the E-RAF gene. How does this enhanced expression of E-RAF gene influence mammary cancer progression remains to be seen. One of the major molecular targets of progesterone bound E-RAF is the collagenase gene. Whether the progesterone bound E-RAF mediated enhancement in collagenase gene expression has any role in mammary cancer metastasis is yet to be examined.

## 9. Multiple intracellular sites for E-RAF action

Recent observation regarding the positive presence of E-RAF in goat uterine mitochondria is indicative of a possible functional role for E-RAF in the mitochondria. Confocal microscopic studies conducted on goat endometrial cells in culture with exposure to varying concentrations of estradiol or progesterone showed that while 3-5nM concentrations of estradiol helped in the nuclear entry of E-RAF, progesterone mediated nuclear entry was found to be effective only in the presence of 15-16nM progesterone. The corresponding effects produced in the presence of different concentrations of cholesterol remains to be seen. The postulate that the enhancement in E-RAF titer in the pregnant uterus is an indirect reflection of the progesterone production in the uterus during the first half of pregnancy takes into account the possibility that mitochondrial steroidogenesis in the uterine cell is under E-RAF control. As mentioned earlier, E-RAF may function as a cholesterol transporter to the mitochondrial steroidogenic site, eventually facilitating the conversion of cholesterol to pregnenolone and progesterone. The nuclear genes influenced by cholesterol-bound E-RAF could well be those the products of expression of which are constituents of the mitochondrial steroidogenic complex like cytochrome P450(Fig.5)

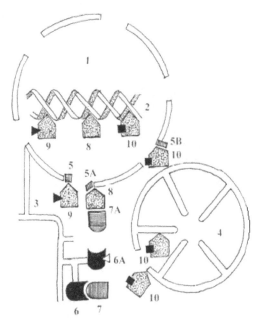

(1) Nucleus (2) Genes (3) Endoplasmic reticulum (4) Mitochondria (5) (5A) and (5B) Nuclear pore complex proteins that bind free E-RAF, progesterone-bound E-RAF and cholesterol bound E-RAF respectively. (6) ap55 (6A) Estradiol-bound ap55 (7) tp66 (7A) tp66-E-RAF complex (8) Free E-RAF (9) Progesterone bound E-RAF (10) Cholesterol bound E-RAF.

Fig. 5. **Mode of action of E-RAF in the target cell.**

The primary site of intracellular location of E-RAF is the endoplasmic reticulum where it remains anchored to the anchor protein 55(ap55) through the mediation of tp66 (transport protein 66) in an estrogen dependent manner.tp66 transports E-RAF to the nucleus, after dissociation from ap55, when the intracellular level of estrogen declines. When bound by cholesterol or progesterone, E-RAF dissociates from tp66 and moves independently to the nucleus. The nuclear entry of E-RAF again is regulated by nuclear pore complex proteins (npcp). Apparently it is the conformation of E-RAF that determines the identity of npcp with which it should interact. There is a distinct possibility that within the nucleus free E-RAF, progesterone bound E-RAF and cholesterol bound E-RAF recognize and regulate the expression of specific sets of genes, possibly influenced by specific acceptor proteins.

Mitochondria appears to be the other target of cholesterol bound E-RAF.The possibility exists that E-RAF functions as a cholesterol transporter to mitochondria, favoring the conversion of cholesterol to pregnenolone and progesterone.This higher titer of E-RAF should be reflected in higher production of uterine progesterone that could eventually contribute to the maintenance of the pregnant uterus during the first half of pregnancy.

## 10. Identification of the estrogen receptor that dimerizes with E-RAF

The experimental observations on the goat uterine E-RAF signals a clear indication that a special class of estrogen receptor dimerised with E-RAF within the nucleus. A DNA cellulose binding assay was developed in which the non-DNA binding estrogen receptor was labeled with $^3$H-estradiol and the binding of the hormone-receptor complex to DNA cellulose in the presence of E-RAF was quantitated. Anuradha et al (1994) reported on the isolation and characterization of a 66kDa, high affinity estrogen binding protein from the goat uterus. The receptor displayed the same affinity to bind estradiol as that of the estrogen receptor $\alpha$ (ER $\alpha$). In view of its inability to bind to DNA on its own, this new estrogen receptor was designated as non-activated estrogen receptor (naER).

A method was developed for the isolation of the non-DNA binding estrogen receptor that dimerized with E-RAF.The method involved preparation of goat uterine cytosol, collection of the DNA-Sepharose unadsorbed fraction, successive ion exchange chromatography over DEAE cellulose and phosphocellulose and finally Hsp 90 Sepharose chromatography in the presence of sodium molybdate, achieving final elution with zero molybdate buffer (Anuradha et al.,1994). While showing its distinctiveness over ER$\alpha$, as a non DNA binding protein, the naER further demonstrated its function as a glycoprotein and a tyrosine kinase (Karthikeyan & Thampan,1996). The tyrosine kinase property was sensitive to the presence of estradiol: the enzyme activity was totally inhibited in the presence of the hormone at concentrations which saturated its binding sites. The observation was a clear indication to the possibility that the naER tyrosine kinase activity can become functional only after naER undergoes a critical structural change within the cell.

Direct biochemical analysis showed that plasma membrane is the primary site of localization of naER (Karthikeyan & Thampan,1996). The possibility of plasma membrane being a site of intracellular localization of estrogen receptor was first proposed by Pietras and Szego (1975,1977) several years ago. Sreeja and Thampan (2004 a,b) demonstrated that naER dissociated from the plasma membrane following exposure to estradiol. This was shown to be an estrogen-specific phenomenon since non-estrogenic steroids failed to bring about the dissociation while the non steroidal estrogen, diethylstilbestrol was as effective as estradiol-17$\beta$ in inducing naER dissociation from the plasma membrane. What was unique in this observation was that the dissociation of naER appeared to be an energy dependent process. The involvement of a $Ca^{++}/Mg^{++}$dependent ATPase in the process was evident. Enhancement of the ATPase activity was dependent on exposure of the membrane to estradiol and the activity was inhibited by the flavanoid, quercetin(Sreeja & Thampan,2004 a).

## 11. Protein protein interactions during naER internalization following estradiol binding

The studies reported from our laboratory (Sreeja & Thampan, 2004 b) have indicated that the internalization of naER from the plasma, following estradiol binding to the receptor was a clathrin-coated vesicle (CCV)-mediated mechanism. A 55 kDa protein of the CCV, apparently carrying the internalization signal (Trowbridge at al, 1993) is the target protein for naER in CCV. The internalized naER interacts with a 58kDa nuclear transport protein, the actin binding p58, that recognizes the nuclear localization signal (NLS) on the receptor. Prior to recognizing p58, the site involved on the naER is bound by Hsp-90.Estradiol binding to naER promotes dissociation of Hsp-90 from the receptor (Anilkumar at al., 2010). Confocal microscopic studies presented in this study showed that in goat endometrial cells in culture exposure of the cells to estradiol resulted in the intracellular movement of both naER and Hsp-90. It was observed that both naER and Hsp-90 entered the nuclei within a matter of 3 hours following the exposure of the cells to estradiol. The functional significance of Hsp-90 in the nuclei remains to be known.naER is transformed into nuclear estrogen receptor II (nERII) within the nucleus. It is evident that this change in identity is associated with a distinct structural change in the protein. Possibly, this transformation that takes place within the nucleus is chaperoned by Hsp-90.

## 12. Nuclear estrogen receptor II (nERII)

Long before naER discovery became a reality, a nuclear receptor that was distinctly different from the classical estrogen receptors had come to my notice. It was observed that when uterine nuclei from ovarectomized rats were exposed to 10nM 3H-estradiol,at 30-37⁰C, the hormone-binding component moved out of the nuclei and reached the outer medium within a span of 5 minutes after hormonal exposure (Thampan,1985;1988). What became apparent in the subsequent studies was that the hormone was bound to a class of ribonucleoproteins (RNP) that moved out of the nuclei following exposure to estradiol. Invivo studies involving ovariectomized rats demonstrated that the RNP that moved out of the nuclei was found associated with cytoplasmic polysomes. The results gave a clear indication to the possibility that a new class of estrogen receptors existed whose primary functional role was in post-transcriptional control mechanisms like splicing, nucleocytoplasmic transport of RNP and the translation.

The subsequent studies reported by our group(Jacob et al.,2006) presented systematic observations on both naER and nERII and concluded that the latter was a transformed form of the former. The observed differences between the two proteins are being listed below(Table 1). The methods employed for purifying the two proteins were identical.

Going back to the observations related to E-RAF function (Thampan,1989), it may be recalled that the estrogen receptor function detected in close proximity to rat uterine nuclear RNA polymerases displayed both naER and nERII characteristics with nERII representing the major share of this activity. The naER existed in dimerisation with E-RAF.Later reports by Karthikeyan and Thampan (1996) showed that nERII tyrosine phosphorylated three subunits of nuclear RNA polymerase II.A re-examination of the 1989 report(Thampan,1989) will reveal that the naER/nERII interaction was not restricted to RNA polymerase II alone. There was very clear evidence to support the hypothesis that the receptor interacted with all four classes of nuclear RNA polymerases. Therefore, it may be speculated that nERII –mediated tyrosine phosphorylation involved specified subunits of all 4 categories of the enzyme.

|                                                          | naER                                | nERII                               |
| -------------------------------------------------------- | ----------------------------------- | ----------------------------------- |
| Sedimentation Value                                      | 4.6S                                | 3.7S                                |
| Stokes radius                                            | 36A⁰                                | 23 A⁰                               |
| Glycoprotein nature                                      | Yes                                 | No                                  |
| Tyrosine kinase activity                                 | Sensitive to exposure to estradiol  | Insensitive to estradiol exposure   |
| Dimerisation with E-RAF                                  | Yes                                 | No                                  |
| Interaction with Hsp-90 in the presence of estradiol     | No                                  | Yes                                 |
| nM estradiol needed for saturation binding               | 20                                  | 30                                  |

The factor responsible for this transformation was subsequently found to be a 61kDa protein, the naER transforming factor (Jaya & Thampan,2000).

Table 1. **Comparison of molecular properties associated with naER and nER II of the goat uterus**

## 13. Does tyrosine phosphorylation of a RNA polymerase subunit favour its dissociation from the core enzyme?

The two models presented here (figures 6 and 7) make an attempt to find an explanation for the observations mentioned above.

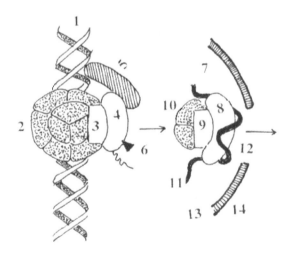

(1) Gene (2) RNA polymerase (3) RNA polymerase subunit that is recognized by naER (4) naER (5) E-RAF (6) estradiol-17β (7) spliceosome (8) nERII (9) RNA polymerase subunit phosphorylated by nERII (10) other subunits dissociated from the RNA polymerase (11) RNA (12) Nuclear pore complex (13) Nucleus (14) cytoplasm.

Fig. 6. naER-nERII transformation during post transcriptional control of gene expression.

The figure on the left displays the interaction of naER-E-RAF heterodimer with genetic elements. While E-RAF recognizes the DNA, naER binds to nuclear RNA polymerase subunits. The figure on the right is a spliceosome -set -up in which the nERII –RNA complex is shown in association with subunits dissociated from RNA polymerase.

nERII is a RNA binding estrogen receptor. Whether naER-E-RAF heterodimer has its binding site on the target gene different from those of the ERα/ERβ mediated gene regulation or whether the action of the heterodimer is independent of the classical estrogen receptor function remains to be clarified. The binding site on the estrogen responsive target gene for E-RAF-naER heterodimer has not yet been identified while there is every likelihood to suggest that it will be different from the estrogen responsive element(ERE).A candidate site could well be AP-1 site in view of an earlier observation that c-fos and E-RAF share immunological similarity. While E-RAF binds to the gene, naER interacts with the nuclear RNA polymerases. Possibly, the naER to nERII transformation could be an event that takes place at the end of the transcription process initiated by the heterodimer. At this stage, nERII dissociates from E-RAF and binds to the RNA (rRNA/mRNA/5S rRNA/tRNA). I wish to propose here that the phosphorylated subunits of the RNA polymerases might dissociate from the core enzyme and move along with nERII during the succeeding stages of gene regulation that witness splicing, nucleocytoplasmic transport and translation.

Sebastian and Thampan (2002 a,b)and Sebastian et al(2004) presented some fascinating observations in this context. Goat uterine nERII was found to be associated with ribonucleoproteins containing U-1 and U-2 snRNA's. Within the snRNP framework nERII interacted with three proteins with molecular masses 32kDa, 55kDa and 60kDa.While p55 and p60 were found to be RNA binding proteins, p32 was found to be involved only in protein-protein interactions with nERII. Whether this protein is the same as SC35 reported by Parnaik in the context of spliceosome assembly (Tripathi & Parnaik,2008) remains to be seen. It was interesting to observe that nERII in association with p32 and p55 formed an effective Ca++/Mg++ activated ATPase that appeared to be directly involved in the nucleocytoplasmic movement of RNP.

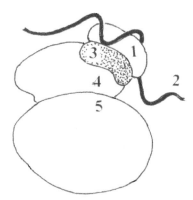

(1) nERII (2) rRNA (3) RNA polymerase I subunit(4)40S ribosomal subunit(5)60S ribosomal subunit.

Fig. 7. **A hypothetical representation for the association of nERII with 40S ribosomal subunit.**

The assumption is that nERII binding to subunits of RNA polymerase I, followed by nERII mediated tyrosine phosphorylation of those subunits results in the dissociation of the subunits from the enzyme along with the rRNA, remaining bound to nERII. The rRNA-nERII-RNA polymerase I subunit complex is shown here as forming an integral part of the 40S subunit of the ribosome.

I wish to speculate here that the subunits dissociated form the RNA polymerases following phosphorylation by nERII could continue their association with nERII and find their involvement in splicing reactions, nucleocytoplasmic transport of RNA and eventually, in translation. If this assumption is correct, future studies on ribosomal subunits should be able to confirm the presence of RNA polymerase I and III subunits in 40S ribosomes. It should also be possible to confirm whether the RNA polymerase II subunits are present in spliceosomes.

## 14. General conclusions and hypothetical possibilities

1. Discussions exclusively on the classical estrogen receptors, ERα and ERβ will serve to uncover only limited information on the role of the receptors in regulating gene expression.
2. There is a distinct possibility that naER-E-RAF heterodimer has a parallel role to play in regulating transcriptional events as has been proposed for ERα and ERβ.
3. nERII is undoubtedly the estrogen receptor that mediates post transcriptional events in gene expression in estrogen target cells.
4. The nERII-mediated events are related to gene expression protocols influenced by all 4 forms of nuclear RNA polymerases.
5. E-RAF targets both the nucleus and the mitochondria. Free E-RAF, progesterone-bound E-RAF and cholesterol bound E-RAF encounter distinct genes that are under regulatory influence. It might function as cholesterol transporter to the mitochondria and facilitate mitochondrial steroidogenesis leading to the production of progesterone. This is, in all possibility, a mechanism projected to take place during pregnancy.
6. The possibility exists that there is an "external"regulator of E-RAF gene expression and also that this regulatory agent is involved in the control of E-RAF gene expression in the pregnant uterus.
7. The possibility for a role for E-RAF in the progression of mammary cancer cannot be ruled out. Studies to be held in the near future are bound to enlighten this possibility.

## 15. Acknowledgement

I wish to acknowledge with gratitude and deep appreciation the contributions of my research students, both past and present. Their observations have made a profound impact on my search into the mysteries of estrogen action.

## 16. References

Anilkumar, P., Vidya, S.K. & Thampan, R.V. (2010) Goat endometrial heat shock protein –90 (Hsp-90). Development of an expedient method for its purification and observations on its intracellular movement. *Protein Expression Purific.*71:49-53.

Anuradha. P., Khan, S. M. Karthikeyan, N. & Thampan, R. V., (1994) The Non-Activated Estrogen Receptor (naER) of the Goat Uterus is a Tyrosine Kinase. *Arch. Biochem. Biophys.* 309:195-204.

Clark,J.H.,Hardin,J.W.,Eriksson,H.,Upchurch,S.&Peck,E.J.,Jr(1979)Heterogeneity of estrogen binding sites in the at uterus,*in* Hamilton,T.H.,Clark,J.H. and Sadler,W.A.(ed),*Ontogeny of receptors and reproductive Hormone Action,*Raven Pres,N.Y.pp65-77.

Clark.J.H.& Peck, E.J.Jr. (1979)*Female sex steroids: Receptors and Function. Monographs in Endocrinology Vol.14,* Springer Verlag, Berlin.

Eriksson,H.,Upchurch,S.,Hardin,J.W.,Peck,E.J.Jr.& Clark,J.H.(1978)Heterogeneity of estrogen receptors in the cytosol and nuclear fractions of the rat uterus.*Biochem.Biophys.Res.Commun.*81:1-7.

Govind A.P., Sreeja S & Thampan R.V. (2003 b): Proteins that mediate the nuclear entry of the goat uterine estrogen receptor activation factor (E-RAF): Identification of a molecular basis for the inhibitory effect of progesterone on estrogen action. *J. Cell. Biochem.* 89:108-119.

Govind A.P., Sreeja. S. & Thampan, R.V. (2003 a): Estradiol dependent anchoring of the goat uterine estrogen receptor activation factor (E-RAF) at the endoplasmic reticulum by a 55 kDa anchor protein (ap55). *J.Cell Biochem.* 89:94-107.

Govind, A. P. & Thampan, R.V. (2003) Membrane associated estrogen receptors and related proteins: Localization at the plasma membrane and the endoplasmic reticulum. *Mol. Cell. Biochem.* 253,233-240.

Green,S. & Chambon,P.(1987)Oestradiol induction of a glucocorticoid responsive gene by a chimeric receptor.*Nature* 325:75-77.

Green,S. & Chambon,P.(1987) A superfamily of potentially oncogenic hormone receptors. *Nature* 324:615-617.

Grody, W.W., Schrader, W.T. & O'Malley, B.W.(1982)Activation, transformation and subunit structure of steroid hormone recptors.*Endocrine Rev.*3:141-172.

Jacob, J., Sebastian, K.S., Devassy, S., Priyadarsini, L., Farook, M.F.,Shameem, A., Mathew, D., Sreeja, S. & Thampan, R.V. (2006) Membrane estrogen receptors: genomic actions and post-transcriptional regulation. *Mol. Cell. Endocrinol.* 246:34-41.

Jacob.J. (2006): Functional Studies on the goat uterine estrogen receptor activation factor.Ph.D.thesis, University of Kerala.

Jaya, P.& Thampan, R.V., (2000) A nuclear transforming factor that converts goat uterine non-activated estrogen receptor to nuclear estrogen receptor II. *Protein Expression Purific.* 20:347-356.

Jensen, E.V.& DeSombre, E.R. (1973) Estrogen Receptor Interaction. *Science* 182:126-134.

Karthikeyan, N & Thampan, R. V., (1994) A DNA Binding (RI) and Non-DNA Binding (RII) Estrogen Receptor in the Goat Uterine Nucleus: Purification and Characterization. *Arch. Biochem. Biophys.* 309: 205-213.

Karthikeyan, N & Thampan, R. V., (1995) The nuclear estrogen receptor RII of the goat uterus: Distinct possibility that the R-II is the deglycosylated form of the non-activated estrogen receptor (naER). *Arch. Biochem. Biophys.* 321,442-452.

Karthikeyan. N & Thampan, R. V., (1996) Plasma Membrane is the primary site of localization of the non-activated estrogen receptor (naER) in the goat uterus: Hormone binding causes receptor internationalization *Arch. Biochem. Biophys.* 325: 47-57.

Kumar,V.,Green,S.,Stack,G.,Berry,M.,Jim,J.R. & Chambon,P(1987)Functional domains of the human estrogen receptor.*Cell* 51:941-950.

Kumar,V.,Green,S.,Staub,A.& Chambon,P.(1986)Co-localization of estradiol binding and putative DNA binding domains of the human estrogen receptor.*EMBO J.*,5:2231-2236.

Mohla, S., DeSombre, E.R. & Jensen, E.V. (1972) Tissue specific stimulation of RNA synthesis by transformed estradiol-receptor complex. *Biochem. Biophys. Res. Commun.* 46:661-667.

Nirlmala, P. B. & Thampan, R. V., (1995) A 55kDa protein of the goat uterus mediates nuclear transport of the estrogen receptor II: Details of the transport mechanism. *Arch. Biochem. Biophys.* 319: 562-569.

Nirmala. P. B. & Thampan, R. V., (1995) A 55kDa protein of the goat uterus mediates nuclear transport of the estrogen receptor I: Purification and Characterization. *Arch. Biochem. Biophys.* 319, 551-561.

Notides,A.C.& Nielson,S.(1974)The macromolecular mechanism of the in vitro 4S to 5S transformation of the uterine estrogen receptor.*J.Biol.Chem.*249:1866-1873.

Pietras, R.J.& Szego, C.M. (1975) Endometrial cell calcium and estrogen. *Nature* 253:357-359.

Pietras,R.J & Szego,C.M(1977)Specific binding sites of estrogen at the outer surfaces of isolated endometrial cells. *Nature* 265:69-72.

Praseetha.S & Thampan, R.V. (2009) Regulatory factors in steroid hormone biosynthesis. *Critical Reviews in Eukaryotic Gene Expression* .19:253-265.

Pratt, W.B. (1990) Interaction of Hsp-90 with steroid receptors. Organizing some diverse observations and presenting the newest concepts. *MolCell. Endocrinol.* 74:C69-C76.

Pratt , W.B. &Toft, D.O.,(1997)Steroid receptor interactions with heat shock protein and immunophilin chaperones . Endocr. Rev.18:306-360

Premkumar, M & Thampan, R. V., (1995) Hormonal control of the rat uterine estrogen receptor activation factor (E-RAF). Biochem. *Mol. Biol. Int.* 37: 1207-1215.

Premkumar,M.,Bhaskar,L, & Thampan. R.V., (1999) Structural characterization of the goat uterine estrogen receptor activation factor using an endogenous calcium activated neutral protease. *Mol. Cell. Endocrinol.* 152:57-64.

Sai Padma, A. & Thampan, R. V. (2000). Interdependence between a 55 kDa protein (p55) and a 12 kDa protein (p12) in facilitating the nuclear entry of goat uterine estrogen receptor under cell-free conditions. *Biol. Chem.*381: 285-294.

Sai Padma, A., Renil, M. & Thampan, R.V. (2000). Protein–protein interactions that precede the nuclear entry of goat uterine estrogen receptor under cell-free conditions. *J.Cell Biochem.*78:650-665.

Sebastian, T, Sreeja, S. & Thampan, R. V. (2004): Import and export of nuclear proteins: Focus on the nucleocytoplasmic movement of two different species of mammalian estrogen receptor. *Mol. Cell. Biochem.* 260:91-102.

Sebastian, T. & Thampan, R.V. (2002) Nuclear estrogen receptor II (nERII) is involved in the estrogen dependent ribonucleoprotein transport in the goat uterus I: Localization of nERII in snRNP .*J.Cell. Biochem.* 84, 217-226.

Sebastian, T. & Thampan, R.V. (2002) Nuclear estrogen receptor II (nERII) is involved in the estrogen dependent ribonucleoprotein transport in the goat uterus II. Isolation and characterization of three snRNP proteins which bind to nER II. *J. Cell. Biochem.* 84: 227-236.

Shyamala, G.& Gorski, J. (1969) Estrogen Receptors in rat uterus. *J. Biol. Chem.* 244:1097-1103.

Sreeja, S & Thampan, R.V. (2004) : Proteins which mediate the nuclear entry of goat uterine non activated estrogen receptor (naER) following naER internalization from the plasma membrane. *Mol. Cell. Biochem.* 259: 141-148.

Sreeja,S & Thampan, R.V. (2004):Estradiol-mediated internalization of the non-activated estrogen receptor from the goat uterine plasma membrane: Identification of the proteins involved. *Mol. Cell. Biochem.* 259: 131-140.

Stanišić, V., Lonard, M.M. & O'Malley, B.W. (2010) Estrogen Receptor- α: molecular mechanisms and interactions with the ubiquitin proteasome system.*Horm.Mol.Biol.Clin.Invest.*1:1-9.

Thampan, R. V., Karthikeyan. N., Premkumar. M & Nirmala. P.B. (1996) Estrogen receptors and receptor-associated proteins of the goat uterus: some new insights. in Sengupta, J. and Ghosh, D.(ed), *Cellular and Molecular Signaling in Reproduction,* New Age International, New Delhi. pp.49-68.

Thampan, R.V., (1985) The Nuclear Binding of Estradiol Stimulates ribonucleoprotein Transport in the Rat Uterus. *J. Biol. Chem.* 260:5420 – 5426.

Thampan, R.V., (1987) A 62 Kilo Dalton Protein Functions as Estrogen Receptor Activation Factor (E-RAF) in the goat uterus. *Mol. Cell. Endocrinol.* 53:119-130.

Thampan, R.V., (1988) Estradiol-Stimulated Nuclear Ribonucleoprotein Transport in the Rat Uterus: A Molecular Basis, *Biochemistry-*27:5019-5026.

Thampan, R.V., (1989) Molecular Aspects of Estrogen Receptor Activation Factor (E-RAF) Function. *Mol. Cell. Endocrinol.* 64:19-34.

Thampan, R.V., & Clark. J.H. (1983) Estrogen Receptor Activation Factor.*in Evolution of Hormone Receptor Systems,* UCLA Symposia in Molecular and Cellular Biology. Vol. 6: 457 –464.

Thampan,T.N.R.V., & Clark.J.H (1981) An Oestrogen Receptor Activator Protein in Rat Uterine Cytosol. *Nature* (London) 290: 152-154.

Thampan. R. V., Zafar, A., Imam, N.S., Sreeja, S., Suma, K. & Vairamani, M. (2000). Cholesterol inhibits the nuclear entry of estrogen receptor activation factor (E-RAF) and its dimerisation with the non-activated estrogen receptor (naER) in goat uterus. *J. Cell. Biochem.* 77: 382-395.

Tripathi, K.& Parnaik,V.K.(2008) Differential dynamics of splicing factor SC35 during the cell cycle.*J. Biosci.* 33: 345–354.

Trowbridge, I.S., Collawan, J.F. &Hopkins, C.R. (1993) Signal dependent membrane protein trafficking in the endocytic pathway.*Annu.Rev.Cell Biol.*9:129-161.

Yamamoto,K.R.(1974)Characterization of the 4S nad 5S forms of the estradiol receptor protein and their interaction with deoxyribonucleic acid,*J.Biol.Chem.*249:7068-7075.

# The Tissue Specific Role of Estrogen and Progesterone in Human Endometrium and Mammary Gland

Karin Tamm[1,2,3], Marina Suhorutshenko[1],
Miia Rõõm[1], Jaak Simm[1] and Madis Metsis[1,2]
*[1]Centre for Biology of Integrated Systems, Tallinn University of Technology, Tallinn,*
*[2]Competence Centre on Reproductive Medicine and Biology, Tartu,*
*[3]Nova Vita Clinic, Tallinn,*
*Estonia*

## 1. Introduction

The purpose of this chapter is to review the tissue-specific role of estrogen (E2) and progesterone (P4) in human endometrium and mammary gland. It is well known that both E2 and P4 are essential for the development and differentiation of human endometrium and mammary gland, but the exact basis for differential tissue-specific signalling of E2 and P4 are still not fully understood. This chapter explores observed functions of two major female steroid hormones and their cognate receptors in normal physiology of human reproductive system but also in assisted reproductive technology and breast cancer treatment.

The normal reproductive physiology requires tightly coordinated action of hypothalamus, pituitary gland, ovaries and endometrium. Also functioning of other endocrine units such as the thyroid and adrenal glands are essential for regular ovulation and cyclic changes. The production of ovarian steroid hormones is coordinated by the hypothalamic-pituitary-gonadal axis which is activated in puberty (Figure 1). The hypothalamus produces and secretes luteinizing hormone-releasing hormone (LHRH), which binds to its receptors in pituitary gland. This causes cascade of biochemical events culminating in the production of two hormones in pituitary gland, luteinizing hormone (LH) and follicle-stimulating hormone (FSH). LH and FSH are secreted into the general blood circulation and attach to receptors on the ovary, where they trigger ovulation and stimulate the production of E2 and P4. Ovarian steroid hormones themselves have direct role in the development of the inner lining of the uterus but they also act as a positive feedback system to hypothalamus and pituitary gland for continuous cyclic changes until the beginning of menopause (Kanis and Stevenson, 1994).

Cholesterol is the building block for all steroid hormones, which is carried into the bloodstream and through a sequence of enzymatic changes is synthesized into final products. In the bloodstream steroid hormones are distributed rapidly throughout the tissues and act on distant targets. This secretory process is called endocrine action and the function of many target tissues as mammary gland, brain, bones, liver and heart are affected by circulating hormones. Steroid hormones can also act very close to their site of secretion

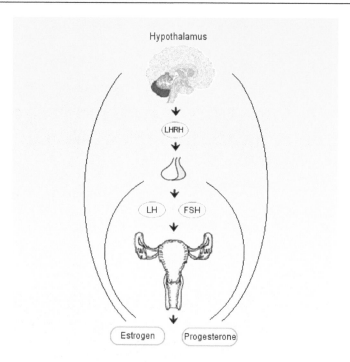

Fig. 1. The female hypothalamic–pituitary–gonadal axis. The hypothalamus produces and secretes luteinizing hormone–releasing hormone (LHRH) into a system of blood vessels that link the hypothalamus and the pituitary gland. LHRH stimulates the pituitary gland by attaching to specific molecules (i.e., receptors). After the coupling of LHRH with these receptors, a cascade of biochemical events causes the pituitary gland to produce and secrete two hormones, luteinizing hormone (LH) and follicle-stimulating hormone (FSH). LH and FSH are two of a class of hormones commonly known as gonadotropins. They are secreted into the general circulation and attach to receptors on the ovary, where they trigger ovulation and stimulate ovarian production of the hormones estrogen and progesterone. These female hormones cause monthly menstrual cycling and have multiple effects throughout the body. In particular, estrogen has profound effects on the skeletal system and is crucial to maintaining normal bone health (Figure adapted from Kanis and Stevenson, 1994).

on adjacent cells and tissues as it happens in gonads, testis and ovaries- paracrine action. Gonads produce only three classes of steroids: progestins, androgens and estrogens where progestins are obligatory precursors of both androgens and estrogens. Likewise, androgens are obligatory precursors of estrogens. Steroidogenesis in the ovary is compartmentalized in a cell-specific manner: the theca cells primarily producing androstenedione and the granulosa cells completing the synthesis of E2. After the ovulation the corpus luteum of the ovary starts to produce P4. Albeit the vast amount of sex steroids are synthesized locally in peripheral tissue, providing individual target tissues with the means to adjust synthesis and metabolism to their local requirements (Venken et al., 2008).

Beside the reproductive system, one of the most widely recognized effects of E2 is the prevention of the osteoporosis. Adequate E2 levels through E2 replacement therapy has shown to prevent or diminish calcium loss from bones in menopausal women (Venken et al., 2008). In the nervous system both estrogens and androgens have been reported to influence verbal fluency, performance of spatial tasks, verbal memory capacity and fine motor skills (Kelly and Ronnekleiv, 2008). The major role for P4 in humans is related to initiation and maintenance of the pregnancy. P4 is essential for milk preparation and secretion in mammary gland and for mediating signals required for sexually responsive behaviour. Recent evidence also supports a role for P4 in the modulation of bone mass (Seifert-Kaluss and Prior, 2010).

NRs function as transcription factors. The biological activities of E2 and P4 are mediated mainly by nuclear receptors (NRs). Binding of a steroid hormone to its cognate receptor results in a conformational change in the nuclear receptor that allows the ligand-receptor complex to bind with high affinity to response elements in DNA and regulate transcription of target genes. In the absence of ligand, NRs are held in a multi-subunit complex containing heatshock proteins such as Hsp90, SP70, HSP40, Hop, and p23 (Wolf et al., 2008). After binding to ligand, these receptors, undergo conformational changes, dissociate themselves from chaperone proteins, dimerize and in some cases translocate into the nucleus (if not already locked into the nucleus) (Bain et al., 2007). The differences in specificity of molecular mechanisms result from receptor subcellular location and binding to genomic DNA as homo- or heterodimers in either head-to-tail or head-to-head orientation to different consensus sequences known as hormone response elements (HREs) (Bain et al., 2007). Upon NR activation a hydrophobic pocket is created in their tertiary structure for interaction with co-activators such as members of the steroid receptor co-activator (SRC) protein family or co-repressors such as NR co-repressor (NCoR) and silencing mediator for retinoic acid and thyroid hormone receptor (SMRT) ( Hall et al., 2005). The recruitment of co-regulators leads to alterations in the rate of gene expression via modification of initiation complex formation process. Two types of estrogen receptors, ERα and ERβ, encoded by separate genes, are found in humans (Enmark etal., 1997; Kuiper and Gustafsson, 1997). P4 signalling is also mediated by two receptors, PRA and PRB, which are encoded by the same gene but transcribed from different promoters, resulting in a PRB that has an additional 164 amino acids at the N-terminus (Wen et al., 1994; Kastner et al., 1990). PRB is a stronger transcriptional activator in most cell types, while PRA acts often as a dominant negative repressor for PRB activity (Tung et al., 1993; Vegeto et al., 1993).

In addition to operating as TFs in the nucleus, NRs have been shown to possess non-genomic action which is usually characterized by a shorter lag time required to elicit a biological response following steroid hormone stimulation. For instance ERs can regulate gene expression independent of estrogen responsive element (ERE) through tethering different TFs and by membrane- initiated ER interference with other intracellular pathways. Examples of motifs recognized by ER other than ERE is the activator protein-1 site (AP-1 site) commonly occupied by the TFs c-Fos/c- Jun B (Björnström and Sjöberg., 2004).

## 2. The role of E2 and P4 in human endometrium

Human endometrium is the inner tissue lining of uterine cavity that undergoes monthly cyclic changes dictated by ovarian steroid hormones E2 and P4 (Figure 2). As endometrium is a regenerative tissue it is subjected to proliferation, secretion and degeneration on monthly basis. Nearly all morphologic and biochemical processes that the uterus undergoes during its acquisition of receptivity are directly or indirectly regulated by ovarian steroid hormones (Lim et al., 2002). The development of human endometrium is divided into follicular and luteal phase. During the follicular phase ovarian E2 is produced with increasing quantities until ovulation, stimulating the proliferation and growth of the epithelial and stromal components of the endometrium. During the luteal phase the increasing amounts of the P4 and secondary maintaining levels of E2 are both involved in the differentiation of the endometrium but P4 reverses the proliferative effects of E2 (Lim et al., 2002). Together, coordinated action of steroid hormones produced by the follicle and corpus luteum prepare the endometrium every month for potential embryo implantation. In the event of embryo implantation P4 predominantly facilitates and permits decidualization of the endometrium and supports maintenance of pregnancy. On the contrary, in the absence of implantation declining levels of E2 and P4 lead to degeneration of the endometrial tissue, which is followed by regeneration during the next cycle. In addition to cell differentiation, P4 plays the key role in the decision of cell survival or death prior to the menstruation. Three proteins related to apoptotic activation in endometrial cells are proto-oncogene p53, FOXO1 (forkhead box-O) and BIM which act as a switches between apoptosis and survival (Brosens and Gellersen, 2006).

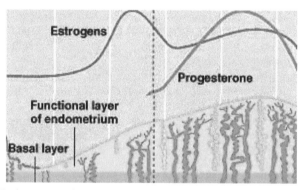

Fig. 2. **E2 and P4 in human endometrium.** E2 causes the growth or proliferation of the endometrium during the first two weeks of the menstrual cycle. After ovulation, the corpus luteum produces P4. This hormone causes the endometrial glands to secrete nutritive substances required by the embryo and to allow it to implant into the endometrial lining (figure adapted from internet http://www.tubal-reversal.net/uterus-menstrual-cycle.htm).

Ovarian steroids mediate their signals through genomic or non-genomic pathways. The genomic signal is passed on by cognate receptors, ERs and PRs, in endometrial cells. As E2 is dominant hormone during the follicular phase of the cycle genes regulated by E2 are also more often related to tissue proliferation. Under the actions of E2 the epithelial cells respond by rapid induction of gene expression that promotes DNA synthesis and cell replication (Lessey et al., 2010). During the luteal phase P4 induces the genes related to differentiation. Clinically used steroid hormone analogues (Tamoxifen, Fluvestrant, Progestin, Mifepristone) could have a suppressive or repressive impact on normal steroid hormone signalling in endometrial cells (Figure 2). The expression of ERs and PRs in spatiotemporal manner is crucial for the successful implantation process (Lessey et al., 2003). Although ERα and ERβ are present in all endometrial cell types throughout the entire menstrual cycle, they are expressed at higher levels during the proliferative phase and show lower activity during the secretory phase because of the suppressive effect of P4. After the proliferative phase P4 takes the E2-primed endometrium towards a state of receptivity. P4, acting through its cognate receptors, is absolutely mandatory for successful implantation and post-implantation embryo survival. PRA and PRB levels are similar during the follicular phase of the menstrual cycle while the PRA is down-regulated at the time of implantation but higher stromal PRB levels during the mid-luteal phase have been reported (Arnett-Mansfield et al., 2004). The expression of the PR gene in endometrial glands is controlled by E2 and P4, where E2 induces PR synthesis and P4 down-regulates the expression of its own receptor (Graham et al., 1990). The actions of P4 counter the effects of P4 in the endometrium through paracrine regulators from the stromal part. Recent studies about small non-protein coding RNAs (microRNA, miRNA) have revealed their important role in gene regulation in endometrium (Kuokkanen et al., 2010; Li et al., 2011). The regulation of specific microRNAs is a mechanism that appears to fine tune gene expression by blocking cell proliferation at the time of implantation P4 dependently (Lessey et al., 2010).

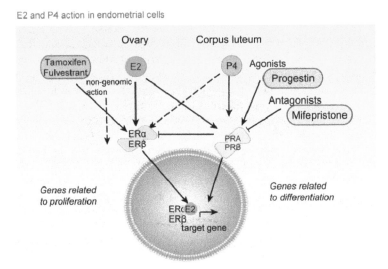

Fig. 3. **E2 and P4 genomic signalling in human endometrial cell.** E2 produced by ovary enters into the cell and binds to its specific receptors ERα or ERβ. Formed complex moves into the cell and has an impact on target gene expression. After the ovulation corpus luteum starts to produce P4 which also diffuses into the endometrial cells and through its receptors regulate gene expression. Steroid hormone analogues (Tamoxifen, Fluvestrant, Progestin, Mifepristone) have a suppressive or repressive impact on ER , PR signalling.

## 2.1 Endometrial gene expression during the time of embryo implantation

In a restricted period, called implantation window (IW), endometrium is most receptive for the embryo attachment. In humans IW is temporally confined to days 20-24 of menstrual cycle (8-10 days after ovulation). During this time period corpus luteum induces high level of P4 and stable level of E2 expression. For successful pregnancy the apposition, adhesion and invasion of developing embryo is needed which can only happen if the endometrium is at the right developmental stage posessing a receptive atmosphere.

There is a certain group of women who repeatedly fail to achieve pregnancy in spite of good quality embryos transferred during IVF (*in vitro* fertilisation) treatments. This has led to the search for better solutions to improve implantation rates. In a molecular level embryo implantation is a dialog between blastocyst and receptive endometrium which is mediated by various growth factors, cytokines, lipid mediators, transcription factors and other putative molecules often regulated by steroid hormones. In recent years, numerous studies applying global gene expression analysis have found a wide range of genes up- or down regulated in human endometrium during the IW (Carson et al., 2002; Kao et al., 2002; Riesewijk et al., 2003; Horcajadas et al., 2004; Krikun et al., 2005; Mirkin et al., 2005; Simon et al., 2005; Punyadeera et al., 2005; Talbi et al., 2006; Horcajadas et al., 2008; Haouzi et al., 2009a,b; Altmäe et al., 2010). Each study has brought out candidate genes believed to be crucial in embryo implantation process but the overlap of potential marker genes between different publications has still remained relatively low. However, today there are already some biomarkers confirmed in separate studies which are pivotial during implantation process. For example, the most potential endometrial marker identified is leukemia inhibitory factor (LIF) and its importance has been proven in animal and human studies (*Stewart et al., 1994;* Arici et al., 1995; Steck et al., 2004). Unfortunately, the development of recombinant human LIF (r-fLIF) has not met the expectations of increasing implantation rates in infertile women (Brinsden et al., 2009). The localization of immune system related molecules like cytokines, IL-6 and IL-11, has been identified in endometrial cells and they have shown coincidental expression changes at the time of high levels of E2 and P4 (Tabibzadeh et al., 1995; Robertson et al., 2000; Vandermolen and Gu, 1996; Cork et al., 2001; Dimitriadis et al., 2000; von Rango et al., 2004). The two integrins, $\alpha4\beta1$ and $\alpha v\beta3$, appear to be good markers of the receptive endometrium in normal fertile women (Lessey et al., 1994). Recognized growth factors related to endometrial receptivity and implantation are transforming growth factor $\beta$ (TGF-$\beta$), epidermal growth factor (EGF), heparin binding-epidermal growth factor (HB-EGF) and inlsulin like growth factor (IGF) (Jones et al., 2006b; Hofmann et al., 1991; Dadi et al., 2007; Lessey et al., 2002; Stavreus-Evers et al., 2002). Growth factors and their respective receptors have shown to enhance embryo development and improve implantation rates in IVF cycles (Kabir-Salmani et al., 2004).

It is more likely that there is no single molecule, which could solve the implantation issue and help patients with recurrent implantation failures. As a complex process implantation seems to depend on many factors, which influence the development of the embryo and endometrial dating in synchronized manner. Moreover, the individual differences and monthly cyclic changes of the regenerative tissue make the search for universal markers relevant to implantation complex.

## 2.2 The influence of the IVF treatment on endometrial receptivity

Since the first announcement of successful IVF treatment in 1978 (Steptoe and Edwards, 1978) assessed fertilization procedures have been increasingly used world-wide. Based on the report by European Society of Human Reproduction and Embryology (ESHRE) in 2008, more than three million babies have been born with the help of IVF (ESHRE 2008).

Nowadays the number of couples seeking for aid to achieve pregnancy is constantly increasing as at least every tenth couple requires infertility treatments. Ovarian stimulation and ovulation induction with gonadotrophin administration has been a success from the 1960s (Fowler and Edwards, 1957). Ovulation induction leads to multi-follicular growth instead of a single follicle in natural cycles escalating possible successful fertilisation. Still, the general success rates for clinical pregnancies have stayed around 30-40% for more than three decades (Department of Health and Human Services Centres for Disease Control and Prevention Report 2001). The focus to develop more effective ovarian stimulation protocols to increase the number of oocytes and embryos obtained from one cycle has by some means overlooked the relevance of supraphysiological levels of ovarian steroid hormones and their collateral effect on the endometrium (Simon et al., 2008). In modern IVF, drugs used to stimulate ovaries during the follicular phase include clomiphene citrate, urinary and recombinant gonadotrophins and gonadotrophin releasing hormone (GnRH) agonists and antagonists (Edwards et al., 2005). The usage of ovarian stimulating drugs often results in shorter luteal phase of the endometrium, which is therefore no longer synchronized with embryo development. The use of GnRH agonists may have a negative effect on implantation. Several studies observing endometrial biopsies from patients undergoing IVF treatment show 1-3 day advancement in endometrial development (Lass et al., 1998; Nikas et al 1999). The formation of pinopodes, considered as morphological markers for receptive endometrium, has also been shifted to day 17 or 18 compared to day 20 in normal cycle (Stavreus-Evers et al., 2001). Elevated concentrations of E2 and subtle P4 increases in the late follicular phase lead to modulated steroid hormone receptor profile (Papanikolau et al., 2005). Histological study has shown down-regulation of the ERs and PRs and pinopode expression in stimulated cycles compared to natural cycles (Develioglu et al., 1999). There is some evidence of a negative impact of supraphysiological steroid levels on endometrium because increased pregnancy rates have been observed in the presence of reduced production of serum E2. This explains the fact that there are higher pregnancy and implantation rates recorded for oocyte recipients versus donors who have only P4 support prior to embryo transfer (Check et al., 1995). A premature reduction in PRs in the early luteal phase has been found after ovarian stimulation. Horcajadas and colleagues have demonstrated that gene expression profiling of the endometrium is different between natural and controlled ovarian stimulation cycles in the receptive phase (Horcajadas et al., 2008).

There are ways to restore the length of luteal phase by stimulating corpus luteum with hCG or by supplementing the luteal phase with steroids, such as E2 and P4 (Smitz et al., 1992). Also, to overcome the side effects caused by high doses of drugs milder stimulation protocols have been developed (Olivennes et al., 2002; Nargund and Frydman, 2007; Pennings and Ombelet, 2007; Ubaldi et al., 2007). The evidence regarding a potentially negative effect of supraphysiological steroid levels on endometrial receptivity (Simon et al., 1995; Devroey et al., 2004), corpus luteum function (Fauser and Devroey, 2003; Beckers et al., 2006), oocyte and embryo quality (Valbuena et al., 2001; Baart et al., 2007) indicate that limited ovarian stimulation and response might have a beneficial effect on implantation potential.

## 2.3 E2 and P4 endometriosis
The ovarian steroid hormones play also a central role in pathogenesis of several uterine disorders, including endometriosis, which is characterized by the presence of endometrial tissue outside the uterine cavity like the peritoneum and ovary. It has been shown that both

eutopic and ectopic endometrial tissues expresses ERs and PRs and they respond to ovarian steroid hormones but the predominance of ERα and PRA receptors have been described in cases of ectopic lesions (Matsuzaki et al., 2001; Attia et al., 2000). Despite the obvious importance of E2/P4 in the development of the endometriosis, the exact aetiology and pathogenesis of it are still unclear. It is predicted that in general endometriosis could affect about 10% of women of reproductive age and up to 25-50% of women seeking infertility treatment. There is still uncertainty whether the decreased fertility is related to reduction of the oocyte/embryo quality or dysregulation of the endometrium (Kim et al., 2007). Aberrant gene expression in endometrium which is suboptimal for implanting blastocyst has been shown by several studies in cases of endometriosis (Giudice et al., 2002; Kao et al., 2003).

Even though endometriosis has been characterized as E2-dependent gynaecological disease, where E2 favours the growth of the tissue, the dysregulation of the P4 response on the molecular level is suggested in endometriosis. It has been noticed that endometriotic tissue does not respond to P4 as normal endometrium does. Altered PR expression or diminished activity predictably results in differential gene expression compared to eutopic tissue (Cakmak et al., 2010). For example, altered P4 signalling can cause unpaired regulation of *HOXA 11, HOXA12* genes in ectopic tissue which are expressed in high levels during the IW in normal tissue (Cakmak et al., 2010). The up-regulation of *HOXA10* and *HOXA11* expression fails to occur in women with endometriosis (Taylor et al., 1999). Recent studies looking for functional miRNA-s have shown up-regulation of miR-21 in eutopic endometrium of women with versus without endometriosis (Luo et al., 2010; Aghajanova et al., 2011).

Hopefully further studies in the future help us understand the molecular mechanisms, which are responsible for the development of endometriosis.

## 3. The role of E2 and P4 in mammary gland

The development and physiology of human mammary gland is also under the strict control of steroid hormones, including E2 and P4. The mammary gland is not completely formed at birth, but begins to develop in early puberty when the primitive ductal structures enlarge and branch (Russo et al., 1987). From that point ovarian E2 and P4 are fundamental for the growth and differentiation of the duct system. There are slight cyclical changes during each menstrual cycle caused by ovarian steroid hormones where E2 is increasing the volume of the tissue and P4 is responsible of the acinar growth of breast tissue. During pregnancy, the mammary gland epithelium experiences its greatest and most rapid proliferation initially as a response to the hormones produced by corpus luteum, following by placental hormones.

Due to difficulties in studying developing mammary gland there is relatively small amount of information about normal ER and PR expression in breast tissue. It has been confirmed that PRs and ERs are found in a minority population (7-10%) of luminal, non-dividing epithelial cells. As E2 is required to induce progesterone receptor (PR) expression it is difficult to separate the effects of P4 alone from E2. However, the obligate role of the ERs and PRs in mammary gland development has been confirmed with knocked out mice studies (Bocchinfuso and Korach, 1997; Humphreys et al., 1997).

### 3.1 E2 and P4 in breast cancer development

Broad spectrum of physiological activity of steroid hormones displays its dark side in cases when cells in steroid hormone guided organs lose their normal responsiveness to hormone.

Third of female malignancies are hormone dependent in their growth. Most prominent leading death causing factors for women under age of 50 are breast cancer and also various cancers of reproductive system. Many factors are involved in the development of breast cancer, including genetics, lifestyle, diet, endogenous hormone status and environment. Demographic risk factors for breast cancer are early age of menarche, nulliparity, late full-term pregnancy, higher social class and increasing age. Known factors with protective effects on breast cancer development are early full-term pregnancy, increasing number of births, longer periods of anovulation and more physical activity (Bernstein et al., 1994). The incidence of this lethal cancer has steadily increased during the last centuries in part due to the better and more widespread screening procedures. Increased ERα expression is one of the earliest changes occurring in the tumorigenic process and is associated with uncontrolled proliferation of the breast tissue (Khan et al., 1994). Some data is showing that ERβ could negatively modulate the effects of ERα but the prognosis for endocrine therapy are still under the question because of the somehow contradictory outcomes (Roger et al., 2001; Speirs et al., 2002). Similarly PR isoform ratio also seems to have a role in breast tumorigenesis as the ration of PRA and PRB has been altered with PRA prevalence (Mote et al., 2002).

Currently, only the expression level of ERα is measured for clinical decision-making and treatment of breast cancer patients as a favourable prognosis in primary tumours. Still, only 50% of ERα-positive tumours respond well to hormonal therapy. Large research programs are dedicated to search for better and more specific clinical breast cancer markers. The significance of ERβ status is still controversial and further analysis of the role it plays in the pathogenesis of breast cancer is required. As more experimental information on E2-mediated signalling accumulates, new possibilities emerge for breast cancer therapy.

### 3.2 Selective ER and PR modulators

Selective ER modulators (SERMs) function through ERs, acting as agonists or antagonists of E2 depending on the target tissue and modulate the signal transduction pathway to E2-responsive genes. The implementation of SERMs in clinical aspects is wide. They are used to treat or prevent breast cancer and osteoporosis, to cure ovulatory dysfunction in women but also for contraceptive purposes. SERMs have an ability to differently regulate many ER-regulated genes (Berrodin et al., 2009; Chang et al., 2010). In general, most SERMs have E2 agonist activity in bone and antagonist activity in the breast, while the activity in the uterus varies among the molecules. The tissue specificity depends on various co-activators (CoA) and co-repressors (CoR) expressed and recruited in different tissues (Riggs et al., 2003). E2 binds to either ERα or ERβ and subsequently binds CoA molecules required to form a transcription complex at EREs located in the promoter region of estrogen-responsive genes. The antiestrogenic action of a SERM results from the inappropriate folding of an ERα or ERβ complex that either cannot recruit CoA molecules or instead recruits CoR molecules. This programmed change in conformation produces antiestrogen action at specific sites like the breast, but estrogen-like effects in the uterus if an excess of CoA molecules is present. SERM–ER complexes may initiate gene transcription to produce an estrogen-like effect, by forming a protein–protein interaction at fos/jun that activates AP-1 sites (Jordan et al., 2001) (Figure 4). Although widely used and with many beneficial effects in treating breast cancer SERMs still battle with several side effects where most common is the stimulation of the endometrium.

Estrogen and SERM signal transduction pathways

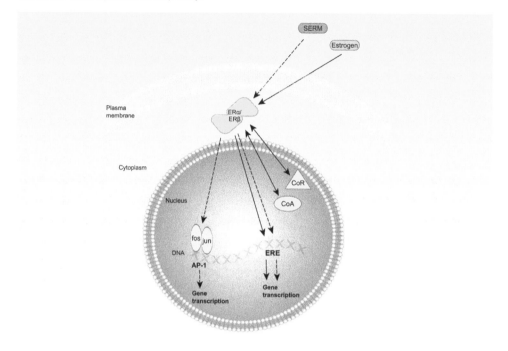

Fig. 4. The signal transduction pathways available to E2 or a SERM to initiate gene transcription. E2 receptors – ERα, ERβ, selective ER modulator-SERM, coactivator –CoA, corepressor CoR, E2 response element-ERE, activating protein -1-AP-1 (Figure adapted from Jordan et al., 2001).

Tamoxifen (TAM), the first SERM available for clinical use, is regarded as a highly effective agent for the prevention and treatment of breast cancer in premenopausal and postmenopausal women. TAM has been used in women to treat breast cancer for over 40 years (Fisher et al., 1998; Fisher et al., 2005). This compound binds with high affinity to ER, thereby blocking the action of native E2. Subsequently it inhibits or modifies the interaction of ER with DNA, which impedes the transcriptional activation of target genes (Berry et al., 2005). TAM strongly counteracts E2 effects, including secretion of several growth factors and growth controlling enzymes, so that a woman's own E2 cannot stimulate growth of the tumor cells. TAM has been a successful drug especially in treating hormone-responsive breast cancer, being one of the main reasons why ER-positive breast cancer patients have a better prognosis compared to those with an ERα-negative breast tumours. Another positive effect was noticed when postmenopausal women's bone density increased after breast cancer treatment (Love et al., 1992). One of the most significant side effects of the treatment with the TAM appears to be its proliferative effect on the endometrium (estrogen-agonistic effect; Buzdar et al., 1998; Bergman et al., 2000). The use of TAM results significant 3.3 fold increase of endometrial cancer (Fisher 2005). The repression of the cell proliferation during breast cancer treatment could lead to endometrial cell proliferation later on (Figure 5). Endometrial pathologies associated with TAM use include hyperplasia, polyps, carcinomas and sarcomas (Cohen et al., 2004). The full mechanism of this paradox remains still undiscovered.

Another well-studied antiestrogen, Raloxifen, has an E2-antagonistic effect similarly to TAM but it is reported to have small or no proliferative effect on uterus (Fugere et al., 2000). Although Raloxifen was developed initially for breast cancer treatment, its use was abandoned in the late 1980s because clinical trials showed no activity in TAM-resistant patients (Buzdar et al, 1998). Today, Raloxifen is used specifically to reduce the risk of osteoporosis in postmenopausal women at high risk for osteoporosis (Jordan et al., 2001, Cohen et al., 2000).

As SERMs have the ability to provide mixed functional ER agonist or antagonist activity, depending on the target tissue, compaunds devoid of agonist activity have been developed. The most known „pure" antiestrogen is Fulverstant (aslo known as ICI 182780) (Bowler et al., 1989; Wakeling et al., 1991). In addition to blocking the ER activity Fulvestrant induces ER degradation by changing its conformation (Dauvois et al., 1993; Gibson et al., 1991; Reese and Katzenellenbogen 1992). This forces the receptor into conformation that it is recognized as being misfolded, which induces its rapid degradation (Wu et al 2005). Fulvestrant is currently licensed for the use in postmenopausal women with ER-positive recurrent disease (Johnston et al., 2010). However, the lack of agonist activity limits its beneficial effects in bone.

SERM might inhibit the ER found in breast cells but activate the ER present in uterine endometrial cells. That would inhibit cell proliferation in breast cells, but stimulate the proliferation of uterine endometrial cells (Figure 5). There are number of decision points that determine the biological response to a SERM, which is linked to its E2-like ability to recruit CoA-s and CoR-s. ER contains a ligand-binding domain, called Activating Function-2 (AF-2), which is essential for the activation of genes that mediate the E2 effect in tissues like breast and uterus. Therefore, the different ligands can induce distinct gene transcription processes. For example, the union of the ligand binding domain with TAM results in partial agonistic effect in the uterus, whereas the same interaction is fully antagonistic in the breast (Perez et al., 2006).

Similarly to anti-estrogens, anti-progestins or Selective Progesterone Receptor Modulators (SPRMs) are developed in order to antagonize the processes activated by P4. Mifepristone (RU-486) acts as a P4 antagonist by competing with endogenous P4 for receptor binding and has three primary pharmacological effects: endometrial, gonadotropic, and adrenocortical (Goldberg et al., 1998). It has 2 to 10 time higher affinity compared to P4 to bind PRs (Brogden et al., 1993). Because PRs are found primarily in reproductive organs, Mifepristone exerts its principal effect on the uterus. More precisely, Mifepristone blocks the effects of natural P4 on the endometrium and decidua. While P4 is supposed to support the pregnancy, anti-P4 leads to degeneration and shedding of the endometrial lining, thereby preventing or disrupting implantation of the conceptus. Mifepristone also increases both uterine production of prostaglandins and uterine sensitivity to the contractile effects of prostaglandins, stimulating uterine contractions. It is postulated that Mifepristone acts directly on the uterine muscle through an entirely separate mechanism, perhaps by increasing gap junctions in the myometrium (Weiss et al., 1993). Tissue culture studies have shown that Mifepristone continues to display procontractile effects on the uterus even when the effects of prostaglandins are neutralized (Brogden et al., 1993). Most research and clinical experience with Mifepristone involves its use as an aborted material. Several studies reported its effectiveness in softening and dilation of the cervix prior to surgical abortion, decrease of pain in women with diagnosed endometriosis and in labour inducement (Goldberg et al., 1998). In the absence of P4, however, Mifepristone can act as a partial agonist (Spitz et al., 1993) and upregulate P4-responsive genes, such as p53, and through this possesses a slight anticarcinogenic effect.

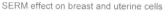

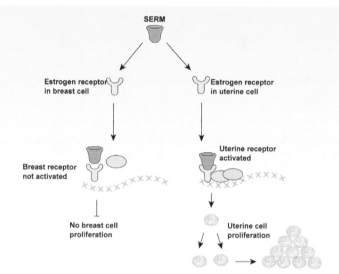

Fig. 5. **The opposite effect of SERM on breast and uterine cell proliferation.** SERM might inhibit the ER found in breast cancer cells but activate the ER present in uterine endometrial cells. A SERM of this type would inhibit cell proliferation in breast cells, but stimulate the proliferation of uterine endometrial cells. (Figure adapted from internet: http://www.cancer.gov/cancertopics/understandingcancer/estrogenreceptors/page14)

### 3.3 The risk for cancer development after IVF treatment

The impact of infertility and fertility treatments on cancer risk has become more and more prevalent since the increasing need to use IVF treatment in current society. Relatively low number of studies has been published to investigate the relation between IVF treatment and developing cancer risk. The administration of high doses of gonadotrophin analogues during the induction of the ovaries and synthetic E2 and P4 preparations in order to support the endometrium has raised the question of a possible contribution of supraphysiological levels of hormones to the development of breast or other cancer types. Previous studies have demonstrated a possible association between infertility treatments and breast cancer for women treated with at least six cycles with clomiphene citrate, or within the first year after starting IVF (Venn et al., 1995, 2001). Also women who start IVF after the age of 30 appear to be at increased risk of developing breast cancer (Katz et al., 2008; Pappo et al., 2008). Other studies have found elevated risk for ovarian cancer too but probably the risk was already higher prior to the first IVF (Källen et al., 2005; Kristiansson et al., 2007). However, there are publications, which have not found a relation between infertility treatments and any cancer development (Potashnik et al., 1999, Doyle et al., 2002; Dor et al., 2002; Lerner-Geva et al., 2010; Brinton et al., 2004). For example, a case-control study (1380 pairs) showed no risk for IVF treatment even among women who carry mutations in breast cancer susceptibility gene 1 (BRCA1) or BRCA2 gene (Kotsopoulos et al., 2008). The common opinion today is that the use of fertility medications does not increase the risk of breast cancer among those with family history of BRCA mutations.

A more recent study, published by Källen and colleagues using Swedish cancer register, showed that there was no or significantly low cancer risk among women udergoing IVF treatment compared to general population. The study included 24 058 women who had been treated with IVF where 1279 women later appeared in the cancer register. For comparison, total of 1 394 061 women in the general population were studied as a control group where 95 775 women had registered cancer (Källen et al., 2011).

The phrase "healthy patient effect" has emerged saying that women who choose IVF treatment might be more aware of risks or more health conscious at the time of conception compared to non-IVF women (Venn et al., 2001). In addition, there are numerous confounding factors which could influence the outcome of the study like the age at the time of the first IVF cycle or the first delivery, the number of the unsuccessful cycles and the follow up time after last IVF treatment. It is obvious that the question needs to be studied in more detail involving large number of women and with attention to precise subgroups.

## 4. Genome-wide E2 and P4 signalling

There are hundreds of studies presenting how expression of a single gene could change upon E2 or P4 treatment in different cell culture. Knock out studies with transgenic animals have confirmed the importance of ERs and PRs in reproductive system and cancer development. To understand the broad role of steroid hormones in humans it is mandatory to study their action in genome-wide level. Recently, the development of large-scale genomic methods to analyse gene expression and factor binding to DNA enable us to study steroid hormone dependent gene expression changes and transcription regulation in the entire genome. As ERs and PRs are acting as TFs they have an ability to regulate the expression of proximal and distal genes by binding hormone responsive elements. Chromatin immunoprecipitation (ChIP) analysis has been broadly used for identification TF binding regions on DNA. ChIP assay can be followed by polymerase chain reaction (PCR), hybridization the probes on a microarray (ChIP-on-chip) or high throughput (HTP)-sequencing (ChIP-Seq) to establish the genomic regions occupied by a specific TF. To understand whether TF binding has a positive or negative impact on gene expression microarrays, sequencing (RNA-Seq) and RT-qPCR are commonly used followed to mRNA extraction.

### 4.1 Genome-wide identification of TF binding regions, ChIP-Seq

ChIP is a technique for assaying protein-DNA interactions *in vivo* (Weinmann et al., 2002). This analysis allows identifying regions of the genome bound directly to ERs or PRs as well as regions bound indirectly via other TFs or co-regulators. During the procedure proteins are cross-linked to DNA and the chromatin is thereafter sonicated to small fragments around 150-1000bp depending on which application is used below. After immunoprecipitation of protein-DNA complexes, the cross-links are reversed and the DNA fragments purified. Extracted DNA could be analyzed with either PCR, ChIP-on-chip or direct sequencing. Regions significantly overrepresented in the immunoprecipitated DNA relative to control DNA are regarded as epigenetically modified or protein-bound, depending on the antibody used (Bock et al., 2008). Computational algorithms are used to infer the information from the array data or sequencing output. ChIP has two main drawbacks. First and the main problem is the specificity of antibodies used. The second problem is aggregation of chromatin that contaminates the purified specific chromatin fraction and raises unspecific background of isolated DNA. In case of ChIP-on-chip ChIP-enriched DNA is spotted on glass slide microarrays (chip) to study how regulatory proteins interact with the genome of living cells (Lin Z et al., 2007, Liu et al., 2008). ChIP-on-Chip has many modifications such as ChIP-linked target site cloning (Lin Z et al., 2007) and ChIP coupled with a DNA selection and ligation (ChIP-DSL) strategy for direct target genes, permitting analysis of fewer cells than required by the conventional ChIP-on-chip method (Kwon et al., 2007). The ChIP-DSL technology is distinct from the latter assay. Besides it being more specific and sensitive, the immunoprecipitated DNA is used to template oligonucleotide ligation, instead of being directly amplified for hybridization, which makes it possible to bypass incomplete decrosslinking. There is also the paired-end ditag (PET) approach, which directly links the 5' terminal tags of genomic sequences with their corresponding 3' terminal tags to form PET ditags and concatenates them for efficient sequencing (Bock et al., 2008).

ChIP-Seq is emerging as the method of choice for genome-wide identification of TF binding sites. The ChIP-Seq involves immunoselecting an enriched population of transcription factor-bound chromatin fragments, which are purified and resolved via next-generation sequencing. Today, several DNA sequencing technologies are available - the ABI SOLiD platform utilizes oligonucleotide ligation and detection methodology (Dietz and Carroll, 2008), the sequencing-by-synthesis methods of 454 Life Sciences and Solexa/Illumina technology utilize, an emulsion based PCR followed by HTP sequencing and reversible terminator sequencing respectively. Also it is possible to sequence on single-molecule sequencing platforms such as the HeliScope by Helicos where, fluorescent nucleotides incorporated into templates can be imaged at the level of single molecules (Figure 6). A typical dataset generated from the Illumina Genome Analyzer yields several million short sequence reads with typical length 36-75 bp. These are aligned to a reference genome, and the resulting trace read placements are used to infer the locations of transcription factor binding in a global fashion. ChIP-seq provides clearly interpretable binding information. Even more, compared to ChIP-on-chip data normalization is not an issue because the sequencing results in absolute read counts (Barski et al., 2007). Also, the repetitive portion of DNA is not a hindrance. One limitation is that the process of mapping tags to the reference genome can bias the analysis toward genomic regions with unique and complex sequence patterns. This is because short sequencing reads that overlap with low-complexity regions or with interspersed repeats stand a higher chance of being discarded for lack of unique genomic alignment (Bock et al., 2008). Even though ChIP-seq shares ChIP-on-chip's dependence on high-quality antibodies, the unparalleled throughput makes ChIP-seq superior for whole genome mapping of DNAprotein interactions. The latest results show that ChIP-Seq method could detect more than 10 000 binding regions for ERα in MCF7 cells (Carroll et al., 2006; Hurtado et al., 2011). Nevertheless, linking the binding regions to the

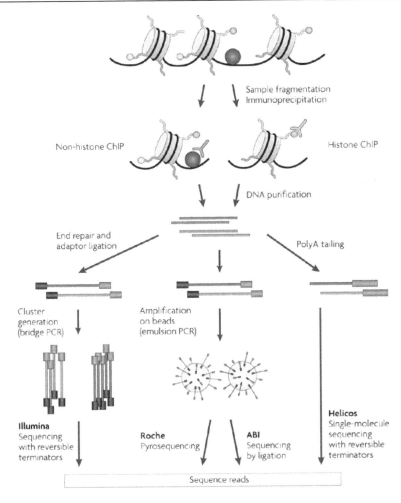

Nature Reviews | Genetics

Fig. 6. **ChIP followed by highthroughput sequencing.** The ChIP process enriches the crosslinked proteins or modified nucleosomes using an antibody specific to the protein or the histone modification of interest. Purified DNA can be sequenced using different next-generation sequencing platforms. On the Illumina Solexa Genome Analyzer (bottom left) clusters of clonal sequences are generated by bridge PCR, and sequencing is performed by sequencing-by-synthesis. On the Roche 454 and Applied Biosystems (ABI) SOLiD platforms (bottom middle), clonal sequencing features are generated by emulsion PCR and amplicons are captured on the surface of micrometre-scale beads. Beads with amplicons are then recovered and immobilized to a planar substrate to be sequenced by pyrosequencing (for the 454 platform) or by DNA ligase-driven synthesis (for the SOLiD platform). On single-molecule sequencing platforms such as the HeliScope by Helicos (bottom right), fluorescent nucleotides incorporated into templates can be imaged at the level of single molecules, which makes clonal amplification unnecessary (adapted from Nature Reviews, Park 2009).

target genes has been an on-going struggle as majority of binding regions can be separated by hundreds of kilobases and in some cases megabases. In many cases the biological functionality of the TF binding is still unrevealed.

Fullwood and colleagues have developed a technique called ChIA-PET (chromatin interaction analysis using paired-end tag sequencing) (Fullwood et al., 2009), which couples chromosome conformation capture (Dekker et al., 2002), a method for identifying interacting chromatin regions, with high-throughput sequencing. The authors found 689 ER-associated chromatin interaction complexes made up of duplexes and more complex interactions. These tend to involve stronger ER-binding events, which are biased toward specific histone marks and other transcriptional regulators more imperative for ER function.

Endometrial cell lines seem to be less hormone responsive compared to MCF7. In our previous study we used ChIP-qPCR to identifying ER and PR targets in two endometrial cell lines. We found 137 target genes for ERs in HEC1A and 83 target genes for PRs in RL95-2 from 382 pre-selected genes. The results confirmed the *in vitro* model of non-receptive (HEC1A) and receptive (RL95-2) endometrium in steroid hormone manner (Tamm et al., 2009).

## 4.2 Expression analysis, RNA-Seq

The transcriptome is the complete set of transcripts in a cell or tissue at a specific developmental stage or physiological condition. Expression microarrays are currently the most widely used methodology for transcriptome analysis. Breast cancer cell line MCF7 is most extensively used cell line in terms of studying E2 responsiveness and ERα localization. The number of genes which could be regulated by E2 has expanded extensively during the last decade from ~100 to ~1500 genes (Frasor et al., 2003, Carroll and Brown, 2006, Kininis et al., 2007, Levenson et al., 2002, Lin et al., 2004, Lin et al., 2007). It is likely that in the near future RNA-Seq, more sensitive technique, will introduce even more genes which show significant change in their activity after E2 or P4 treatment. Gene expression studies investigating endometrial receptivity using human biopsy samples have searched for genes differentially expressed in follicular and luteal phase (Kao et al., 2002; Carson et al., 2002; Riesewijk et al., 2003; Mirkin et al., 2005). The highest number of regulatory genes was brought out in Carson´s study with 323 up-regulated and 370 down-regulated genes comparing follicular phase to the luteal phase. As mentioned before, the overlap of genes identified in different publications is relatively low. The difference could be due to variations is study design and limiting factors of microarray analysis. Microarray is hybridization-based approach, which involves incubating fluorescently labelled cDNA with custom made microarrays. Prominent limitations with this method include hybridization, cross-hybridization artefacts, different data analysis and low coverage of all possible genes in large genomes (Casneuf et al., 2007). Comparing expression levels across different experiments is often difficult and requite complicated normalization methods. The newer and potentially more comprehensive way to measure the whole active transcriptome is by direct ultra-high-throughput sequencing named RNA-Seq. The resulting sequence reads are individually mapped to the source genome and counted to obtain the number and density of reads corresponding to RNA from each known exon, splice event or new candidate gene (Mortazavi et al., 2008). RNA-Seq uses recently developed deep-sequencing technologies where RNA is converted to a library of cDNA fragments with adaptors attached to one or both ends. Each molecule is sequenced from single end or paired end. The reads are typically 30-400bp, depending on the DNA-sequencing technology used. Similarly to ChIP extracted

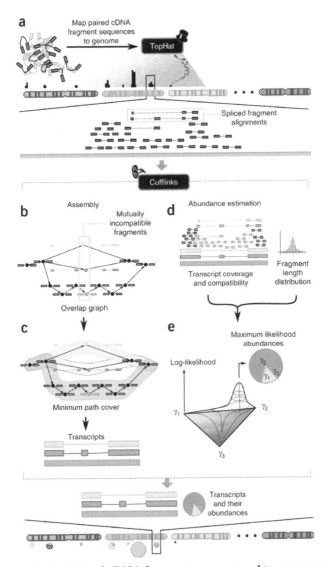

Fig. 7. RNA-Seq method. a) Paired cDNA fragments are mapped to genome using TopHat software b) Each pair of fragment is treated as a single alignment and the abundances of the aasembled transcripts are estimated (b-e). First the fragments from distinct spliced mRNA isoforms are identified (b). Isoforms are then assembled from the overlap graph (c) and transcript abundance is estimated (d). Cufflinks estimates transcript abundances using a statistical model in which the probability of observing each fragment is a linear function of the abundances of the transcripts from which it could be originated. The program numerically maximizes a function that assigns a likelyhood to all possible sets of relative abundances of different isoforms (e), producing the abundances that best explain the observed fragments (adapted from Trapnell et al., 2010).

RNA can be used with Illumina, Applied Biosystems SOLiD and Roche 454 Life Science platforms (Wang et al., 2009, Rev). RNA-Seq has very low, if any, background signal because cDNA sequences can be mapped to unique regions of the genome. It does not have any upper limit of quantification like DNA microarrays which lack sensitivity for genes expressed either at low or very high levels. Like other HTP Sequencing technologies, RNA-seq faces several bioinformatics challenges in data processing.

The analysis of RNA-Seq data starts from raw cDNA sequences, usually having lengths of 40-70bp, depending on the platform. The general goal is to find which sites in human genome the RNA was transcribed from and determine the expression levels of these transcripts. Additionally, RNA-Seq data can be used to study expression levels of alternative splicing isoforms.

The usual analysis consists of three main steps:

1. Map each RNA sequence to the human genome. Mapping program has to enable spliced alignments because the sequences can come from separated exons. For this a fast and open source tool TopHat can be used (Trapnell et al., 2009)

2. Count mappings to every site and measure the expression level of the sites. The expression level is usually measured in Fragments Per Kilobase of exon per Million fragments mapped (FPKM) which permits comparison of results across experiments. FPKM of a site shows how frequently the mapped fragments fall on that site. This analysis is possible using Cufflinks software, which can measure FPKM for whole genes and also for specific spliced isoforms (Trapnell et al., 2010)

3. Compare experiments and find genes (or spliced isoforms) that have statistically significant different FPKM across experiments. This is also possible using commercial or open source software as Cufflinks.

More detailed explanation of the analysis is depicted in the Figure 7.

## 5. Conclusion

This chapter summarised the current knowledge of E2 and P4 action in human endometrium and mammary gland. To understand both sides of steroid hormone action - in normal physiology and especially in pathology it is important to understand the molecular intracellular events of E2 and P4 in tissue-type manner. The same hormones could have different or even opposite effects in different tissues. Thus, attention should be applied to steroid hormones' or their analogues' possible side effects before using them in clinical treatments. Questions still remain about the aberrations of the endometrium leading to implantation failure, endometriosis and other dys-regulations. Even though studies of breast cancer development continuously unravel new information about the mechanisms leading from normal to malignant tissue proliferation, breast cancer is still the most fatal cancer type among women. The number of couples seeking for aid to achieve fertility is constantly increasing and thus a better understanding of factors needed for successful treatment and possible side effects is crucial.

We would like to punctuate the importance of the next generation sequencing technologies which we believe are the key in understanding hormone dependent action in whole organism. With today's knowledge of nearly entire human genome sequence and the development of new technologies based on HTP sequencing it has become possible to define all targets for the TF in vivo and establish entire transcriptome in a single experiment. Data analysis is still complicated in a way and needs excellent computational skills but the data collected today will become the knowledge of tomorrow.

## 6. Acknowledgment

This work has been supported by the Tallinn University of Technology (Tareted project no. B611), Estonian Ministry of Education and Science (Targeted project no. SF0180044s09) and Enterprise Estonia (Grant no. EU30200).

## 7. References

Altmäe, S., Martínez-Conejero, J.A., Salumets, A., Simón, C., Horcajadas, J.A. & Stavreus-Evers A. *Endometrial gene expression analysis at the time of embryo implantation in women with unexplained infertility.* Mol Hum Reprod. 2010 Mar;16(3):178-87. Epub 2009 Nov 22.

Arici, A., Engin, O., Attar, E. & Olive DL. (1995) *Modulation of leukemia inhibitory factor gene expression and protein biosynthesis in human endometrium.* J Clin Endocrinol Metab. 1995 Jun;80(6):1908-15.

Arnett-Mansfield, R.L., DeFazio, A., Mote, P.A. & Clarke CL. (2004) *Subnuclear distribution of progesterone receptors A and B in normal and malignant endometrium.* J Clin Endocrinol Metab. 2004 Mar;89(3):1429-42.

Attia, G.R., Zeitoun, K., Edwards, D., Johns, A., Carr, B.R. & Bulun, S.E. (2000). Progesterone receptor isoform A but not B is expressed in endometriosis. *J. Clin. Endocrinol. Metab*, 85, 2897–2902.

Baart, E.B., Martini, E., Eijkemans, M.J., Van Opstal, D., Beckers, N.G., Verhoeff, A., Macklon, N.S. & Fauser, B.C. (2007). Milder ovarian stimulation for in-vitro fertilization reduces aneuploidy in the human preimplantation embryo: a randomized controlled trial. *Hum. Reprod.*, 22, 980-988.

Bain, DL., Heneghan, A.F, Connaghan-Jones, KD. & Miura MT (2007). *Nuclear receptor structure: implications for function.* Annu Rev Physiol. 2007;69:201-20. Review.

Barski, A., Cuddapah, S., Cui, K., Roh, TY., Schones, DE., Wang, Z., Wei, G., Chepelev, I. & Zhao K. (2007) *High-resolution profiling of histone methylations in the human genome.* Cell. 2007 May 18;129(4):823-37.

Beckers, N.G., Platteau, P., Eijkemans, M.J., Macklon, N.S., de Jong, F.H., Devroey, P. & Fauser, B.C. (2006). The early luteal phase administration of oestrogen and progesterone does not induce premature luteolysis in normo-ovulatory women. *Eur. J. Endocrinol.*, 155, 355-363.

Bergman, L., Beelen, ML., Gallee, MP., Hollema, H., Benraadt, J. and van Leeuwen, FE. (2000*) Risk and prognosis of endometrial cancer after tamoxifen for breast cancer.* Comprehensive Cancer Centres' ALERT Group. Assessment of Liver and Endometrial cancer Risk following Tamoxifen. Lancet 2000;356: 881–887.

Bernstein, L., Hanisch, R., Sullivan-Halley, J. & Ross, R.K. (1995) *Treatment with human chorionic gonadotropin and risk of breast cancer.* Cancer Epidemiol Biomarkers Prev. 1995 Jul-Aug;4(5):437-40.

Berrodin, T.J., Chang, K.C., Komm, B.S., Freedman, L.P. & Nagpal S. (2009) *Differential biochemical and cellular actions of Premarin estrogens: distinct pharmacology of bazedoxifene-conjugated estrogens combination.* Mol Endocrinol. 2009 Jan;23(1):74-85. Epub 2008 Nov 26.

Berry, M., Metzger, D. and Chambon, P. (1990) *Role of the two activating domains of the oestrogen receptor in the cell-type and promoter-context dependent agonistic activity of the anti-oestrogen 4- hydroxytamoxifen.* EMBO J. 1990;9: 2811-2818.

Björnström, L. & Sjöberg, M. (2004*) Estrogen receptor-dependent activation of AP-1 via nongenomic signalling.* Nucl Recept. 2004 Jun 14;2(1):3.

Bocchinfuso, W.P. & Korach KS. (1997) *Mammary gland development and tumorigenesis in estrogen receptor knockout mice.* J Mammary Gland Biol Neoplasia. 1997 Oct;2(4):323-34.

Bock, C. & Lengauer T. (2008). *Computational epigenetics.* Jan 1;24(1):1-10. Epub 2007 Nov 17. Bioinformatics.

Bowler, J., Lilley, T.J., Pittam, J.D. and Wakeling, A.E. (1989) *Novel steroidal pure antiestrogens.* Steroids 1989;54:71-99.

Brinsden, P.R., Alam, V., de Moustier, B. & Engrand P. (2009) *Recombinant human leukemia inhibitory factor does not improve implantation and pregnancy outcomes after assisted reproductive techniques in women with recurrent unexplained implantation failure.* Fertil Steril. 2009 Apr;91(4 Suppl):1445-7. Epub 2008 Aug 16.

Brinton, L.A., Scoccia, B., Moghissi, K.S., Westhoff, C.L., Althuis, M.D., Mabie, J.E. & Lamb EJ. (2004) *Breast cancer risk associated with ovulation-stimulating drugs.* Hum Reprod. 2004 Sep;19(9):2005-13. Epub 2004 Jun 24.

Brogden, R.N., Goa, K.L. & Faulds D. (1993) *Mifepristone: a review of its pharmacodynamic and pharmacokinetic properties, and therapeutic potential.* Drugs. 1993;45:384-409.

Brosens, J.J. & Gellersen, B. (2006) *Death or survival--progesterone-dependent cell fate decisions in the human endometrial stroma.* J Mol Endocrinol. 2006 Jun;36(3):389-98. Review.

Buzdar, A. (1998) *The place of chemotherapy in the treatment of early breast cancer.* British Journal of Cancer 1998; 78

Cakmak, H.& Taylor, H.S. (2010). Review. Molecular mechanisms of treatment resistance in endometriosis: the role of progesterone-hox gene interactions. *Semin. Reprod. Med.,* 1 (January, 28), 69-74.

Carroll, JS. & Brown M. (2006) *Estrogen receptor target gene: an evolving concept.* Mol Cell Biol. 2007 Jul;27(14):5090-104. Epub 2007 May 21.

Carson, DD., Lagow, E., Thathiah, A., Al-Shami, R., Farach-Carson, MC., Vernon, M., Yuan, L., Fritz MA. & Lessey. BA. (2002) *Changes in gene expression during the early to midluteal (receptive phase) transition in human endometrium detected by high-density microarray screening.* Mol Hum Reprod. 2002 Sep;8(9):871-9.

Casneuf, T., Van de Peer, Y. & Huber W. *In situ analysis of cross-hybridisation on microarrays and the inference of expression correlation.* BMC Bioinformatics. 2007 Nov 26;8:461.

Chang, Y., Lee, J.J., Chen, W.F., Chou, D.S., Huang, S.Y. & Sheu JR. (2010) *A novel role for tamoxifen in the inhibition of human platelets.* Transl Res. 2011 Feb;157(2):81-91. Epub 2010 Nov 30.

Check, J.H., O'Shaughnessy, A., Lurie, D., Fisher, C. & Adelson, H.G. (1995). Evaluation of the mechanism for higher pregnancy rates in donor oocyte recipients by comparison of fresh with frozen embryo transfer pregnancy rates in a shared oocyte programme. *Hum. Reprod.*, 10, 3022–3027.

Cohen, F. J., Watts, S., Shah, A., Akers, R., and Plouffe, L., Jr. (2000) *Uterine effects of 3-year raloxifene therapy in postmenopausal women younger than age 60.* Obstet. Gynecol. 2000; 95: 104–110.

Cohen, I. (2004) *Endometrial pathologies associated with postmenopausal tamoxifen treatment.* Gynecology and Oncology 2004;94: 256–266.

Cork, B.A., Li, T.C., Warren, M.A. & Laird SM. (2001) *Interleukin-11 (IL-11) in human endometrium: expression throughout the menstrual cycle and the effects of cytokines on endometrial IL-11 production in vitro.* J Reprod Immunol. 2001 Apr;50(1):3-17.

Dadi, T.D., Li, M.W. & Lloyd K.C. (2006) *Development of mouse embryos after immunoneutralization of mitogenic growth factors mimics that of cloned embryos.* Comp Med. 2006 Jun;56(3):188-95.

Dauvois, S., White, R. and Parker, M.G. (1993) *The antiestrogen ICI 182780 disrupts estrogen receptor nucleocytoplasmic shuttling.* Journal of Cell Science 1993; 106: 1377-1388.

Dekker, J., Rippe, K., Dekker, M. & Kleckner N (2002) *Capturing chromosome conformation.* Science. 2002 Feb 15;295(5558):1306-11.

Department of Health and Human Services Centres for Disease Control and Prevention Report 2001

Develioglu, O.H., Hsiu, J.G., Nikas, G., Toner, J.P., Oehninger, S. and Jones, H.W. Jr (1999). Endometrial estrogen and progesterone receptor and pinopode expression in stimulated cycles of oocyte donors. *Fertil. Steril.*, 71, 1040-1047.

Devroey, P., Bourgain, C., Macklon, N.S. & Fauser, B.C. (2004). Reproductive biology and IVF: ovarian stimulation and endometrial receptivity. *Trends Endocrinol. Metab.*, 15, 84-90.

Dietz, SC. & Carroll, JS. (2008) *Interrogating the genome to understand oestrogen-receptor-mediated transcription.* Expert Rev Mol Med. 2008 Apr 1;10:e10. Review.

Diez-Perez, A. (2006) *Selective Estrogen Receptor Modulators.* Arq Bras Endocrinol Metab 2006;50/4:720-734.

Dimitriadis, E., Salamonsen, L.A. & Robb L. (2000) *Expression of interleukin-11 during the human menstrual cycle: coincidence with stromal cell decidualization and relationship to leukaemia inhibitory factor and prolactin.* Mol Hum Reprod. 2000 Oct;6(10):907-14.

Dor, J., Lerner-Geva, L., Rabinovici, J., Chetrit, A., Levran, D., Lunenfeld, B., Mashiach, S. & Modan B. (2002) *Cancer incidence in a cohort of infertile women who underwent in vitro fertilization.* Fertil Steril. 2002 Feb;77(2):324-7.

Doyle, P., Maconochie, N., Beral, V., Swerdlow, A.J. & Tan SL. (2002) *Cancer incidence following treatment for infertility at a clinic in the UK.* Hum Reprod. 2002 Aug;17(8):2209-13.

Duan, L., Glass, CK., Rosenfeld MG. & Fu XD (2007) *Sensitive ChIP-DSL technology reveals an extensive estrogen receptor alpha-binding program on human gene promoters.* Proc Natl Acad Sci U S A. 2007 Mar 20;104(12):4852-7. Epub 2007 Mar 14.

Edwards, R.G. (2005) Historical significance of gonadotrophins in assisted reproduction. *Reprod. BioMed Online*, 10, 3

Enmark. E., Pelto-Huikko, M., Grandien K., Lagercrantz, S., Lagercrantz, J., Fried, G., Nordenskjöld, M. & Gustafsson, JA. (1997) *Human estrogen receptor beta-gene structure, chromosomal localization, and expression pattern.* J Clin Endocrinol Metab. 1997 Dec;82(12):4258-65.

Fauser, B.C. & Devroey, P. (2003). Reproductive biology and IVF: ovarian stimulation and luteal phase consequences. *Trends. Endocrinol. Metab.*, 14, 236-242.

Fisher, B., Costantino, JP., Wickerham, DL., Redmond, CK., Kavanah, M., Cronin, WM., Vogel, V., Robidoux, A., Dimitrov, N., Atkins, J., Daly, M., Wieand, S., Tan-Chiu, E., Ford, L. & Wolmark N. (1998) *Tamoxifen for prevention of breast cancer: report of the National Surgical Adjuvant Breast and Bowel Project P-1 Study.* J Natl Cancer Inst. 1998; 90 (18): 1371-1388.

Fisher, B., Costantino, JP., Wickerham, DL., Redmond, CK., Kavanah, M., Cronin, WM., Vogel, V., Robidoux, A., Dimitrov, N., Atkins, J., Daly, M., Wieand, S., Tan-Chiu, E., Ford, L. & Wolmark, N. (2005) *Tamoxifen for the Prevention of Breast Cancer: Current Status of the National Surgical Adjuvant Breast and Bowel Project P-1 Study.* J Natl Cancer Inst 2005;97(22):1652-1662.

Frasor, J., Danes, JM., Komm, B., Chang, KC., Lyttl,e CR. & Katzenellenbogen BS. (2003) *Profiling of estrogen up- and down-regulated gene expression in human breast cancer cells: insights into gene networks and pathways underlying estrogenic control of proliferation and cell phenotype.* Endocrinology. 2003 Oct;144(10):4562-74. Epub 2003 Jul 10.

Fugere, P., Scheele, W. H., Shah, A., Strack, T. R., Glant, M. D., and Jolly, E. (2000) *Uterine effects of raloxifene in comparison with continuous-combined hormone replacement therapy in postmenopausal women.* Am. J. Obstet. Gynecol. 2000;182: 568-574.

Fullwood, MJ., Liu, MH., Pan, YF., Liu, J., Xu, H., Mohamed, YB., Orlov, YL., Velkov, S., Ho, A., Mei, PH., Chew, EG., Huang, PY., Welboren, WJ., Han, Y., Ooi, HS., Ariyaratne, PN., Vega, VB., Luo, Y., Tan, PY., Choy, PY., Wansa, KD., Zhao, B., Lim, KS., Leow, SC., Yow, JS., Joseph, R., Li, H., Desai, KV., Thomsen, JS., Lee, YK., Karuturi, RK., Herve, T., Bourque, G., Stunnenberg, HG., Ruan, X., Cacheux-Rataboul, V., Sung, WK., Liu, ET., Wei, CL., Cheung, E. & Ruan, Y. (2009) *An oestrogen-receptor-alpha-bound human chromatin interactome.* Nature. 2009 Nov 5;462(7269):58-64.

Gibson, M.K., Nemmers, L.A., Beckman, W.C. Jr., Davis, V.L., Curtis, S.W. and Korach, K.S. (1991) *The mechanism of ICI 164,384 antiestrogenicity involves rapid loss of estrogen receptor in uterine tissue.* Endocrinology 1991;129:2000-2010.

Giudice, L.C., Telles, T.L., Lobo, S. & Kao, L. (2002). The molecular basis for implantation failure in endometriosis: on the road to discovery. *Ann. N Y Acad. Sci.*, 955, 252-264.

Goldberg, J.R., Plescia, M.G. & Anastasio, G.D. (1998) *Mifepristone (RU 486). Current Knowledge and Future Prospects.* Arch Fam Med. 1998;7:219-222.

Graham, R.A., Seif, M.W., Aplin, J.D., Li, T.C., Cooke, I.D., Rogers, A.W. & Dockery P. (1990) *An endometrial factor in unexplained infertility.* BMJ. 1990 Jun 2;300(6737):1428-31.

Hall, JM. & McDonnell DP (2005). *Coregulators in nuclear estrogen receptor action: from concept to therapeutic targeting.* Mol Interv. 2005 Dec;5(6):343-57. Review.

Haouzi, D., Assou, S., Mahmoud, K., Tondeur, S., Rème, T., Hedon, B., De Vos, J. & Hamamah S. (2009b) *Gene expression profile of human endometrial receptivity: comparison between natural and stimulated cycles for the same patients.* Hum Reprod. 2009 Jun;24(6):1436-45. Epub 2009 Feb 26.

Haouzi, D., Mahmoud, K., Fourar, M., Bendhaou, K., Dechaud, H., De Vos, J., Rème, T., Dewailly, D. & Hamamah S. (2009) *Identification of new biomarkers of human endometrial receptivity in the natural cycle.* Hum Reprod. 2009 Jan;24(1):198-205. Epub 2008 Oct 3.

Hofmann, G.E., Scott, R.T. Jr., Bergh, P.A. & Deligdisch L. (1991) *Immunohistochemical localization of epidermal growth factor in human endometrium, decidua, and placenta.* J Clin Endocrinol Metab. 1991 Oct;73(4):882-7.

Horcajadas, J.A., Mínguez, P., Dopazo, J., Esteban, F.J., Domínguez, F., Giudice, L.C., Pellicer, A. & Simon, C. (2008). *J. Clin. Endocrinol. Metab.,* 93, 4500–4510.

Horcajadas, J.A., Mínguez, P., Dopazo, J., Esteban, F.J., Domínguez, F., Giudice, L.C., Pellicer, A. & Simón C. (2008) *Controlled ovarian stimulation induces a functional genomic delay of the endometrium with potential clinical implications.* J Clin Endocrinol Metab. 2008 Nov;93(11):4500-10. Epub 2008 Aug 12

Horcajadas, J.A., Riesewijk, A., Martín, J., Cervero, A., Mosselman, S., Pellicer, A. & Simón C. (2004) *Global gene expression profiling of human endometrial receptivity.* J Reprod Immunol. 2004 Aug;63(1):41-9.

Humphreys, R.C., Lydon, J., O'Malley, B.W. & Rosen JM. (1997*) Mammary gland development is mediated by both stromal and epithelial progesterone receptors.* Mol Endocrinol. 1997 Jun;11(6):801-11.

Johnston, S.J. & Cheung, K.L. (2010) *Fulvestrant – a novel endocrine therapy for breast cancer.* Curr Med Chem 2010, 17:902–914.

Jones, R.L., Stoikos, C., Findlay, J.K. & Salamonsen, L.A. (2006) *TGF-beta superfamily expression and actions in the endometrium and placenta.* Reproduction. 2006 Aug;132(2):217-32. Review.

Jordan, C. (2001) *Selective Estrogen Receptor Modulator: A Personal Perspective.* Cancer Res 2001; 61: 5683–5687

Jordan, VC., Gapstur, S. & Morrow M. (2001) *Selective Estrogen Receptor Modulation and Reduction in Risk of Breast Cancer, Osteoporosis, and Coronary Heart Disease.* Review. Journal of the National Cancer Institute 2001; Vol. 93, No. 19: 1449-57.

Kabir-Salmani, M., Shiokawa, S., Akimoto, Y., Sakai, K. & Iwashita M. (2004) *The role of alpha(5)beta(1)-integrin in the IGF-I-induced migration of extravillous trophoblast cells during the process of implantation.* Mol Hum Reprod. 2004 Feb;10(2):91-7.

Källén, B., Finnström, O., Lindam, A., Nilsson, E., Nygren, K.G. & Olausson PO. (2011) *Malignancies among women who gave birth after in vitro fertilization.* Hum Reprod. 2011 Jan;26(1):253-8. Epub 2010 Nov 18.

Källén, B., Finnström, O., Nygren, K.G. & Olausson PO. (2007) *In vitro fertilization (IVF) in Sweden: risk for congenital malformations after different IVF methods.* Birth Defects Res A Clin Mol Teratol. 2005 Mar;73(3):162-9.

Kanis, JA. & Stevenson, JC. (1994). Effect of estrogen therapy on bone density in elderly women. N Engl J Med 1994 Mar 10;330(10):715; author reply 716

Kao, L.C., Germeyer, A., Tulac, S., Lobo, S., Yang, J.P., Taylor, R.N., Osteen, K., Lessey, B.A. & Giudice, L.C. (2003). Expression profiling of endometrium from women with endometriosis reveals candidate genes for disease-based implantation failure and infertility. *Endocrinol.*, 144, 2870–2881

Kao, L.C., Tulac, S., Lobo, S., Imani, B., Yang, J.P., Germeyer, A., Osteen, K., Taylor, R.N., Lessey, B.A. & Giudice LC. (2002). *Global gene profiling in human endometrium during the window of implantation.* Endocrinology. 2002 Jun;143(6):2119-38.

Kao, LC., Tulac, S., Lobo, S., Imani, B., Yang, JP., Germeyer, A., Osteen, K., Taylor, RN., Lessey, BA. & Giudice LC. (2002) *Global gene profiling in human endometrium during the window of implantation.* Endocrinology. 2002 Jun;143(6):2119-38.

Kastner, P., Krust, A., Turcotte, B., Stropp, U., Tora, L. Gronemeyer, M.A. & Chambon, P. (1990) Two distinct estrogen-regulated promoters generate transcripts encoding the two functionally different human progesterone receptor forms A and B. *Embo. J., 9(5), 1603–1614.*

Kastner. P., Bocquel. MT., Turcotte, B., Garnier, JM., Horwitz, KB., Chambon P. & Gronemeyer H. (1990) *Transient expression of human and chicken progesterone receptors does not support alternative translational initiation from a single mRNA as the mechanism generating two receptor isoforms.* J Biol Chem. 1990 Jul 25;265(21):12163-7.

Katz, D., Paltiel, O., Peretz, T., Revel, A., Sharon, N., Maly, B., Michan, N., Sklair-Levy, M. & Allweis T. (2008) *Beginning IVF treatments after age 30 increases the risk of breast cancer: results of a case-control study.* Breast J. 2008 Nov-Dec;14(6):517-22. Epub 2008 Oct 14.

Kelly, MJ. & Rønnekleiv OK. (2008). *Membrane-initiated estrogen signaling in hypothalamic neurons.* Mol Cell Endocrinol. 2008 Aug 13;290(1-2):14-23. Epub 2008 Apr 30. Review.

Khan, S.A., Rogers, M.A., Obando, J.A. & Tamsen A. (1994) *Estrogen receptor expression of benign breast epithelium and its association with breast cancer.* Cancer Res. 1994 Feb 15;54(4):993-7.

Kim, J.J., Taylor, H.S., Lu, Z., Ladhani, O., Hastings, J.M., Jackson, K.S., Wu, Y., Guo, S.W. & Fazleabas AT. (2007). Altered expression of HOXA10 in endometriosis: potential role in decidualization. *Mol. Hum. Reprod.*, 5 (May, 13), 323-32.

Kininis, M., Chen, BS., Diehl, AG., Isaacs, GD., Zhang, T., Siepel, AC., Clark, AG. & Kraus WL. (2006) *Genomic analyses of transcription factor binding, histone acetylation, and gene expression reveal mechanistically distinct classes of estrogen-regulated promoters.* Mol Endocrinol. 2006 Aug;20(8):1707-14. Epub 2006 Jan 5. Review.

Kotsopoulos, J., Librach, C.L., Lubinski, J., Gronwald, J., Kim-Sing, C., Ghadirian, P., Lynch, H.T., Moller, P., Foulkes, W.D., Randall, S., Manoukian, S., Pasini, B., Tung, N., Ainsworth, P.J., Cummings, S., Sun, P. &Narod, S.A. Hereditary Breast Cancer Clinical Study Group. *Infertility, treatment of infertility, and the risk of breast cancer among women with BRCA1 and BRCA2 mutations: a case-control study.* Cancer Causes Control. 2008 Dec;19(10):1111-9. Epub 2008 May 29.

Krikun, G., Schatz, F., Taylor, R., Critchley, H.O., Rogers, P.A., Huang, J. & Lockwood CJ. (2005) *Endometrial endothelial cell steroid receptor expression and steroid effects on gene expression.* J Clin Endocrinol Metab. 2005 Mar;90(3):1812-8. Epub 2004 Dec 21.

Kristiansson, P., Björ, O. & Wramsby H. (2007) *Tumour incidence in Swedish women who gave birth following IVF treatment.* Hum Reprod. 2007 Feb;22(2):421-6. Epub 2006 Oct 27.

Kuiper, GG. & Gustafsson, JA. (1997) *The novel estrogen receptor-beta subtype: potential role in the cell- and promoter-specific actions of estrogens and anti-estrogens.* FEBS Lett. 1997 Jun 23;410(1):87-90. Review.

Kuokkanen, S., Chen, B., Ojalvo, L., Benard, L., Santoro, N. & Pollard JW. (2010) *Genomic profiling of microRNAs and messenger RNAs reveals hormonal regulation in microRNA expression in human endometrium.* Biol Reprod. 2010 Apr;82(4):791-801. Epub 2009 Oct 28.

Kwon, YS., Garcia-Bassets, I., Hutt, KR., Cheng, CS., Jin, M., Liu, D., Benner, C., Wang, D., Ye, Z., Bibikova, M., Fan, JB.,

Lass, A., Peat, D., Avery, S. & Brinsden, P. (1998). Histological evaluation of endometrium on the day of oocyte retrieval after gonadotrophin-releasing hormone agonist-follicle stimulating hormone ovulation induction for invitro fertilization. *Hum. Reprod.,* 13, 3203-3205.

Lerner-Geva, L., Rabinovici, J. & Lunenfeld B. (2010) *Ovarian stimulation: is there a long-term risk for ovarian, breast and endometrial cancer?* Womens Health (Lond Engl). 2010 Nov;6(6):831-9. Review.

Lessey, B.A. (1994) *The use of integrins for the assessment of uterine receptivity.* Fertil Steril. 1994 May;61(5):812-4.

Lessey, B.A. (2003) *Two pathways of progesterone action in the human endometrium: implications for implantation and contraception.* Steroids. 2003 Nov;68(10-13):809-15. Review

Lessey, B.A. (2010) *Fine tuning of endometrial function by estrogen and progesterone through microRNAs.* Biol Reprod. 2010 Apr;82(4):653-5. Epub 2010 Feb 3.

Lessey, B.A., Gui, Y., Apparao, K.B., Young, S.L. & Mulholland J. (2002) *Regulated expression of heparin-binding EGF-like growth factor (HB-EGF) in the human endometrium: a potential paracrine role during implantation* Mol Reprod Dev. 2002 Aug;62(4):446-55.

Levenson, AS., Svoboda, KM., Pease, KM., Kaiser, SA., Chen, B., Simons, LA., Jovanovic, BD., Dyck. PA. & Jordan VC. (2002) *Gene expression profiles with activation of the estrogen receptor alpha-selective estrogen receptor modulator complex in breast cancer cells expressing wild-type estrogen receptor.* Cancer Res. 2002 Aug 1;62(15):4419-26.

Li, R., Qiao, J., Wang, L., Li, L., Zhen, X., Liu, P. & Zheng X. (2011) *MicroRNA array and microarray evaluation of endometrial receptivity in patients with high serum progesterone levels on the day of hCG administration.* Reprod Biol Endocrinol. 2011 Mar 6;9:29.

Lim, H., Song, H., Paria, B.C., Reese, J., Das, S.K. & Dey SK. (2002). *Molecules in blastocyst implantation: uterine and embryonic perspectives.* Vitam Horm. 2002;64:43-76. Review.

Lin, Z., Reierstad, S., Huang, CC. & Bulun SE. (2007) *Novel estrogen receptor-alpha binding sites and estradiol target genes identified by chromatin immunoprecipitation cloning in breast cancer.* Cancer Res. 2007 May 15;67(10):5017-24.

Lin, CY., Ström, A., Vega, VB., Kong, SL., Yeo, AL., Thomsen, JS., Chan, WC., Doray, B., Bangarusamy, DK., Ramasamy, A., Vergara, LA., Tang, S., Chong, A., Bajic, VB., Miller, LD., Gustafsson, JA. & Liu ET. (2004) *Discovery of estrogen receptor alpha target genes and response elements in breast tumor cells.* Genome Biol. 2004;5(9):R66. Epub 2004 Aug 12.

Lin, CY., Vega, VB., Thomsen, JS., Zhang, T., Kong, SL., Xie, M., Chiu, KP., Lipovich, L., Barnett, DH., Stossi, F., Yeo, A., George, J., Kuznetsov, VA., Lee, YK., Charn, TH., Palanisamy, N., Miller, LD., Cheung, E., Katzenellenbogen, BS., Ruan, Y., Bourque, G., Wei, CL. & Liu ET. (2007) *Whole-genome cartography of estrogen receptor alpha binding sites.* PLoS Genet. 2007 Jun;3(6):e87. Epub 2007 Apr 17.

Liu, Y., Gao, H., Marstrand, TT., Ström, A., Valen, E., Sandelin, A., Gustafsson, JA. & Dahlman-Wright K. *The genome landscape of ERalpha- and ERbeta-binding DNA regions.* Proc Natl Acad Sci U S A. 2008 Feb 19;105(7):2604-9. Epub 2008 Feb 13.

Love, R.R. (1992) *Tamoxifen prophylaxis in breast cancer.* Oncology (Williston Park). 1992 Jul;6(7):33-8; discussion 38-40, 43. Review.

Matsuzaki, S., Murakami, T., Uehara, S., Canis, M., Sasano, H. & Okamura, K. (2001). Expression of estrogen receptor alpha and beta in peritoneal and ovarian endometriosis. *Fertil.Steril.,* 75, 1198–1205.

Mirkin, S., Arslan, M., Churikov, D., Corica, A., Diaz, JI., Williams, S., Bocca, S. & Oehninger S. (2005) *In search of candidate genes critically expressed in the human endometrium during the window of implantation.* Hum Reprod. 2005 Aug;20(8):2104-17. Epub 2005 May 5.

Mortazavi, A., Williams, BA., McCue, K., Schaeffer, L. & Wold B. (2008) Mapping and quantifying mammalian transcriptomes by RNA-Seq. Nat Methods. 2008 Jul;5(7):621-8. Epub 2008 May 30.

Mote, P.A., Bartow, S., Tran, N. & Clarke CL. (2002) *Loss of co-ordinate expression of progesterone receptors A and B is an early event in breast carcinogenesis.* Breast Cancer Res Treat. 2002 Mar;72(2):163-72.

Nargund, G. & Frydman, R. (2007). Towards a more physiological approach to IVF. *Reprod. Biomed Online,* 14, 550–552.

Nikas, G., Develioglu, O.H., Toner, J.P. and Jones, H.W. Jr (1999). Endometrial pinopodes indicate a shift in the window of receptivity in IVF cycles. *Hum. Reprod.,* 14, 787-792.

Olivennes, F., Fanchin, R., Ledee, N., Righini, C., Kadoch I.J. & Frydman, R. (2002). Perinatal outcome and developmental studies on children born after IVF. *Hum. Reprod. Update,* 8, 117–128.

Papanikolaou, E.G., Bourgain, C., Kolibianakis, E., Tournaye, H., Devroey, P. (2005). Steroid receptor expression in late follicular phase endometrium in GnRH antagonist IVF cycles is already altered, indicating initiation of early luteal phase transformation in the absence of secretory changes. *Hum. Reprod.,* 20, 1541–1547.

Pappo, I., Lerner-Geva, L., Halevy, A., Olmer, L., Friedler, S., Raziel, A., Schachter, M. & Ron-El, R. (2008) *The possible association between IVF and breast cancer incidence.* Ann Surg Oncol. 2008 Apr;15(4):1048-55. Epub 2008 Jan 23.

Park, PJ. (2009) *ChIP-seq: advantages and challenges of a maturing technology.* Nat Rev Genet. 2009 Oct;10(10):669-80. Epub 2009 Sep 8.

Pennings G & Ombelet W. (2007). Coming soon to your clinic: patient-friendly ART. *Hum. Reprod.*, 22, 2075–2059.

Potashnik, G., Lerner-Geva, L., Genkin, L., Chetrit, A., Lunenfeld, E. & Porath A. (1999) *Fertility drugs and the risk of breast and ovarian cancers: results of a long-term follow-up study.* Fertil Steril. 1999 May;71(5):853-9.

Punyadeera, C., Dassen, H., Klomp, J., Dunselman, G., Kamps, R., Dijcks, F., Ederveen, A., de Goeij, A. & Groothuis P. (2005) *Oestrogen-modulated gene expression in the human endometrium.* Cell Mol Life Sci. 2005 Jan;62(2):239-50.

Reese, J.C. and Katzenellenbogen, B.S. (1992) *Examination of the DNA-binding ability of estrogen receptor in whole cells: implications for hormone-dependent transactivation and the actions of antiestrogens.* Mol. Cell. Biol. 1992;12:4531-4538.

Riesewijk, A., Martín, J., van Os, R,, Horcajadas, JA., Polman, J., Pellicer, A., Mosselman, S. & Simón C. (2003) *Gene expression profiling of human endometrial receptivity on days LH+2 versus LH+7 by microarray technology.* Mol Hum Reprod. 2003 May;9(5):253-64.

Riggs, B.L. & Hartmann, L.C. (2003) *Selective estrogen-receptor modulators -- mechanisms of action and application to clinical practice.* N Engl J Med. 2003 Feb 13;348(7):618-29. Review. No abstract available. Erratum in: N Engl J Med. 2003 Mar 20;348(12):1192.

Robertson, S.A., Mau, V.J., Young, I.G. & Matthaei KI. (2000) *Uterine eosinophils and reproductive performance in interleukin 5-deficient mice.* J Reprod Fertil. 2000 Nov;120(2):423-32.

Roger, P., Sahla, M.E., Mäkelä, S., Gustafsson, J.A., Baldet, P. & Rochefort H. (2001) *Decreased expression of estrogen receptor beta protein in proliferative preinvasive mammary tumors.* Cancer Res. 2001 Mar 15;61(6):2537-41.

Russo, J., Calaf, G., Roi, L. & Russo IH. (1987) *Iinfluence of age and gland topography on cell kinetics of normal human breast tissue.* J Natl Cancer Inst. 1987 Mar;78(3):413-8.

Seifert-Klauss, V. & Prior, JC (2010). *Progesterone and bone: actions promoting bone health in women.* J Osteoporos. 2010 Oct 31;2010:845180.

Simon, C. (2008) *New perspectives in medically assisted procreation.* Gynecol Endocrinol. 2008 Sep;24(9):485.

Simon, C., Cano, F., Valbuena, D., Remohi, J. & Pellicer, A. (1995). Clinical evidence for a detrimental effect on uterine receptivity of high serum oestradiol concentrations in high and normal responder patients. *Hum Reprod*, 10, 2432-2437.

Simon, C., Oberyé, J., Bellver, J., Vidal, C., Bosch, E., Horcajadas, J.A., Murphy, C., Adams, S., Riesewijk, A., Mannaerts, B. & Pellicer A. *Similar endometrial development in oocyte donors treated with either high- or standard-dose GnRH antagonist compared to treatment with a GnRH agonist or in natural cycles.* Hum Reprod. 2005 Dec;20(12):3318-27. Epub 2005 Aug 5.

Smitz, J., Devroey, P., Faguer, B., Bourgain, C., Camus, M. & Van Steirteghem, A.C. (1992). A prospective randomized comparison of intramuscular or intravaginal natural progesterone as a luteal phase and early pregnany supplementation. *Hum. Reprod.,* 7, 168–175.

Speirs, V., Carder, P.J. & Lansdown MR. (2002) *Oestrogen receptor beta: how should we measure this?* Br J Cancer. 2002 Sep 9;87(6):687; author reply 688-9.

Spitz, I.M. & Bardin, C.W. (1993) *Mifepristone (RU 486): a modulator of progestin and glucocorticoid action.* N Engl J Med. 1993;329:404-412.

Stavreus-Evers, A., Aghajanova, L., Brismar, H., Eriksson, H., Landgren, B.M. & Hovatta O. (2002) *Co-existence of heparin-binding epidermal growth factor-like growth factor and pinopodes in human endometrium at the time of implantation.* Mol Hum Reprod. 2002 Aug;8(8):765-9.

Stavreus-Evers, A., Nikas, G., Sahlin, L., Eriksson, H. & Landgren BM. (2001) *Formation of pinopodes in human endometrium is associated with the concentrations of progesterone and progesterone receptors.* Fertil Steril. 2001 Oct;76(4):782-91.

Steck, T., Giess, R., Suetterlin, M.W., Bolland, M., Wiest, S., Poehls, U.G., & Dietl J. (2004) *Leukaemia inhibitory factor (LIF) gene mutations in women with unexplained infertility and recurrent failure of implantation after IVF and embryo transfer.* Eur J Obstet Gynecol Reprod Biol. 2004 Jan 15;112(1):69-73.

Steptoe, P.C. & Edwards, R.G. (1978). *Birth After the Reimplantation of a Human Embryo.* The Lancet, 312 (8085), 366.

Stewart, C.L. (1994) *Leukaemia inhibitory factor and the regulation of pre-implantation development of the mammalian embryo.* Mol Reprod Dev. 1994 Oct;39(2):233-8. Review.

Strathy, J.H., Molgaard, C.A., Coulam, C.B. & Melton, L.J. (1982). Endometriosis and infertility: a laparoscopic study of endometriosis among fertile and infertile women. *Fertil. Steril.,* 6 (Dec, 38), 667-72.

Tabibzadeh, S., Kong, Q.F., Babaknia, A. & May LT. (1995) *Progressive rise in the expression of interleukin-6 in human endometrium during menstrual cycle is initiated during the implantation window.* Hum Reprod. 1995 Oct;10(10):2793-9.

Talbi, S., Hamilton, A.E., Vo. KC., Tulac, S., Overgaard, M.T., Dosiou, C., Le Shay, N., Nezhat, C.N., Kempson, R., Lessey, B.A., Nayak, N.R. & Giudice LC. *Molecular phenotyping of human endometrium distinguishes menstrual cycle phases and underlying biological processes in normo-ovulatory women.* Endocrinology. 2006 Mar;147(3):1097-121. Epub 2005 Nov 23.

Tamm, K., Rõõm, M., Salumets, A. & Metsis M (2009) *Genes targeted by the estrogen and progesterone receptors in the human endometrial cell lines HEC1A and RL95-2.* Reprod Biol Endocrinol. 2009 Dec 24;7:150.

Taylor, H.S., Bagot, C., Kardana, A., Olive, D. & Arici, A. (1999). HOX gene expression is altered in the endometrium of women with endometriosis. *Hum. Reprod.,*14, 1328–1331.

Trapnell, C., Pachter, L. & Salzberg SL (2009) *TopHat: discovering splice junctions with RNA-Seq.* Bioinformatics. 2009 May 1;25(9):1105-11. Epub 2009 Mar 16.

Trapnell, C., Williams, BA., Pertea, G., Mortazavi, A., Kwan, G., van Baren, MJ., Salzberg, SL., Wold BJ. & Pachter L. (2010) *Transcript assembly and quantification by RNA-Seq reveals unannotated transcripts and isoform switching during cell differentiation.* Nat Biotechnol. 2010 May;28(5):511-5. Epub 2010 May 2.

Tung. L., Mohamed, MK., Hoeffler, JP., Takimoto, GS. & Horwitz, KB. (1993) *Antagonist-occupied human progesterone B-receptors activate transcription without binding to progesterone response elements and are dominantly inhibited by A-receptors.* Mol Endocrinol. 1993 Oct;7(10):1256-65. Erratum in: Mol Endocrinol 1993 Nov;7(11):1378.

Ubaldi F, Rienzi L, Baroni E, Ferrero S, Iacobelli M, Minasi MG, Sapienza F, Romano S, Colasante A, Litwicka K. & Greco, E. (2007). Hopes and facts about mild ovarian stimulation. *Reprod Biomed Online*, 14, 675–681.

Valbuena, D., Martin, J., de Pablo, J.L., Remohi, J., Pellicer, A. & Simon, C. (2001). Increasing levels of estradiol are deleterious to embryonic implantation because they directly affect the embryo. *Fertil. Steril.*, 2001;76:962-968.

Vandermolen, D.T. & Gu Y. (1996) *Human endometrial interleukin-6 (IL-6): in vivo messenger ribonucleic acid expression, in vitro protein production, and stimulation thereof by IL-1 beta.* Fertil Steril. 1996 Nov;66(5):741-7.

Vegeto, E., Shahbaz, MM., Wen, DX., Goldman, ME., O'Malley, BW. & McDonnell DP. (1993) *Human progesterone receptor A form is a cell- and promoter-specific repressor of human progesterone receptor B function.* Mol Endocrinol. 1993 Oct;7(10):1244-55.

Venken, K., Callewaert F., Boonen, S. & Vanderschueren D (2008). *Sex hormones, their receptors and bone health.* Osteoporos Int. 2008 Nov;19(11):1517-25. Epub 2008 Apr 5.

Venn, A., Jones, P., Quinn, M. & Healy D. (2001) *Characteristics of ovarian and uterine cancers in a cohort of in vitro fertilization patients.* Gynecol Oncol. 2001 Jul;82(1):64-8.

Venn, A., Watson, L., Lumley, J., Giles, G., King, C. & Healy D. (1995) *Breast and ovarian cancer incidence after infertility and in vitro fertilisation.* Lancet. 1995 Oct 14;346(8981):995-1000.

von Rango, U., Alfer, J., Kertschanska, S., Kemp, B., Müller-Newen, G., Heinrich, P.C., Beier, H.M. & Classen-Linke I (2004) *Interleukin-11 expression: its significance in eutopic and ectopic human implantation.* Mol Hum Reprod. 2004 Nov;10(11):783-92. Epub 2004 Oct 1.

Wakeling, AE., Dukes, M. and Bowler, J. (1991) *A potent specific pure antiestrogen with clinical potential.* Cancer Res. 1991;51:3867-3873.

Wang, Z., Gerstein, M. & Snyder M. (2009) *RNA-Seq: a revolutionary tool for transcriptomics.* Nat Rev Genet. 2009 Jan;10(1):57-63. Review.

Weinmann, AS. & Farnham PJ. (2002). *Identification of unknown target genes of human transcription factors using chromatin immunoprecipitation.* Methods. 2002 Jan;26(1):37-47.

Weiss, BD. (1993) *RU 486: the progesterone antagonist.* Arch Fam Med. 1993;2:63-70.

Wen, DX., , YF., Mais, DE., Goldman, ME. & McDonnell, DP. (1994) *The A and B isoforms of the human progesterone receptor operate through distinct signaling pathways within target cells.* Mol Cell Biol. 1994 Dec;14(12):8356-64.

Wolf, IM., Heitzer, MD., Grubisha, M. & DeFranco DB (2008). *Coactivators and nuclear receptor transactivation.* J Cell Biochem. 2008 Aug 1;104(5):1580-6. Review.

Wu, Y.L., Yang, X., Ren, Z., McDonnell, D.P., Norris, J.D., Willson, T.M. & Greene, G.L. (2005) *Structural basis for an unexpected mode of SERM-mediated ER antagonism.* Mol Cell 2005, 18:413–424.

# Part 2

# Pathophysiology of Steroid Hormones

# 4

# Cryptorchidism and Steroid Hormones

Marzena Kamieniczna[1], Anna Havrylyuk[2] and Maciej Kurpisz[1]
*[1]Institute of Human Genetics Polish Academy of Sciences,*
*[2]Danylo Halytsky Lviv National Medical University,*
*Department of Clinical Immunology and Allergology,*
*[1]Poland*
*[2]Ukraine*

## 1. Introduction

Two important functions of testis are production of spermatozoa and synthesis of steroids. These functions depend on anatomical, hormonal and constitutional homeostasis and begin during the first stage of gestation. Cryptorchidism can be defined as an abnormal localization of one or both testes. It's the failure of one or both testes descent into the scrotal sac. The third trimester in humans is crucial for the testis descent. When the testis is not found in normal location it may be palpable or nonpalpable. The palpable testis may be cryptorchid, ectopic or retractile. Non-palpable testis may be cryptorchid, atrophic or absent. Cryptorchidism occurs when the testis fails to descend into its normal postnatal location and may be found in the abdomen, in the inguinal canal or just reaching the external ring (prescrotal) (Nguyen 1999). Before sex determination, both female and male embryonic gonads are located in the same high intra-abdominal position. During mammalian development, the cranial suspensory ligament (CLS) and the caudal ligament (or gubernaculum) is responsible for a sexual dimorphic position of the testis and ovary. In males, regression of the CLS, along with the outgrowth of the gubernaculum and its migration to the scrotum, results in the extraabdominal position of the testis (Agoulnik 2005). Androgens induce regression of the cranio-suspensory ligament to release the testis to descent. The inguinoscrotal descent of the normal testicle takes place between 26 and 35 weeks of gestation. In preterm males with cryptorchidism the testes may descent postnatally (Berkowitz 1993, Cortez 2008). Cryptorchidism is one of the most common urogenital disorders in boys. Cryptorchidism can occur as an isolated disorder or may be associated with other congenital anomalies. The intraabdominal temperature is dangerous for germ cells and cryptorchidism may be a risk factor for male infertility and for testicular malignancy in adulthood. The decrement in intratesticular temperature in adult males is 2-4°C lower compared with body temperature (Thonneau 1998). This temperature difference is necessary to maintain spermatogenesis. The lower temperature in the scrotum is essential for normal spermatogenesis. Dangerous effects of increased temperature on spermatogenesis are well documented. For undescended testis abnormal spermatogenesis may be related with degenerative changes connected with high temperature (Mieussed 1993). This condition affects both morphology and function of the Sertoli and Leydig cells of the testis (Farrer 1985) The association of cryptorchidism with testicular cancer is also well documented (Giwercman 1989). The prevalence of cryptorchidism among boys is 2-4% in full - term male birth and 2-8.4% among boys with premature births. The incidence of cryptorchidism is significantly increased in premature males (Berkowitz 1993). Presently we observe an increased trend in the incidence of congenital cryptorchidism. Sometimes statistics includes testis in a high scrotal position (as normal descent) or cryptorchid testis may spontaneously descent in the first months after birth, therefore the incidence of cryptorchidism decreases from 1% to 0.5% by age of 1 year due to spontaneous descent (Barthold 2003). In earlier studies it has been speculated that the late spontaneous testicular descent occurs in more than half (Boisen 2004) or 70% of newborns with cryptorchidism. On the contrary the data obtained by Wenzler et al. (Wenzler 2004) showed that in patients with cryptorchidism spontaneous testicular descent occurs infrequently during the first year of life. They found that in patients with cryptorchidism before 12 months only 6.9% of the cryptorchid testicles reached the acceptable scrotal location at age of 1 year or later (Wenzler 2004). There are large regional differences in incidence of cryptorchidism. The study on the prevalence of congenital cryptorchidism in Demmark and Finland was also performed and much higher incidence of congenital cryptorchidism in Denmark was found. In Denmark an increase in reproductive health problems is explained by environmental factors, including endocrine disrupters and a lifestyle (Boisen 2004). In the meantime the incidence of cryptorchidism has increased in many countries. In two comparable British studies the incidence of cryptorchidism delivered at term boys approximately doubled between the 1950s and the 1980s. (Toppari 2001). However the report by Cortes (2008) has shown that the incidence of cryptorchidism in Denmark has not changed and is similar to the previous reports obtained in the 1950s. They have pointed out the general difficulties to compare the frequency of cryptorchidism as reported in different publications, since the definition of cryptorchidism is not yet uniform (Cortes 2008). The International Clearinghouse for Birth Defects Monitoring System has collected data on cryptorchidism, but they are unreliable, because of a discrepancy with the data from cohort studies (Toppari 2001). The present incidence may be even higher than reported one because of under-reporting tendency (Kaleva 2005).

Cryptorchidism is a risk factor for male infertility in adulthood and for the male health (testicular cancer). Cryptorchidism uni- or bilateral is associated with degenerative changes in Sertoli cells and germ cells and is the most common etiologic factor of azoospermia (Hadziselmovic 2001). 89% of untreated cryptorchid patients with bilateral maldescent develop azoospermia and 32% treated medically or 46% boys treated surgically develop azoospermia (Hadziselimovic 2001). Hormonal treatment with human chorionic gonadotropin (HCG) or gonadotropin releasing hormone may be given initially for cryptorchidism. Very often a surgical intervention is needed to protect function of seminiferous tubules and to prevent degenerative changes in Sertoli and germ cells saving the man's future fertility potential.

## 2. Pathogenesis of cryptorchidism

The etiology of cryptorchidism remains mostly unclear (Foresta 2008). The main risk factor is preterm birth, low birth weight, disrupted endocrine regulations, several gene defects and environmental factors (endocrine disruptors). Preterm birth and small size for gestational age are risk factors for cryptorchidism (Pierik 2004). Cryptorchidism is considered to be indirectly related to birth weight. The incidence of cryptorchidism is about 20-25% in infants with birth weight less than 2.5 kg (Scorer 1964). Androgens play a crucial role in the development of male external genital organs and testicular descent. Hormonal dysregulation can be one out of many etiological factors of cryptorchidism (Suomi 2006). Testicular descent is at least partly dependent on fetal testicular testosterone, which in turn is initiated and maintained by human chorionic gonadotropin produced by the placenta (Biggs 2002). An increased risk of cryptorchidism in cases with placental abnormalities is noted (Biggs 2002). The increasing incidence of reproductive abnormalities in human males may be associated with increased estrogen exposure during gestation. The increased expression of estradiol in the syncytiotrophoblast may have impact on testicular descent (Hadziselmovic 2000). Industrial and agricultural chemicals acting as endocrine disrupters might have a deleterious effect on normal male sexual differentiation. These chemicals may occur in our close environments of work and life, drinking water, a food. Humans can also be exposed to natural phytoestrogens through consumption of food products derived from the plants (Toppari 1996, Sultan 2001). Various groups of chemicals, including pesticides and phthalate esters, have been identified as being weakly estrogenic or antiandrogenic (Sharpe 2003). Ferlin has proposed a distinction between intrinsic and extrinsic causes of cryptorchidism. In the first group frequently displayed bilateral cryptorchidism is associated with progressive testicular damage and icreased risk of infertility or testicular damage. In these cases early orchidopexy may reduce the risk of these consequences but does not eliminate it definitely. Genetic alterations are more frequent in this group (Klinefelter syndrome, RXFP2 gene mutations) (Ferlin 2008). In the group with extrinsic causes of cryptorchidism (low birth weight, prematurity, maternal diabetes or preeclampsia during pregnancy) a spontaneous descent in the first months of age is noted. The early orchidpexy can reduce almost completely risk of testicular damage (Trisnar 2009). The possible genetic background of cryptorchidism still remains unresolved and genetics causes are rarely found (Ferlin 2008).

The following genetic abnormalities may be associated with cryptorchidism:
- - mutations in the gene coding for insulin-like factor 3,

The mutation R102C was detected in a boy with unilateral persistent cryptorchidism (Ferlin 2008). The other mutation (T86M) was detected in a boy with bilateral cryptorchidism and spontaneous descent in the first months of age (Ferlin 2008).
- mutations in INSL3 receptor gene (RXFP2).
- mutations in the gene coding for receptor for insulin-like factor 3, INSL3/LGR8,
- mutations in the androgen receptor gene,
- chromosomal alterations in Klinefelter syndrome.

Familial occurrence – cryptorchidism is heritable susceptibility.

Seasonal variation in the incidence of cryptorchidism suggest that environmental factors may have the importance in its etiology. Cryptorchidism can be often the consequence of testicular dysgenesis, a developmental disorder of the gonads due to disruption of embryonal programming and gonadal development during fetal life. Testicular dysgenesis syndrome (TSD) can result in maldescent, reduced fertility and an increased risk for malignant development, increased frequency of incomplete descent of a testis into the scrotum and hypospodias (Skakkebaek 2001). TSD can arise due to environmental factors including endocrine disrupters (potential endocrine disruptors in diet, in place of occupation; lifestyle, dietary phytoestrogens, present in food, water, air) or genetic defects.

The contalateral testis in men with unilateral testis cancer (Berthelsen 1983) or unilateral cryptorchidism (Kaki 1999) can be often damaged as well. There is also clear confirmation of testicular dysgenesis syndrome. Fetal exposure to endocrine disruptors (EDs) with estrogen-like or antiandrogen-like activity has been suggested as a cause for TDS (Sharpe 1993).

Environmental or genetic defects can influence Leydig cell function and result in androgen insufficiency which may cause testicular maldescent (Skakkebaek 2001).

Uterine exposure to environmental endocrine disruptors can have also deleterious effects on male reproductive system development in embryos. Environmental endocrine disruptors (EEDs) are defined as exogenous substances witch can disrupt endocrine homeostasis and reproduction. EEDs include xenoestrogens, synthetic hormones, natural hormones or substances affecting endocrine signaling (Vidaeff 2005).

Chemicals have been found to possess either weak estrogenic, anti-androgenic or other hormonal activities, which are often referred to as endocrine disrupters. Fetal or perinatal exposure to endocrine disrupters results in disturbed sexual differentiation, urogenital malformations and decreased reproductive health in adult life (Sharpe 1993).

The significantly increased risk of bilateral cryptorchidism in boys whose mothers smoked heavily during pregnancy may indicate that heavy maternal smoking can be included in the pathogenesis of cryptorchidism (Throup 2005). Altered hormonal levels in smokers may have a casual role in cryptorchidism. Paternal pesticide exposure may be also associated with cryptorchidism. The investigation of circulating androgens bioactivity in 3-month-old boys suggests that infant boys are exposed to biological effects of androgens during the postnatal activation of the hypothalamic-pituitary-testicular axis, and the degree of the exposure may result in testis location superior to the scrotum (Raivio 2003)

## 3. Hormonal regulation of testicular descent

Testicular descent is hormonally regulated. Regulation of testicular descent is not yet completely understood. There are various forms of cryptorchidism (congenital with or without spontaneous descent, mild versus severe, acquired). These forms may reflect distinct hormonal patterns which differ in each situation (Suomi 2006). Apart from anatomical configuration and hormonal stimulation, genetic control of testis descent is very important. Major regulators of testicular descent are insulin-like factor 3 and testosterone. Testes migrate from initial intraabdominal position into the scrotal sac in two distinct hormonally regulated phases. During the first transabdominal phase (androgen independent) (10-23th week gestation) the CLS (cranial suspensory ligament) regresses while the gubernaculum shortens and develops caudal segment into the gubernaculum bulge. The second inguinoscrotal phase (depends on androgens) is normally completed by the 35th week – the gubernaculum extends caudally into the scrotum and involutes, following the passage of the testis through the inguinal canal.

The first phase of testis descent (transabdominal) is regulated essentially by insulin-like factor 3 (INSL3), a peptide, product of the pre- and postnatal Leydig cells. INSL3 controls the passage through its receptor Lgr8 (leucine-rich-containing repeats G protein-coupled receptor). Genetic disruption of the Insl3 gene or its receptor (Lgr8) in mice has led to high intraabdominal cryptorchidism (Adham 2004). In the second phase (inguinoscrotal) androgens (testosterone) are the major mediators of testis descent (Foresta 2008). The inguinoscrotal phase is at least partly dependent on fetal testicular testosterone secretion, which in turn is initiated and maintained by human chorionic gonadotropin produced by placenta. In mutation analysis of the human homologs of INSL3, LGR8 or HOXA10 genes in patients with cryptorchidism there were rarely found mutations or polymorphisms (Bogatcheva 2005, Bertini 2004).

For a normal descent and testicular development of the testes, a normal hypothalamo-pituitary-gonadal axis is essential. Certain androgens:estrogens ratio is required for physiological function of the testis. Steroid hormones act through specific receptors: ARs, ERα, ERβ.

Insl-3 is under estrogenic control. Mutations in ins-3 gene showed a low incidence at 1.3% in patients with cryptorchidism. Estrogens may affect insl-3 expression and may have a role in regulation of testicular descent (Tomboc, 2000).

**Androgen receptors (ARs)** mediate the biological effects of both T and 5α-dihydrotestosterone. AR mutations are not a frequent cause of isolated cryptorchidism (Ashim 2004, Ferlin 2006, Ferlin 2008). AR mutations in men with history of cryptorchidism are connected rather with infertility. The AR is highly polymorphic due to a glutamine repeat (CAG) and a glycine repeat (GGN). Polymorphic CAG and GGN segments regulate AR function. A clear associations were observed between shorter CAG repeats and disorders dependent on enhanced androgen action. Longer CAG repeats have been associated with undescended testes, idiopathic hypospadias and decreased sperm counts. In result of combined analysis of CAG and GGC repeat lengths the stronger association with cryptorchidism was found (Ferlin 2005). The CAG repeat length has been also assessed in males with cryptorchidism, but no association between CAG repeat length and undescended testes was found in Japanese population (Sasagawa 2000) or Caucasian population (Aschim 2004). It was indicated rather association between GGN length and cryptorchidism or hypospadias (Aschim 2004). Median GGN lengths were significantly higher (24 vs. 23) among subjects with cryptorchidism, compared with controls and subjects with hypospadias. GGN length 23 is the most prevalent in males from general population. A majority of individuals with cryptorchidism demonstrated GGN numbers of 24 or more (Aschim 2004).

## 4. Hypothalamic-pituitary-testicular axis

Androgens regulate testicular descent, but androgen action alone is not sufficient for normal testicular descent. A proper hypothalamus-pituitary-testis axis function together with normal synthesis and action is a prerequisite for normal testicular descent. Various defects in this axis may result in cryptorchidism (Toppari 2007). Regulation of androgen production depends on hCG (placental human chorionic gonadotropin) and LH (pituitary luteinizing hormone) actions. INSL3 (insulin-like hormone-3) is the main regulator of gubernaculum development and testicular descent. Reduced levels of INSL3 may cause cryptorchidism (Toppari 2007). INSL3 production is also related to LH levels. Cryptorchid boys have normal testosterone and elevated LH levels (Toppari 2007). The first postnatal months of boys are characterized by activation of the hypothalamic-pituitary-testicular axis that results in the well depicted surge of reproductive hormones. Serum testosterone levels at that time are high, but infants do not display signs of virilization, and subsequently there is only indirect evidence that circulating androgens during the surge are biologically active. Three-month-old boys are exposed to biological effects of androgens during the postnatal activation of the hypothalamic-pituitary-testicular axis, and this exposure may be reduced in boys with at least 1 testis located superior to the scrotum. Functional integrity of the HPG axis is fundamental for testicular descent. Gonadotropin-releasing hormone (GnRH) regulates the production of pituitary gonadotropins FSH and LH. Gonadotropins FSH and LH are the main regulators of postnatal testicular activity. LH stimulates Leydig cells to produce testosterone while FSH regulates Sertoli cell functions (Toppari 2006). Human fetal testis binds hCG and physiological levels hCG stimulate testosterone production at least from 14 weeks of gestation (Huhtaniemi 1977). LH becomes more important regulator of fetal testosterone synthesis in the late pregnancy (Quinton 2001). The high percentage of cryptorchidism cases resolves spontaneously during the period of high serum gonadotropin and steroid hormone levels at the age of 1-3 months (Anderson 1998).

**Testosterone** is one of the main regulators of testiculat descent. It is the main androgen in the circulation, mainly protein-bound, either strongly to sex hormone binding globulin (SHGB), or loosely to albumin. Only about 2% of this hormone is unbound; this is called free testosterone and is considered to be the most biologically active form of testosterone. In the target tissue testosterone can either bind directly to the androgen receptor (AR) or, if the tissue expresses the enzyme 5a-reductase, can be converted to dihydrotestosterone (DHT). Testosterone is produced by Leydig cells and low testosterone level is a consequence of a reduced ability of the Leydig cells to synthesize T.

Impaired testosterone biosynthesis or distinct increase in testosterone metabolism is observed in cryptorchidism. Aromatase may convert androgens into estradiol. Testosterone is converted by aromatase CYP 19 to estradiol in many tissues of healthy men. The development of internal male genitalia is testosterone dependent, and 5α-dihydrotestosterone (synthesized from T by the enzyme 5α-reductase 2) is essential for normal external masculinization. DHT is produced from circulating testosterone, which is manufactured by the fetal testis under stimulation of hCG.

**Estrogens** Estrogens are necessary for maintaining functional integrity of the male reproductive tract. Estrogens and ERα are important for fertility. Excess of estrogens can affect function of the cells of male reproductive system. The excess of estrogens was reported to be associated with cryptorchidism, epididymal defects, impaired fertility. Estradiol however is an essential hormone for male reproduction. The maternal and placental estradiol is elevated in children with cryptorchidism. The increased expression of estradiol in the syncytiotrophoblast may have an impact on testicular descent (Hadziselmovic 2000). Low estrogen levels in mothers may mean that a placental defect increases the risk of cryptorchidism (Mc Glynn 2005). Estrogens are synthesized in the male reproductive system by at least four different cell types: Leydig cells, Sertoli cells, germ cells and epithelial cells of the epididymis. Estrogens are synthesized in a cortex of the adrenal gland, too. In the immature testis, the main source of estrogens are Sertoli cells.

In horse and mouse *in vivo* cryptorchidism is associated with the increase in conversion of androgens to estrogens in the testis (Hejmej 2008), epididymal duct and the prostate. Increase in testosterone metabolism rather than an impairment of testosterone production is proposed to explain incidence of cryptorchidism. Testicular descent is significantly inhibited by estradiol. The estrogen effect might be mediated through suppression of fetal Leydig cell development, with resulting decrease of androgens and INSL3 production.

## 5. Estrogen receptor α, ERs

The association of cryptorchidism with a specific haplotype of the estrogen receptor 1 gene was reported (Yoshida 2005). The specific haplotype AGATA located within the 3' end of human ESRI1 is associated with cryptorchidism in the Japanese population. The AGATA haplotype was frequently found to be significant in cryptorchid children. Homozygosity for the AGATA haplotype was found only among cryptorchid boys (Yoshida 2005). ERα and PR (progesterone receptor) expressed in paratesticular tissues are important for normal testicular descent. ERα was overexpressed in boys with undescended testis previously treated with human chronic gonadotropin (Przewratil 2004).

The analysis of the whole AGATA haplotype is possible by testing only the SNP12 (the tag SNP for the AGATA haplotype). Results obtained by Galan indicated that SNP 12 is the tag SNP for the AGATA haplotype also in Caucasians, but is not connected with cryptorchodism and infertility. Surprisingly ESR1 SNP12 may have a protective effect on cryptorchidism in the Italian populations, since it was found more frequently among healthy populations (Galan 2007).

**Progesterone** influences spermiogenesis, sperm capacitation/acrosome reaction and testosterone biosynthesis in the Leydig cells. The detection of progesterone receptor (PR) isoforms have a diagnostic value in prostate cancer (Oettel 2004). The position of the undescended testis did not appear to influence progesterone metabolism (Läckgren 2008). PRs density was higher in paratesticular tissues (cremaster muscle and processus vaginalis) obtained from boys with undescended testis compared to the control group (Przewratil 2005)

## 6. Steroid hormones, male immune system and reproductive system

Steroid hormones especially testosterone, progesteron and estradiol can modulate the immune system. The relationship between the immune system and reproduction is very strict. The immune response may be involved in reproductive processes what may interfere with fertility. A role of estrogens and testosterone in (auto)antibody production was proved. Estrogens increase, while testosterone decreases antibody production. Immune disorders have been formulated to take part in etiology of cryptorchidism.

The significant associations of cryptorchidism with HLA class I antigens were found. Some associations of HLA class I alleles (HLA-A11, A23, A29) with cryptorchidism were explained by their crossreactivity with receptors for LH and hCG present on fetal Leydig cells and/or interference with the hormone-binding sites through a mechanism of "molecular mimicry" (Martinetti 1992). Most likely the "molecular mimicry" between hormonal receptors and HLA surface antigens may also play a role in etiopathogenesis of cryptorchidism. The human major histocompatibility complex class II HLA molecules, by presenting antigens to helper T cells, play a decisive role in induction of antibody production (Chen 2008). Antisperm antibodies (AsA) in serum samples from prepubertal boys with testicular failure were substantially reported (Lenzi 1991, Kurpisz 1996, Sinisi 1998). We have investigated the frequency of HLA class II alleles to recognize possible genetic predisposition for antisperm antibodies development in prepubertal boys with diagnosed cryptorchidism. We have found, a strong correlation between the presence of some HLA-antigens in patients with unilateral and bilateral cryptorchidism, and a formation of antisperm antibodies. We have observed that boys suffering from bilateral cryptorchidism differed from controls in their HLA-DRB1*11 frequency. Associations of cryptorchidism with some HLA-DRB1 and HLA-DQB1 alleles, very rare in Caucasians, were described only for a Japanese population (Tsuji 2000). No correlation with HLA class II polymorphism, however, was observed in a study of Italian population. We have observed strong difference between cryptorchidism with history of infertility within these families and healthy controls, showing a high risk for HLA-DRB1*11 bearers. This result may suggest that sporadic and familial cryptorchidism may have different genetic background. HLA-DRB1*11 was also, albeit weakly, associated with bilateral cryptorchidism. Predisposition to produce anti-sperm antibodies seems to be only weakly associated with HLA class II genes.

Autoimmune reactions, particular directed to testicular elements and/or spermatozoa have been found to be often associated with cryptorchidism. Antisperm immunization has been proposed as possible additional factor associated with late surgery in prepubertal boys with cryptorchidism. Cryptorchidism in young boys can induce immune reactions against sperm-specific antigens. Future fertility status thus may be endangered, because antisperm antibodies can impair fertility at different levels. The relationship between the presence of antisperm antibodies and male infertility has been documented in large number of earlier studies (Krause 2009). There are some reports on high frequency of antisperm antibodies (AsA) in infertility patients who have suffered in the past from cryptorchidism. In healthy men seminiferous epithelium is anatomically sequestered from the systemic immunity. There exist multiple elements of active tolerance. An increased ability for induction of antisperm antibodies in men has been observed in various testicular pathologies: varicocele, testicular torsion, vasectomy and genital tract infections. An induction of antisperm antibodies in adult males may take place because of a break in the anatomical "blood-testis" barrier or because of the failure of an immunosuppressive mechanism providing tolerance to sperm. Sometimes, such antibodies can arise without a known reason. Pathologic conditions within the urogenital tract may predispose to antisperm antibody formation. In prepubertal boys, testicular failures may cause an activation of destructive to testes humoral immune response, because the anatomical testicular barrier is then not completely formed and immunosupression not fully activated due to the absence of male germ cells. Diminished levels of testosterone observed in prepubertal boys may be an additional reason for inefficient immunosupresion at young age and may contribute to the rise of autoantibody development (Jones 1994). It is difficult to argue whether it is mainly anatomical sequestration or rather active immunosuppresion playing a dominant role in preserving intact spermatogenic differentiation. It was earlier reported that 20-60% of individuals with a history of maldescended testis have circulating antisperm antibodies and most of them demonstrates oligoasthenozoospermia (Urry 1994). Evaluating the immune status of prepubertal boys with testicular failures, we have previously found detectable levels of AsA predominantly in boys with pathology of both gonads (Kurpisz 1996). One possible explanation for the induction of immune response to spermatozoa (testis) may be an increase of testicular temperature in boys with cryptorchidism, which may initiate the degenerative changes in spermatogenesis and alter testicular functions. A unique exposure of membrane antigens on testicular cells can be thus noted. Changes in the Leydig cells function may provoke the disturbances in the levels of locally secreted hormones, e.g. diminished levels of testosterone. Altogether, this multifactorial machinery may create a "vicious circle" that will perpetuate intratesticular inflammation leading to the inhibition of spermatogenesis that was to be triggered at the onset of puberty.

## 7. Final remarks

Cryptorchidism is one of the most common urogenital disorders found in postnatal boys. Main predisposing factor are: preterm birth, dysfunctional endocrine regulations, gene defects and environmental factors (endocrine disruptions). It is believed that testicular descent is hormonally regulated and although genetic, contribution is observed, the number of genes/mutations responsible for testis descent is relatively rare. Changed environment in testis located in abdomen may induce pathological reactions mainly resulted in immune response induction. This, however, seems to be a secondary phenomenon. Despite this, once triggered immune response may persist and underlie future infertility in adulthood. Early surgical intervention in cryptorchidism can be therefore recommended.

# 8. References

Agoulnik, A.I. Cryptorchidism: An estrogen spoil? (2005). *Journal of Clinical Endocrinology & Metabolism*, 90, 4975-4977.

Anderson AM, Toppari J, Haavisto AM, Petersen JH, Simell T, Simell. (1998). Longitudinal reproductive hormone profiles in infants: peak of inhibin B levels in infant boys exceeds levels in adult men. *Journal of Clinical Endocrinology & Metabolism*, 83, 675-681.

Aschim EL, Nordenskjöld A, Giwercman A, Lundin KB, Ruhayel Y, Haugen TB, Grotmol T Giwercman YL. (2004). Linkage between cryptorchidism, hypaspodias, and GGN repeat length in the androgen receptor gene. *Journal of Clinical Endocrinology & Metabolism*, 89, 5105-5109.

Bartholg J, Gonzalez R. (2003). The epidemiology of congenital cryptorchidism, testicular ascent and orchidopexy. *Journal of Urology*, 170, 2396-2402.

Bertini V, Bertelloni S, Valetto A, Lala R Foresta C, Simi P. (2004). Homeobox HOXA10 gene analysis in cryptorchidism. *Journal of Pediatric Endocrinology & Metabolism*, 17, 41-45.

Bogatcheva NV, Agoulnik AI. (2005). INSL3/LGR8 role in testicular descent and cryptorchidism. *Reproductive BioMedicine Online*, 10, 49-54.

Boisen KA, Kaleva M, Main KM, Virtanen HE, Haavisto AM, Schmidt IM, Chellakooty M, Damgaard IN, Mau C, Reunanen M, Skakkebaek NE, Toppari J. (2004). Difference in prevalence of congenital cryptorchidism in infants between two Nordic countries. *Lancet*, 363, 1264-1269.

Chen X, Jensen PE. (2008). MHC class II antigen presentation and immunological abnormalities due to deficiency of MHC class II and its associated genes. *Experimental and Molecular Pathology*, 85: 40-44.

Cortes D, Kjellberg EM, Breddam M, Thorup J. (2008). The true incidence of cryptorchidism in Denmark. *Journal of Urolology*, 179, 314-318.

Domagała A, Kamieniczna M, Kurpisz M. (2000). Sperm antigens recognized by antisperm antibodies present in sera of infertile adults and prepubertal boys with testicular failure. *International Journal of Andrology*, 23; 150-155.

El Houtate B, Rouba H, Sibai H, Barakat A, Chafik A, Chadli E, Imken L, Bogatheva N, Feng S, Agoulnik A, McElreavey K. (2007). Novel mutations involving the INSL3 gene associated with cryptorchidism. *Journal of Urolology*, 177, 1947-1951.

Farrer JH, SikkaSC, Xie HW, Constantinide D, Raifer J. (1985). Impaired testosterone biosynthesis in cryptorchidism. *Fertility and Sterility*, 44, 125-132.

FerlinA, Vinanzi C, Garolla A. (2006). Male infertility and androgen receptor gene mutations: clinical features and identification of seven novel mutations. *Clinical Endocrinology*, 65, 606-610.

Ferlin A, Zuccarello D, Zuccarello B, Chirico MR, Zanon GF, Foresta C. (2008). Genetic alterations associated with cryptorchidism. *JAMA* 300, 2271-2276.

Ferlin A, Garolla A, Bettella A, Bartoloni L, Vinanzi C, Roverato A, Foresta C. (2005). Androgen receptor gene CAG and GGC repeat lengths in cryptorchidism. *European Journal of Endocrinology*, 152, 419-425.

Foresta C, Zuccarello D, Garolla A, FerlinA. (2008). Role of hormones, genes, and environment in human cryptorchidism. *Endocrine Reviews*, 29, 560-580.

Galan JJ, Guarducci E, Nuti F, Gonzales A, Ruiz M, Ruiz A, Krausz C. (2007). Molecular analysis of estrogen receptor alpha gene AGATA haplotype and SNP12 in European populations: potential protective effect for cryptorchidism and lack of association with male infertility. *Human Reproduction*, 22, 444-449.

Giwercman A, Bruun E, Frimodt-Moller C, Skakkebaek N. (1989). Prevalence of carcinoma in situ and other histopathological abnormalities in testis of men with a history of cryptorchidism. *Journal of Urology*, 142, 998-1001.

Hadźiselimović F, Geneto R, Emmons L. (2000). Elevated placental estradiol: a possible etiological factor of human cryptorchidism. *Journal of Urology*, 164, 1694-1695.

Hadziselimowic F, Herzog B. (2001). Importance of early postnatal germ cell maturation for fertility of cryptorchid males. *Hormone Research*, 55, 6-10.

Hejmej A, Bilińska B. (2008). The effects of cryptorchidism on the regulation of steroidogenesis and gap junctional communication in equine testes. *Endocrinologia Polska*, 59, 112-118.

Huhtaniemi IT, Korenbrot CC, Jaffe RB. (1977). HCG binding and stimulation of testosterone biosynthesis in the human fetal testis. *Journal of Clinical Endocrinology & Metabolism*, 4; 963-967.

Jones WR. (1994). Gamete immunology. *Human Reproduction*, 9, 828-841.

Kaki T, Sofikitis N. (1999). Effects of unilateral cryptorchidism on contralateral epididymal sperm quality, quantity and fertilizing capacity. *Yonago Acta Medica*, 42, 79-86.

Kaleva M, Toppari J. (2005). Cryptorchidism: an indicator of testicular dysgenesis? *Cell Tissue Research*, 322, 167-172.

Krause WK, Naz RK. (2009) Immune infertility. Springer-Verlag Berlin Heidelberg.

Kurpisz M, Kasprzak M, Mazurkiewicz I. (1996). The easy formation of antisperm antibodies In prepubertal boys and the difficult humoral response in severe-combined immunodeficiency mice. *Fertility and Sterility*, 66, 805-808.

Läckgren G, Berg A. (2008). In vitro metabolism of progesterone by the human undescended testis. *International Journal of Andrology*, 6, 423-432.

Lenzi A, Gandini L, Lombardo F, Cappa M, Nardini P, Ferro F. (1991). Antisperm antibodies in young boys. *Andrologia*, 23L 233-235.

Martinetti M, Maghnie M, Salvaneschi L, Di Ninno N, Daielli C, Palladini G, Guccia M. (1992). Immunogenetic and hormonal study of cryptorchidism. *Journal of Clinical Endocrinology & Metabolism*, 74, 39-42.

McGlynn K, Graubard B, Nam J, Stanczyk F,Longnecker M, Klebanoff M. (2005). Maternal hormone levels and risk of cryptorchism among populations at high and low risk of testicular germ cell tumors. *Cancer Epidemiology, Biomarkers & Prevention* 14, 1732-1737.

Mieussed R, Fouda PJ, Vayse P, Guitard J, Moscovici J, Juskiewenski S. (1993). Increase in testicular temperature in case of cryptorchidism in boys. *Fertility and Sterility*, 59, 1319-1321.

Nguyen HT, Coakley F, Hricak H. (1999). Cryptorchidism: strategies in detection. *European Radiology*, 9, 336-343.

Oettel M, Mukhopadhyay AK. (2004). Progesterone: the forgotten hormone in men? *Aging Male*, 7, 236-257.

Quinton R, Duke VM, Robertson A, Krik JM, Matfin G, de Zoysa PA. (2001). Idiopathic gonadotropin deficiency: genetic questions addressed through phenotypic characterization. *Clinical Endocrinology*, 55, 163-174.

Pierik FH, Burdorf A, Deddens JA, Juttmann RE, Weber R. (2004). Maternal and paternal risk factors for cryptorchidism and hypospodias: A case-control study in newborn boys. *Environmental Health Perspectives*, 112, 1570-1576.

Przewratil P, Paduch D, Kobos J, Niedzielski J. (2004). Expression of estrogen receptor α and progesterone receptor in children with undescended testicle previously treated with human chorionic gonadotropin. *Journal of Urolology*, 172, 1112-1116.

Raivio T, Toppari J, Kaleva M, Virtanen H, Haavisto AM, Dunkel L, Jänne OA. (2003). Serum androgen bioactivity in cryptorchid and noncryptorchid boys during the postnatal reproductive hormone surge. *Journal of Clinical Endocrinology & Metabolism*, 88, 2597-2599.

Sinisi AA, Pasquali P, Papparella A, Valente A, Orio F, Esposito D, Cobellis G, Cuomo A, Angelone G, Martone A, Fioretti GP, Bellastella A. (1998). Antisperm antibodies in cryptorchidism before and after surgery. *Journal of Urology*, 160:1835-1837.

Skakkebaek N, Rajpert-De Meyts E, Main K. (2001). Testicular dysgenesis syndrome: an increasingly common develpomental disorder with environmental aspects. *Human Reproduction*, 16, 972-978.

Thonneau P, Ducot B, Bujan L. Mieusset R, Spira A. (1996). Heat exposure as a hazard to male infertility. *Lancet*, 347, 204-205.

Thorup J, Cortes D, Petersen BL. (2006). The incidence of bilateral cryptorchidism is increased and the fertility potential is reduced in sons born to mothers who have smoked during pregnancy. *Journal of Urology*, 176, 734-737.

Tomboc M, Lee P, Mitwally M, Schneck F, Bellinger M, Witchel S. (2000). Insulin-like 3/relaxin like factor gene mutations are associated with cryptorchidism. *Journal of Clinical Endocrinology & Metabolism*, 85 4013-4018.

Toppari J, Kaleva M, Virtanen HE. (2001) Trends in the incidence of cryptorchidism and hypospodias, and methodological limitations of registry-based data. *Human Reproduction Update*, 7, 282-286.

Toppari J, Kaleva M, Virtanen HE, Main KM, Skakkebaek NE. (2007). Luteinizing hormone in testicular descent. *Molecular and Cellular Endocrinology*, 269, 34-37.

Toppari J, Virtanen H, Skakkebaek NE, Main KM. (2006). Environmental effects on hormonal regulation of testicular descent. *Journal of Steroid Biochemistry & Molecular Biology*, 102, 184-186.

Toppari J, Larsen JC, Christiansen P, Giwercman A, Grandjean P. (1996). Male reproductive health and environmental xenoestrgens. *Environmental Health Perspectives*, 104: 741-803.

Trisnar B, Res Muravec. (2009). Fertility potential after unilateral and bilateral orchidopexy for cryptorchidism. *World Journal of Urology*, 27, 513-519.

Sasagawa I, Suzuki Y, Tateno T, Nakada T, Murowa K, Ogata T. (2000). CAG repeat length of the androgen receptor gene in Japanese males with cryptorchidism. *Molecular Human Reproduction*, 6, 973-975.

Scorer CG. (1964). The descent of the testis. *Archives of Disease in Childhood*, 39, 605-609.

Sharpe RM, Skakkebaek NE. (1993). Are oestrogens involved in falling sperm counts and disorders of the male reproductive tract? *Lancet*, 341, 1392-1396.

Sultan C, Paris F, Terouanne B, Balaguer P, Georget V, Poujol N, Jeandel C, Lumbroso S, Nikolas J. (2001). Disorders linked to insufficient androgen action in male children. *Human Reproduction Update*, 7: 314-322.

Suomi AM, Main Km, Kaleva M, Schmidt IM, Chellakooty M, Virtanen HE. (2006). Hormonal changes in 3-month-old cryptorchid boys. *Journal of Clinical Endocrinology & Metabolism*, 91, 953-958.

Tsuji Y, Misuto M, Yasunami R, Sakata K, Shibahara H, Koyama K. (2000). HLA-DR and HLA-DQ gene typing of infertile women possessing sperm-immobilising antibody. *Journal of Reproductive Immunology*, 46, 31-38.

Urry RL, Carrell DT, Starr NT, Snow BW, Middleton RG. (1994). The incidence of antisperm antibodies in infertility patients with a history of cryptorchidism. *Journal of Urology*, 151, 381-383.

Wenzler DL, Bloom DA, Park JM. (2004). What is the rate of spontaneous testicular descent in infants with cryptorchidism? *Journal of Urology*, 171, 849-851.

Vidaeff A, Sever LE. (2005). In utero exposure to environmental estrogens and male reproductive health: a systematic review of biological and epidemiologic evidence. *Reproductive Toxicology*, 20, 5-20.

Yoshida R, Fukami M, Sasagawa I, Hasegawa T, Kamatani N, Ogata T. (2005). Association of cryptorchidism with a specific haplotype of the estrogen receptor α gene: implication for the susceptibility to estrogenic environmental endocrine disruptors. *Journal of Clinical Endocrinology & Metabolism*, 90, 4716-4721

# 5

# DHEA and Impaired Glucose Tolerance Clinical and Basic Study

Hajime Ueshiba
*Department of Internal Medicine, Toho University School of Medicine, Tokyo, Japan*

## 1. Introduction

Dehydroepiandrosterone (DHEA) is either secreted directly from the adrenal cortex or is converted from DHEA sulfate (DHEA-S) in the peripheral organs. DHEA and DHEA-S are the most abundant adrenal androgens in blood, however their its physiological roles still remain unclear. Some recent studies have shown that DHEA and DHEA-S exert beneficial effects on conditions such as diabetes mellitus, atherosclerosis, obesity, tumors and osteoporosis (Coleman et al.,1982; Gorden et al.,1988; Cleary,1991). In this chapter, the relationships between DHEA or DHEA-S and diabetes mellitus (DM) or impaired glucose tolerance (IGT) are described.

## 2. Clinical and basic study

### 2.1 Clinical study

Abnormalities of secretion and metabolism of many steroid hormones occur in DM. In poorly controlled type 1 DM, serum concentrations of DHEA and DHEA-S decrease (Couch,1992) while plasma ACTH and cortisol levels increase in type 2 DM (Hashimoto et al.,1993). Low levels of DHEA and DHEA-S in type 2 DM are associated with hyperinsulinemia(Hubert et al.,1991; Nesler et al.,1989; Schriock et al.,1988; Smith et al.,1987;). We analyzed serum DHEA and DHEA-S levels in poorly controlled type 2 DM.

### 2.1.1 Subjects and methods

The subjects were type 2 diabetic patients seen regularly at the outpatient clinic of Toho University Hospital. We chose 130 patients, whose blood glucose control had been poor (more than 10% in HbA1c). Their medication was managed by diet only or with sulfonylurea, and patients under insulin therapy were excluded. The patient group consisted of 74 men and 56 women between the ages of 40-69yr. Age-matched normal subjects served as the control group. Informed consent was obtained from each subject before the study.

Blood samples were obtained from patients with type 2 diabetes mellitus and normal subjects between 9 and 10 a.m. after an overnight fast. From patients with type 2 diabetes mellitus, blood samples were obtained before and 6 months after the treatment. Serum levels of DHEA, DHEA-S and immunoreactive insulin (IRI), fasting plasma glucose (FPG) and HbA1c were measured. Steroid hormones were determined by the previously reported

HPLC/RIA method(Ueshiba et al.,1991) except DHEA-S which was measured using RIA kit(Mitsubisi Chemical Co., Tokyo, Japan), FPG by glucose oxidase method, HbA1c by HPLC, IRI by commercial kits (Daiichi, Tokyo, Japan). Data are showed as mean ± SD. Variables were compared by Bonferroni's analysis and p-values less than 0.05 were considered to indicate statistical significance.

### 2.1.2 Results

Serum levels of DHEA and DHEA-S were low in both male and female patients with type 2 DM across the entire age range studied, compared to the age-matched normal subjects (Fig.1). IRI was high in all groups before the treatment (Table1). Following a 6-month treatment, FPG and HbA1c improved and IRI decreased in most patients (Table1). In parallel with the improvement of FPG and HbA1c, blood concentrations of DHEA and DHEA-S levels increased to within the normal range in all the groups (Fig.1).

| | Number | FPG(mg/dl) | HbA1c(%) | IRI($\mu$U/ml) |
|---|---|---|---|---|
| **Male 40 years** | | | | |
| Before treatment | 22 | 183±16 | 11.6±1.2 | 11.8±3.9 |
| After treatment | 22 | 111±14 | 7.2±0.6 | 8.7±2.1 |
| Normal | 20 | 93±7 | 5.2±0.3 | 5.9±2.3 |
| **Male 50 years** | | | | |
| Before treatment | 29 | 172±18 | 11.7±1.2 | 12.4±3.7 |
| After treatment | 29 | 106±14 | 6.8±0.6 | 8.4±1.5 |
| Normal | 25 | 94±5 | 5.1±0.3 | 6.1±2.1 |
| **Male 60 years** | | | | |
| Before treatment | 23 | 176±19 | 11.4±1.1 | 13.3±4.1 |
| After treatment | 23 | 108±14 | 6.7±0.6 | 8.9±3.4 |
| Normal | 20 | 90±7 | 5.2±0.2 | 5.8±1.8 |
| **Female 40 years** | | | | |
| Before treatment | 17 | 172±16 | 12.0±1.1 | 11.9±3.2 |
| After treatment | 17 | 108±12 | 7.0±0.6 | 9.3±2.8 |
| Normal | 15 | 94±7 | 5.1±0.2 | 5.4±1.5 |
| **Female 50 years** | | | | |
| Before treatment | 23 | 166±16 | 11.6±0.8 | 12.3±3.8 |
| After treatment | 23 | 112±15 | 7.1±0.4 | 8.1±2.4 |
| Normal | 20 | 92±7 | 5.1±0.3 | 4.8±1.6 |
| **Female 60 years** | | | | |
| Before treatment | 16 | 175±19 | 11.9±1.2 | 11.6±2.8 |
| After treatment | 16 | 107±9 | 6.8±0.5 | 7.9±2.7 |
| Normal | 15 | 93±5 | 5.3±0.3 | 4.7±1.8 |

Table 1. Clinical characteristics of type 2 diabetic patients before and after treatment and in age-matched normal subjects.

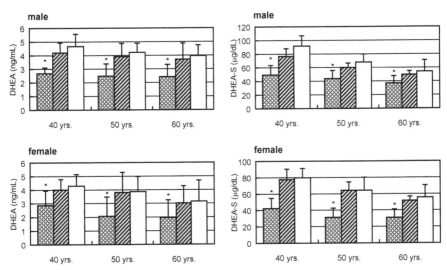

*P< 0.05 compared with values after treatment and with normal values

Fig. 1. Serum DHEA and DHEA-S levels in male and female type 2 diabetic patients before (stippled bars) and after (hatched bars) treatment and in age-matched normal subjects (opena bars).

### 2.1.3 Discussion

In this study we demonstrated that serum DHEA and DHEA-S levels decreased markedly with poor control of type 2 DM and increased to age-matched normal values with the improvement of FPG and HbA1c after 6 months' treatment with diet and/or sulfonylurea. Barrett-Connor showed that DHEA and DHEA-S levels were also low in patients with non-insulin-dependent diabetes mellitus (Barrett-Connor, 1992), but she did not measure the changes of these steroid hormones after treatment. Markedly reduced levels of DHEA and DHEA-S in type 2 DM with poor therapeutic control with slightly increased plasma IRI are consistent with an association between DHEA synthesis and/or metabolism and insulin. Nestler et al. showed that insulin reduces serum DHEA and DHEA-S by increasing the metabolic clearance rate of DHEA in men or inhibiting their productin (Nestler,1992). The metablic clearance rate of DHEA is reported to be increased two- to fivefold in obesity and insulin-resistant, hyperinsulinemic state (Nestler,1995). The infusion of a high dose of insulin reduces serum DHEA levels suggesting the involvement of the inhibition of adrenal 17,20lyase activity. The administration of metformin which inhibits hepatic glucose production and enhances peripheral tissue sensitivity to insulin, to healthy normal weight men and to obese men with hypertension but without diabetes mellitus decreased serum insulin levels and increased serum DHEA-S levels in obese men with hypertension and in healthy controls (Nestler,1995). However, Yamauchi et al. reported that serum DHEA and DHEA-S are low even in patients with impaired glucose tolerance and low insulin response (Yamauchi,1996), and therefore the decrease in serum DHEA levels may not exclusively arise from the hyperinsulinemic state. Hyperglycemia may reduce 17,20-lyase activity and consequently serum DHEA may decrease. The improvement of plasma glucose control parallels the recovery of 17,20-lyase activity.

## 2.2 Basic study

The guinea pig utilizes a similar mechanism of adrenal steroidogenesis to that of humans. In a guinea pig model in which impaired glucose tolerance is induced by streptozotocin (STZ) treatment, we measured serum levels of DHEA, DHEA-S and c-peptide to determine if these were related to serum glucose levels.

### 2.2.1 Materials and methods

All experiments were performed using Hartley male guinea pigs with a body weight of 500-600 g. Experimental protocols followed the Principals of Laboratory Animal Care and were approved by the Ethics Committee of Toho University School of Medicine. Until experiments began, guinea pigs were housed in groups of three in metabolism cages in a temperature-controlled room with a 12h light/dark cycle. They had free access to tap water and guinea pig chow.

Under intra-abdominal anaesthesia (pentobarbital sodium 30mg/Kg), streptozotocin (STZ) was administrated to 12 guinea pigs intra-abdominally. After 4 weeks, a glucose tolerance test (50% glucose, 1g/Kg, intra-abdominal route) was performed. Impaired glucose tolerance (IGT) was defined as a blood glucose level of more than 300 mg/dl after 3 hrs. Six control guinea pigs had intra-abdominal saline only.

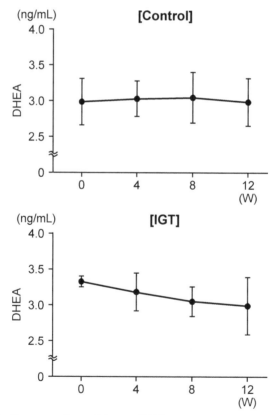

Fig. 2. Changes in Concentrations of Serum DHEA

Blood samples were taken from intra-orbital vessels after 12 hrs starvation. Serum DHEA, DHEA-S, fasting plasma glucose (FPG) and serum c-peptide were measured in each group at four time points: before STZ administration; after 4 weeks; after 8 weeks; and after 12 weeks. Simultaneously glucose tolerance tests were performed. From 15 weeks of STZ administration DHEA-S(Mylis) (20mg/Kg) was administrated via the intra-abdominal route three times per week in three IGT group guinea pigs and three control group animals. After 4 weeks, 8 weeks and 12 weeks of DHEA-S administration, blood samples were taken by the same method and glucose tolerance tests were also performed.

Data are expressed as mean±SD. Statistical analysis was performed using ANOVA with Bonferroni's correction. A value of $p < 0.05$ was considered statistically significant.

### 2.2.2 Results

Concentrations of serum DHEA showed no significant change during observation in the control group, however there was a tendency towards decrease in the IGT group (Fig. 2). Concentrations of serum DHEA-S also had no significant change in the control group. However, in the IGT group, concentrations of serum DHEA-S decreased significantly from 39.0±4.2 μg/dl (before STZ administration) to 27.5±5.0 μg/dl (after 8 weeks)($p < 0.05$)(Fig. 3).

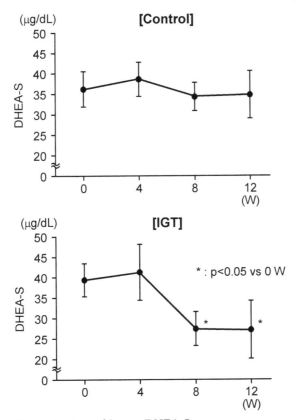

Fig. 3. Changes in Concentrations of Serum DHEA-S

Blood glucose levels three hours after DHEA-S administration showed no significant change between guinea pigs with DHEA-S and those without DHEA-S in the control group. In the IGT group, three hour blood glucose levels had improved from 333.7±24.5 mg/dl (before) to 190.7±89.8 mg/dl (after 4 weeks) (Fig. 4). However FPG showed no significant change between the control group and the IGT group. The result was similar after DHEA-S administration.

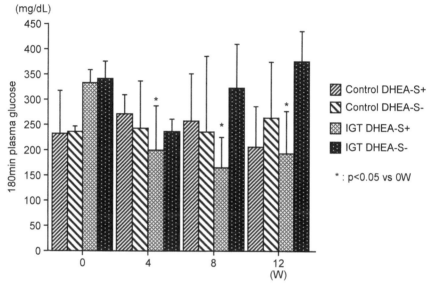

Fig. 4. Changes in 3 hour blood glucose level

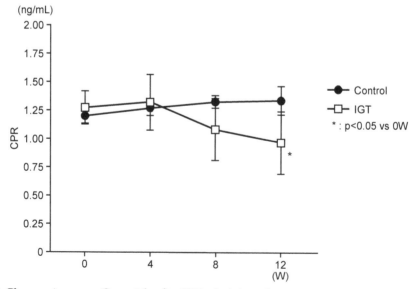

Fig. 5. Changes in serum C-peptide after STZ administration

Serum c-peptide levels showed no significant change during observation in the control group. However in the IGT group, these levels decreased significantly from 1.280±0.144 ng/ml (before) to 0.965±0.272 ng/ml (after 12 weeks)(Fig. 5 ). Serum c-peptide levels after DHEA-S administration were not significantly different between guinea pigs with DHEA-S and those without DHEA-S in both the control group and the IGT group. C-peptide levels continued to be significantly lower in the IGT group than in the control group (P<0.05) (Fig. 6).

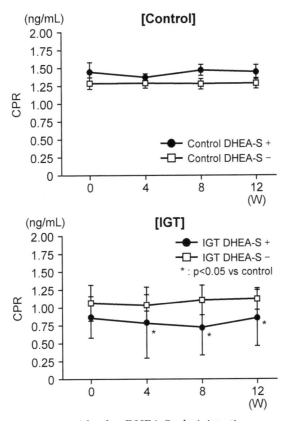

Fig. 6. Changes in serum c-peptide after DHEA-S administration

### 2.2.3 Discussion

Coleman et al.(1982). first reported that DHEA had an effect on lowering blood glucose in animal experiments. Since this report, there have been many reports that DHEA and DHEA-S are related to insulin or blood glucose levels. However, their exact role has not been determined (Gansler et al.,1985; Farah et al.,1992; Barrett-Connor,1992; Yamaguchi et al.,1998). Some of these reports described the use of rats and mice in animal experiments, but few studies used guinea pigs which have a similar mechanism of adrenal steroidogenesis to that of humans (Strott et al.,1981; Hyatt et al.,1983) In our guinea pig models in which impaired glucose tolerance is induced by STZ treatment , serum levels of DHEA and DHEA-S were decreased. We measured serum c-peptide instead of serum insulin because there were no reports of serum insulin measurements in guinea pigs (Massey&Smyth,1975; Rosenzweig et al.,1980; Gracia-Webb et al.,1983; Schlosser et al.,1987). Guinea pigs in the IGT group showed a significant decrease in serum c-peptide levels and it was speculated that this was not hyper-insulinemia. In IGT group guinea pigs, blood glucose levels improved after DHEA-S administration, however serum c-peptide levels were still significantly decreased. There was no correlation between serum c-peptide levels and DHEA or DHEA-S levels. In the STZ-induced model of diabetes, adult rats ranged from mild type 2 diabetes to type 1 diabetes depending upon STZ dose (Ho RS et al.,1988). In this experiment, fasting blood glucose levels in STZ-administered guinea pigs were not significantly different from those in control group. However, serum c-peptide levels were decreased and this state was thought to be approaching type 1 diabetes.

Similar to clinical data, it was thought that hyperglycemia itself suppressed DHEA and DHEA-S after prolonged hyperglycemia independent of serum insulin levels in the absence of hyperinsulinemia. In IGT group guinea pigs, serum c-peptide was still decreased after DHEA-S administration, however blood glucose levels improved significantly. It was thought that DHEA-S itself was involved in this improvement of blood glucose levels. In the hyperglycemic state in humans, the mechanism of decrease of DHEA and DHEA-S levels is not still clear. It has been reported that DHEA levels are low in situations of life-threatening stress(Parker et al., 1985; Wade et al.,1988). Long duration hyperglycemia in this experiment is a form of excessive stress. It was speculated that histological changes in the adrenal gland may occur. The zona fasciculata which secretes cortisol necessary to maintain life may become enlarged and the zona reticularis which secretes DHEA and DHEA-S may shrink. In addition to reports of the mechanism of the improvement of impaired glucose tolerance by DHEA and DHEA-S, further studies reported a number of other effects. These included acceleration of glucose uptake in cells, increasing sensitivity in insulin sensitive tissue and suppressing the activities of G6Pase and FBPase, the enzymes of glyconeogenesis in the liver(McIntosh & Berdanier,1991; Nakashima et al.,1995) However, many points remained unclear.

## 3. Conclusion

These experiments suggest that the relationship between blood glucose levels and DHEA or DHEA-S is close. It is therefore possible that DHEA-S may become a therapeutic agent for diabetes mellitus in the future.

## 4. References

Barrett-Connor, E. (1992). Lower endogenous androben levels and dyslipidemia in men with non-insulin-dependent diabetes mellitus. *Annals of Internal Medicine*, 117, 807-811.

Cleary, MP. (1991). The antiobesity effect of dehydroepiandrosterone in rats. *Proc Soc Exp Biol Med*, 196, 8-16.

Coleman, DL. Leiter, EH. Schwizer, RW. (1982). Therapeutic effects of dehydroepiandrosterone (DHEA) in diabetic mice. *Diabetes*, 31, 830-833.

Couch, RM. (1992). Dissociation of cortisol and adrenal androgen secretion in poorly controlled insulin-dependent diabetes mellitus. *Acta Endocrinologica*, 127, 115-117.

Farah, MJ. Givens, JR. Kitabchi, AE. (1992). Bimodel correlation between the circulating insulin level and the production rate of dehydroepiandrosterone: Positive correlation in controls and negative correlation in the polycystic ovary syndrome with acanthosis nigricans. *Journal of Clinical Endocrinology and Metabolism,* 70, 1075-1081.

Gansler, TS. Muller, S. Cleary, MP. (1985). Chronic administration of dehydroepiandrosterone reduces pancreatic β-cell hyperplasia and hyperinsulinemia in genetically obese Zucker rats. *Proceedings of the Society for Experimental Biology and Medicine,* 180, 155-162.

Gordon, GB. Bush, DE. Weisman, HF. (1988). Reduction of atherosclerosis by administration of dehydroepiandrosterone: A study in the hypercholesterolemic New Zealand White rabbit with aortic intimal injury. *H Clin Invest,* 82, 712-720.

Gracia-Webb, P. Bottomly, S. Bonser, AM. (1983). Instability of C-peptide reactivity in plasma and serum stored at -20℃. *Clinica Chimica Acta,* 129, 103-106.

Hashimoto, K. Nishioka, T. Takao, T. Numata, Y. (1993). Low plasma corticotropin-releasing hormone(CRH) levels in patients with non-insulin dependent diabetes mellitus(NIDDM). *Endocrine Journal,* 40, 705-709.

Ho RS et al.(1988). In-vIvo and in-vitro glucose metabolism in a low-dose streptozotocin rat model of noninsulin-dependent diabetes. In: Frontiers in Diabetes Research - Lessons from Animal Diabetes (ed by Shafrir E, Renold AE) p288-294, John Libbey, London, Paris.

Hubert, GD. Schriock, ED. Givens, JR. Buster, JE. (1991). Supression of circulating4Androstenedione and dehydroepiandrosterone sulfate during oral glucose tolerance in normal females. *J Clin Endocrinol Metab,* 73, 781-784.

Hyatt, PJ. Bhatt, K. Tait, JF. (1983). Steroid biosynthesis by zona fasciculata and zona reticularis cells purified from the mammalian adrenal cortex. *Journal of steroid Biochemistry,* 19, 953-959.

Massey, DE. Smyth, DG. (1975). Guinea pig proinsulin. *Journal of Biological Chemistry,* 250, 6288-6290.

McIntosh, MK. Berdanier, CD. (1991). Antiobesity effects of dehydroepiandrosterone are mediated by futile substrate cycling in hepatocytes of BHE/cdb rats. *American Institute of Nutrition,* 121, 2037-2043.

Nakashima, N. Haji, M. Sakai, Y et al. (1995). Effect of dehydroepiandrosterone on glucose uptake in cultured human fibroblasts. *Metabolism,* 44, 543-548.

Nesler, JE. Usiskin, KS. Barlascini, CO. Welty, DF. Clore, JN. Blackard, WG. (1989). Supression of serum dehydroepiandrosterone sulfate levels by insulin: An evaluation of possible mechanisms. *J Clin Endocrinol Metab,* 69 , 1040-1046.

Nestler, JE. McClanahan, MA. Clore, JN. Blackard, WG. (1992). Insulin inhibits adrenal 17, 20-lyase activity in men. *J Clin Endocrinol Metab,* 74, 362-367.

Nestler, JE. Beer, NA. Jakubowicz, DJ. Beer, RM. (1994). Effects of a reduction in circulating insulin by metformin on serum dehydroepiandrosterone sulfate in nondiabetic men. *J Clin Endocrinol Metab,* 78, 549-554.

Nestler, JE. (1995). Regulation of human dehydroepiandrosterone metabolism by insulin. *Ann N Y Acad Sci,* 774, 73-81.

Parker, LN. Levin, ER. Lifrak, ET. (1985). Evidence for adaptation to severe illness. *Journal of Clinical Endocrinology and Metabolism,* 60, 947-952.

Rosenzweig, JL. Lesniak, MA. Samuels, BE et al. (1980). Insulin in the extrapancreatic tissues of guinea pigs differs markedly from the insulin in their pancreas and plasma. *Trans Assoc Amer Physicians,* 93. 263-278.

Schlosser, MJ. Kapeghian, JC. Verlangieri, AJ. (1987). Selected physical and biochemical parameters in the streptozotocin-treated guinea pig: insights into the diabetic guinea pig model. *Life Sciences*, 41, 1345-1353.

Schriock, ED. Buffington, CK. Hubert, GD. Kurtz, BR. Kitabchi, AE. Buster, JE et al. (1988). Divergent correlation of circulating dehydroepiandrosterone sulfate and testosterone with insulin levels and insulin receptor binding. *J Clin Endocrinol Metab*, 66, 1329-1331.

Smith, S. Ravnikar, VA. Barbieri, RL. (1987). Androgen and insulin response to an oral glucose challenge in hyperandrogenic women. *Fertil Sterril*, 48, 72-77.

Strott, CA. Goff, AK. Lyons, CD. (1981). Functional differences between the outer and inner zones of the guinea pig adrenal cortex. *Endocrinology*, 109, 2249- 2252.

Ueshiba, H. Segawa, M. Hayashi, T. Miychi, Y. Irie, M. (1991). Serum steroid hormones in patients with Cushing's syndrome determined by a new HPLC/RIA method. *Clin Chem*, 37, 1329-1333.

Wade, CE. Lindberg, JS. Cockrell, JL et al. (1988). Upon-admission adrenal steroidogenesis is adapted to the degree of illness in intensive care unit patients. *Journal of Clinical Endocrinology and Metabolism*, 67, 223-227.

Yamaguchi, Y. Tanaka, S. Yamakawa T et al. (1998). Reduced serum dehydroepiandrosterone levels in diabetic patients with hyperinsulinaemia. *Clinical Endocrinology*, 49, 377-383.

Yamauchi, A. Takei, I. Nakamoto, S. Ohashi, N. Kitamura, Y. Tokui, M et al. (1996). Hyperglycemia decreased dehydroepiandrosterone in Japanese male with impaired glucose tolerance and low insulin response. *Endocrine Journal*, 43, 285-290.

# 6

# 17β-Hydroxysteroid Dehydrogenase Type 3 Deficiency: Diagnosis, Phenotypic Variability and Molecular Findings

Maria Felicia Faienza and Luciano Cavallo

*Department of Biomedicine of Developmental Age, University of Bari,*
*Italy*

## 1.Introduction

The steroid hormones are lipophilic compounds with low molecular weight, derived from cholesterol, which play a crucial role in differentiation, development and physiological functions of many tissues. They are synthesized primarily by endocrine glands, such as the gonads, the adrenal glands and the feto-placental unit during pregnancy. In addition, the central nervous system (CNS) seems to be able to synthesize a number of biologically active steroids, termed "neurosteroids", with autocrine or paracrine functions (Baulieu, 1991). The circulating steroid hormones act both on peripheral target tissues and on the CNS, coordinating physiological and behavioral responses with specific biological purposes, e.g. reproduction. Thus, they influence the sexual differentiation of the genitalia and their functional state in adulthood, the development of secondary sexual characteristics, and sexual behavior. Unlike the lower mammals in which the ovaries and testes are the exclusive source of androgens and estrogens, in humans the adrenals cortex secretes large amount of inactive steroid precursors. These adrenal steroid precursors exert their functions in target tissues after conversion into active estrogens and/or androgens. This phenomenon which describes the conversion and action of steroid hormones within peripheral target tissues has been called "intracrinology" (Labrie, 1991, 2000).

The rate of formation of each sex steroid hormone depends on the level of expression of the specific enzymes that synthesize androgens and estrogens in each cell of each tissue (Labrie et al., 1998; Stewart § Sheppard, 1992).

The final step in the biosynthesis of active steroid hormones is catalyzed by members of the family of 17β–hydroxysteroid dehydrogenase (17β–HSD), which comprises different enzymes involved in steroidogenesis.

## 2. 17β–hydroxysteroid dehydrogenases

The 17β-hydroxysteroid dehydrogenases (17β-HSDs) belong to the short-chain dehydrogenase reductase (SDR) protein superfamily, which also includes the 3β-hydroxysteroid dehydrogenase (3β–HSD). These enzymes regulate the levels of bioactive steroid hormones in many tissues and they are expressed not only in genital tissues, which are the primary target, but also in peripheral blood. The 17β-HSDs, along with other steroid metabolizing enzymes such as aromatase, steroid sulfatase, 3β-HSD and 5α-reductase are able to produce their own hormones at the peripheral cells (intracrine activity). In steroidogenic tissues (the gonads and adrenal cortex) they catalyze the final step in androgens, estrogens and progesterone byosinthesis; in peripheral tissues, they convert active steroid hormones into their metabolites, and regulate hormone binding to their nuclear receptor. So far, 14 17β–HSDs have been characterized in mammals, which show little amino acid homology but that are all members of the SDR family, with the exception of 17β-HSD type 5 (17β-HSD5) which is an aldo-keto reductase (Lukacik et al., 2006; Luu The, 2001; Prehn et al., 2009). These isoenzymes differ as regards tissue-specific expression, catalytic activity, substrate and cofactors specificity (NAD/NADH $vs$ NADP/NADPH), and subcellular localization (Payne § Hales, 2004). Although $in$ $vitro$ they act both as reductase or as oxidase enzymes, $in$ $vivo$ they work in a predominat one-way, or reductive or oxidative, converting inactive 17-ketosteroids in their active 17β-hydroxy forms (Khan et al., 2004). Thus, they can be grouped into $in$ $vivo$ oxidative enzymes (17β-HSD types 2, 4, 6, 8, 9, 10, 11 and 14) and $in$ $vivo$ reductive enzymes (17β-HSD types 1, 3, 5 and 7).

## 2.1 Family members of 17β-HSDs

The main function of 17β–HSD type 1 (17β–HSD1), which has its highest concentration in the ovaries and placenta, is the catalytic reduction of estrone to estradiol (Luu The et al., 1989). 17β-HSD type 2 (17β-HSD2) plays a major role in the inactivation of the sex steroid hormones by oxidizing estradiol and testosterone (T) to estrone and Δ4-Androstenedione (Δ4-A), respectively (Wu et al., 1993), and has a broad tissue distribution (Casey et al., 1994). 17β-HSD type 3 (17β-HSD3) plays a predominant role in male T production from Δ4-A (Geissler et al., 1994). Although this enzyme is found primarily in the testes, it is also present in adipose tissue, brain, sebaceous glands and bone. 17β-HSD type 4 (17β–HSD4) is expressed in the liver (Adamski et al., 1996) and in the peroxisomes (Markus et al., 1995); this isoenzyme plays a major function in the metabolism of fatty acids, as has been described in murine models, while it has a minor role in the metabolism of steroids. In humans, mutations of the gene encoding for 17β–HSD4 isoenzyme lead to serious illness and death within the first year of life (Moller et al., 2001). 17β-HSD type 5 (17β–HSD5), which is highly expressed in the testes, prostate, adrenals and liver, is believed to play a major role in the conversion of Δ4-A to T and therefore could explain the virilization obtained in patients affected with alterations of 17β-HSD3. 17β-HSD type 7 (17β-HSD7) has been shown to play a role in metabolism of cholesterol (Marijanovic Z et al., 2003). 17β–HSD type 8 (17β-HSD8) has been linked to a recessive form of polycystic kidney disease (Fomitcheva et al., 1998). Several of the 17β–HSD enzymes show overlap with enzymes involved in lipid metabolism (Tab.1).

Since most of the 17β-HSD enzymes are steroid metabolizing enzymes, they are possible drug targets in many cancers, such as breast and prostate cancer, as well as common diseases, such as obesity and metabolic syndrome.

## 2.2 The role of 17β-HSDs

In a study conducted to observe the tissue-specificity of the transcriptional profiles of the 17β-HSDs, the expression of 17β-HSDs type 1, 2, 3, 4, 5, 7 and 10 was observed both in the genital skin fibroblasts (both scrotal and foreskin) and in the peripheral blood, with the

| Type of 17β-HSD (Gene Name) | Locations | Functions | Cofactor/ reactions | Gene location |
|---|---|---|---|---|
| 17β-HSD type 1 (HSD17B1) | liver, ovary, mammary glands and placenta | catalyzes the interconversion of E1 to E2 | NADPH/ reduction | 17q21.2 |
| 17β-HSD type 2 (HSD17B2) | placenta, liver, intestine, endometrium, kidney, prostate, pancreas | inactivates both E2 into E1 and T into Δ4-A | NAD+/ oxidation | 16q23.3 |
| 17β-HSD type 3 (HSD17B3) | mainly testes, adipose tissue, brain, sebaceous glands and bone | converts Δ4-A to T | NADPH/ reduction | 9q22.32 |
| 17β-HSD type 4 (HSD17B4) | liver, heart, prostate, testes, lung, skeletal muscle, kidney, pancreas, thymus, ovary, intestine, placenta and breast cancer lines | inactivates both E2 into E1, and 5-diol into DHEA-β; oxidation of FA | NAD+/ oxidation | 5q23.1 |
| 17β-HSD type 5 (AKR1C3) | placenta, testes, prostate, adrenals and liver | converts Δ4-A to T in peripheral tissues; bile acid production and detoxification; eicosanoid synthesis | NADPH/ reduction | 10p15.1 |
| 17β-HSD type 6 (HSD17B6/RODH) | not determined | only retinoid metabolism identified in humans | NAD+/ oxidation | 12q13.3 |
| 17β-HSD type 7 (HSD17B7) | not determined | cholesterol synthesis; catalyzes the interconversion of E1 to E2 | NADPH/ reduction | 10p11.2 1q23 |
| 17β-HSD type 8 (HSD17B8) | widespread, liver, kidney, ovary, testes | possible role in fatty acid metabolism; inactivates both E2 into E1 and androgens | NAD+/ oxidation | 6p21.32 |
| 17β-HSD type 9 (HSD17B8/RDH5) | not determined | only retinoid metabolism identified in humans | not determined | 12q13.2 |
| 17β-HSD type 10 (HSD17B10) | widespread, liver, CNS, kidney, testes | oxidation of fatty acids; catalyzes the synthesis of DHT from 5α-androstane-3α, 17βdiol; oxidation of the 21OH groups on C21 steroids | NAD+/ oxidation | Xp11.22 |

| Type of 17β-HSD (Gene Name) | Locations | Functions | Cofactor/ reactions | Gene location |
|---|---|---|---|---|
| 17β-HSD type 11 (HSD17B11) | steroidogenic tissues, pancreas, liver, kidney, lung and heart | converts 5α-androstane-3α, 17βdiol to androsterone; lipid metabolism | NAD+/ oxidation | 4q22.1 |
| 17β-HSD type 12 (HSD17B12) | not determined | fatty acid synthesis; 3-ketoacyl-CoA reductase | NADPH/ reduction | 11p11.2 |
| 17β-HSD type 13 (HSD17B13) | not determined | enzymatically not characterized | not determined | 4q22.1 |
| 17β-HSD type 14 (HSD17B14) | CNS, kidney | inactivates both E2 into E1 and T into Δ4A; β oxidation of FA | NAD+/ oxidation | 19q13.33 |

E 1 = Estrone; E2 = 17β-estradiol; 5-diol = androst-5-ene 3α; DHEA = dihydroepiandrosterone; NADPH/NADP+ = nicotinamide adenine di nucleotide phosphate; Δ4-A = androstenedione; T = testosterone; FA = fatty acids

Table 1. The different types of identified 17β-HSD with corresponding locations and function

exception of the 17β-HSD-2 which was not seen in peripheral blood (Hoppe et al., 2006). All 17β-HSDs except 17β–HSD1 showed a significantly higher mRNA concentration in the foreskin compared to the scrotal tissue, demonstrating a tissue-specific local control of steroid hormone synthesis and action in addition to systemic effects (Hoppe et al., 2006). It has been demonstrated that the expression of 17β-HSD5 increases with aging in scrotal skin fibroblasts and in peripheral blood mononuclear cells, while the 17β-HSD3 mRNA expression is higher in the younger age subjects (Hammer et al., 2005; Hoppe et al., 2006). This implicates that 17β-HSD3 has a more important role in childhood, which later is taken over by the 17β-HSD5 after puberty.

It was also demonstrated the existence of a large inter individual variability of the enzymatic transcription patterns (Hoppe et al., 2006). Microarray investigation of multiple blood samples taken on different days from the same individual showed time-dependent differences in gene clustering. The nature and extent of inter individual and temporal variation in gene expression patterns in specific cells and tissues is an important and relatively unexplored issue in human biology (Whitney et al., 2003). In light of such intra- and inter individual variability, basal and after stimulation levels of the steroid hormones can vary a within wide range in normal subjects.

## 2.3 17β-hydroxisteroid dehydrogenase type 3

17β-hydroxisteroid dehydrogenase type 3 (17β-HSD3) isoenzyme catalyzes the reductive conversion of the inactive C-19 steroid, Δ4-A, into the biologically active androgen, T, in the Leydig cells of the testes (Payne § Hales, 2004). This protein shows a 23% sequence homology with the other 17β-HSD isoenzymes, utilizes NAPDH as cofactor and it seems to be prevalently expressed in the fetal and adult testes. Extragonadal tissues such as bone, adipose tissue, sebaceous glands and brain have also been shown to express this enzyme

(Lukacik et al., 2006). It is encoded by *HSD17B3* gene which maps to chromosome 9q22; it is 60 kb in length and contains 11 exons. The cDNA encodes a protein of 310 amino-acids with a molecular mass of 34.5 kDa and no apparent membrane-spanning domain (Andersson et al., 1996).

It has been demonstrated that *HSD17B3* gene is constitutively suppressed and its transcription begins only upon removal of suppressors that act on the Alu repeat region located upstream of the translation site start of the gene promoter region (Xiaofei et al., 2006).

*HSD17B3* gene alterations affecting the enzyme function have been associated with a rare form of 46,XY disorder of sexual development (DSD), termed 17β-hydroxisteroid dehydrogenase deficiency (Geissler et al., 1994).

## 3. Development of the male genitalia

The development of the male internal and external genitalia in an XY fetus requires a complex interplay of many critical genes, enzymes and cofactors (Hannema § Hughes, 2007). Wolffian ducts (mesonephric ducts) and mullerian ducts (paramesonephric ducts) are both present in early fetal life in the bipotential embryo. The wolffian ducts are the embryological structures that form the epididymis, vas deferens and seminal vesicles. T is produced by Leydig cells as early as 8 weeks of gestation and acts on the androgen receptor to stabilize the wolffian ducts (Tong et al., 1996). T and its 5α-reduced end product, dihydrotestosterone (DHT), induce the formation of male external genitalia, including the urethra, prostate, penis and scrotum (Wilson, 1978). The mullerian ducts should regress in a male with the presence of the mullerian inhibiting substance produced by Sertoli cells in the testes. In addition, multiple other factors are necessary for the male phenotype to be congruent with a 46,XY genotype. The enzyme 17β–HSD3 is present almost exclusively in the testes and converts Δ4-A to T. The 5α -reductase type 2 enzyme is needed to convert T to DHT. In order for T and DHT to exert their androgenic role, there must be an intact androgen receptor. The lack of any one of these critical factors, including 17β–HSD3, can lead to a child with a DSD.

### 3.1 Disorders of sexual development

Disorders of sexual development (DSDs) are congenital conditions in which development of chromosomal, gonadal or anatomical sex is atypical (Houk et al., 2006; Hughes et al., 2006). These disorders are classified into three major categories: sex chromosome DSD, 46,XX DSD and 46,XY DSD. This designation was proposed to replace the former term of pseudohermaphroditism, according to the consensus statement on management of intersex disorders (Hughes et al., 2006). 46,XY DSD are a heterogeneous group of clinical conditions characterized by 46,XY karyotype, either normal or dysgenetic testes and female or ambiguous phenotype of external (and possibly internal) genitalia (Hughes et al., 2006). This disorder can have several etiologies, but more frequently is due to a disruption in androgen production and/or action. Defects in androgen action and metabolism include mutations in the androgen receptor gene (complete, partial or mild androgen insensivity syndrome-AIS and Kennedy syndrome), or in the steroid 5α-reductase type 2 gene, encoding the enzyme which convert T into DHT in the uro-genital tract (Quigley et al., 1995; Wilson et al., 1993). Instead, disorders of androgens biosynthesis are rare and usually due to alteration of enzyme involved in the conversion of cholesterol to T, such as the steroidogenic acute regulatory (stAR) protein, the steroidogenic enzyme P450ssc, 3β–HDS type 2, 17α–hydroxylase/17-20 lyase and 17β-hydroxysteroid dehydrogenase type 3 (17β-HSD3) (Gobinet et al., 2002; Miller et al., 2005), (Fig.1)

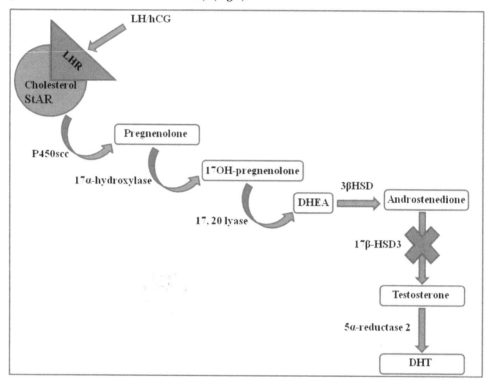

Fig. 1. Steroidogenic pathway and role of 17β- HSD3

## 4. 17β-hydroxysteroid dehydrogenase type 3 deficiency

17β-hydroxysteroid dehydrogenase type 3 (17β-HSD3) deficiency (OMIM #264300), originally described as 17-ketosteroid reductase deficiency (Saez et al., 1971), is an autosomal recessive disorder which represents the most common defect of the biosynthesis of T in 46,XY DSD (Bertelloni et al., 2004; Mendonca et al., 2000). This disorder is due to an impaired conversion of Δ4-A into T in the testes (Bertelloni et al., 2009; Faienza et al., 2008). Deficiency in the 17β-HSD3 enzyme can be caused by either homozygous or compound heterozygous mutations in the *HSD17B3* gene (Geissler et al., 1994). Mutations in the *HSD17B3* gene confer a spectrum of 46,XY disorders of sexual organ development ranging from completely undervirilized external female genitalia (Sinnecker type 5), predominantly female (Sinnecker type 4), ambiguous (Sinnecker type 3), to predominantly male with micropenis and hypospadias (Sinnecker type 2) (Boehmer et al., 1999; Sinnecker et al., 1996). The most frequent presentation of 17β-HSD3 deficiency is a 46,XY individual with female external genitalia, labial fusion and a blind ending vagina, with or without clitoromegaly (Sinnecker types 5 and 4).

## 4.1 Epidemiology and demographic

The DSD affect 1 in 5,000 to 5,500 people (0.018%) (Parisi et al., 2007; Thyen et al., 2006). Although the precise incidence of 17β-HSD3 deficiency is unknown, a nation-wide survey in the Netherlands showed a minimal incidence of 17β-HSD3 deficiency of about 1:147.000 newborns, with a frequency of heterozygotes of 1 in 135 (Boehmer et al., 1999). The frequency of complete androgen insensitivity syndrome (CAIS) from the same population was 1 in 99,000, which indicates that the frequency of 17β-HSD3 deficiency is 0.65 times that of CAIS (Boehmer et al., 1999). 17β-HSD3 deficiency is rare in Western countries, whereas in areas of high consanguinity, such as among the Gaza Strip Arab population, the incidence of 17β-HSD3 deficiency has been reported to be 1 in 100–300 people (Rosler et al., 1996, 2006). Of the known cases of 17β-HSD3 deficiency, most of the patients have been reported in Europe, Asia, Australia and South America, whereas only 11 cases have been reported in the United States (Mains et al., 2008; Moeller § Adamski, 2009). In a recent study from a gender assessment team in the United States that looked at DSD over a 25-year period, no patient with 17β-HSD3 deficiency was diagnosed (Paris et al., 2007). Moreover, in the United Kingdom DSD database, patients with 17β-HSD3 represent about the 4% of the total 46,XY DSD subjects (13/322) (Hughes, 2008). Probably the rate of 17β-HSD3 deficiency in the United States is not so low, but many cases are misdiagnosed. In one study, patients who were later confirmed to have 17β-HSD3 deficiency were initially misdiagnosed with AIS, and the rate of misdiagnosis was calculated to be 67% (Faisal et al., 2000). The risk of misdiagnosis is especially problematic because the clinical findings in 17β-HSD3 deficiency may mimic AIS in childhood and 5α-reductase deficiency in puberty (Lee et al., 2007). Thus, correct diagnosis should be made early so that treatment, management and genetic counseling can be specifically directed toward 17β-HSD3 deficiency (Hiort et al., 2003; Johannsen et al., 2006).

## 4.2 Clinical features

The characteristic phenotype of 17β-HSD3 deficiency is a 46,XY individual with testes and male wolffian-duct derived urogenital structure (e.g. epydidymus, vas deferens and seminals vesicles), but with undervirilization of the external genitalia. Patients show a phenotypic variability ranging from undervirilization of the external genitalia with or without clitoromegaly and/or labial fusion, to complete female external genitalia and a blind-ending vagina; testes may be situated in the abdomen or in the inguinal channels or in the labia majora (Grumbach et al., 1998). Gynecomastia, likely as consequence of high Δ4-A levels and its conversion to estrogens in peripheral tissues, is not usually present (Andersson et al, 1996; Balducci et al., 1985; Mendonca et al., 2000). Two late-onset variants of uncertain pathophysiology, one of which is characterized by gynecomastia in boys (Rogers et al., 1985; Castro-Magana et al., 1993) and the other by polycystic disease in woman have been described (Pang et al., 1987).

### 4.2.1 Birth

Patients with mutations in the *HSD17B3* gene may go unnoticed at birth as they commonly have female external genitalia (Balducci et al., 1985; Lee et al., 2007; Rosler et al., 1996). These children are usually assigned the female gender and grow up as such, and the diagnosis may be missed until adolescence (Andersson et al., 1996; Balducci et al., 1985; Bohmer et al., 1999; Faienza et al., 2007; Lee et al., 2007; Mendonca et al., 2000; Rosler et al., 2006).

Those subjects who come to medical attention in childhood have some degree of virilization or inguinal hernia with testes present along the inguinal canals or labioscrotal folds (Andersson et al., 1996; Bohmer et al., 1999; Lee et al., 2007). Less often patients have ambiguous external genitalia (Can et al., 1998; Eckstein et al., 1989), male genitalia with a micropenis (Ulloa-Aguirre et al., 1985) or hypospadias (Andersson et al., 1996). In these patients, the male sex is assigned at birth and they are raised accordingly (Rosler et al., 1996).

The degree of virilization can vary from Sinnecker stage 5 to stage 2 as mentioned above. This is speculated to be due to the partial activity of 17β-HSD3 in the testes and extratesticular T conversion by other members of the family, such as 17β-HSD5 (Lee et al., 2007; Qiu et al., 2004).

On examination, a separate urethral and vaginal opening is noted in many subjects, although a short urogenital sinus is reported in some (Bertelloni et al., 2006; Lee et al, 2007). Blind ending vagina that have length ranging from 1 to 7 cm has been reported in this condition (Faienza et al., 2007; Mendonca et al., 2000).

Although these findings are not specific for 17β-HSD-3 deficiency and can be seen in other 46,XY DSD, they should raise suspicion for 17β– HSD3 deficiency.

## 4.2.2 Pubertal

At the time of puberty, patients initially reared as females who have not undergone gonadectomy may have primary amenorrhea and varying degrees of virilization, including development of male body habitus, increased body hair and deepening of the voice (Faienza et al., 2007; Lee et al., 2007; Mains et al., 2008; Mendonca et al., 2000; Rosler et al., 1992; Rosler et al., 1996;). The clitoris can enlarge to as much as 5–8 cm in length due to peripheral conversion of T (Balducci et al., 1985; Mendonca et al., 2000;), but still remains smaller than a normal-sized penis and may be affected by chordee (Farkas § Rosler, 1993).

The paradox of the failure of intrauterine virilization but virilization in puberty remains an enigma not fully explained. A limited capacity of the extragonadal tissues to convert Δ4-A to T in embryonic life might explain the lack of virilization at birth (Ulloa-Aguirre et al., 1985). This might then be overcome at puberty, when the levels of Δ4-A are more elevated and thus activate the peripheral conversion into T. It has been demonstrated that in these subjects more than 90% of circulating T derives from peripheral conversion of Δ4-A into T by other isoenzymes (Andersson et al., 1996; Goebelsmann et al.,1973). There is abundant evidence of the presence of 17β-HSDs and other enzymes involved in androgen formation in a large series of human tissues, particularly liver, skin and adipose tissue (Martel et al., 1992).

This extragonadal activity is presumable under different genetic control (17β-HSD type 1, 2 or 5 encoding gene) which is apparently unimpaired in these patients (Andersson et al., 1996; Luu-The et al., 1989).

Moreover, there seems to be a correlation between the type of mutation and the percentage of enzyme inactivation. There are several reports showing a residual enzymatic activity (15-20%) in cultured mammalian cells carrying the R80Q mutation, after several hours of incubation with the substrate (androstenedione). On the contrary, most missense mutations seems to severely impair the enzyme activity (Andersson et al., 1996; Geissler et al., 1994;).

A late onset form of 17β-HSD3 deficiency causing breast development was reported in up to 6% of the patients with idiopathic pubertal gynecomastia (Castro-Magana et al., 1993).

It appeared to be related to the functional inactivity of 17β-HSD3 during puberty and increased aromatization of Δ4-A to produce excessive estrogens; however, the *HSD17B3* gene was not studied for defects in this study (Balducci et al., 1985; Bertelloni et al., 2009b).

### 4.2.3 Prenatal

Recently, the first case of prenatally identified 17β-HSD3 deficiency was reported in a child with discordance between 46,XY karyotype and female external genitalia with phallic structure (Bertelloni et al., 2009b).

### 4.3 Endocrine findings

The phenotype of 17β-HSD3 deficiency is clinically indistinguishable from that of AIS or 5α -reductase 2 deficiency. In fact, the majority of the subjects had a misdiagnosis of AIS or 5α-reductase deficiency before adequate assessment, and these two latter DSD represent the principal differential diagnoses in infancy and adolescence, respectively (Balducci et al., 1985; Bertelloni et al., 2009a; Lee et al., 2007) (Fig. 2). 17β-HSD3 however, can be reliably diagnosed by systematic endocrine evaluation (Fig. 2) and the diagnosis confirmed by molecular genetics study.

The characteristic hormonal profile of 17β-HSD3 deficiency is of increased concentrations of Δ4-A and reduced levels of T (Faisal et al., 2000). In particular, a diagnostic hallmark of 17β-HSD3 deficiency is a decreased serum T/Δ4-A ratio (<0.8-0.9) after human corionic gonadotropin (hCG) stimulation in prepubertal subjects, while baseline values seems to be informative in early infancy and adolescence (Rosler et al., 1996). A normal ratio above 0.8 after hCG stimulation raises the suspicion of other diagnoses such as androgen receptor mutation. An elevated T/DHT raises the suspicion of a 5α-reductase type 2 deficiency. However, low basal T/Δ4-A ratio is not specific for 17β-HSD3 deficiency, being sometimes also found in patients with other defects in T synthesis or with Leydig cell hypoplasia. The clinical phenotype of Leydig cell hypoplasia may also resemble that of 17β-HSD3 deficiency before puberty, but the absence of all testicular androgens (baseline and after hCG stimulation) and the lack of pubertal development or isosexual pubertal arrest should allow to differentiate between them (Bertelloni et al., 2009a).

A diagnostic tool could be represented by the urinary ketosteroid analysis performed by means gas chromatography tandem mass spectrometry, a high sensitive technique for the detection of anabolic steroid residues in urine (Van Poucke et al., 2005).

The DHT levels in 17β- HSD-3 deficiency can be decreased, normal or high, while the dehydroepiandrosterone (DHEA) levels are typically high (Mendonca et al., 2000).

Elevated serum LH and FSH levels at baseline and after GnRH test administration, indicating the impairment of the pituitary regulatory control by gonadal hormones, have been found in these subjects (Mendonca et al., 2000). Increased serum LH causes elevated Δ4-A levels, allowing the formation of some T either in extra glandular tissues or in the testes, when some residual enzyme activity is present (Andersson et al., 1996). Elevation of FSH may also be due to a damage to the spermatogenic tubules as a result of long term cryptorchidism as documented in histological specimens from adult subjects. However, FSH levels have been reported to be normal in some subjects (Van Poucke et al., 2005; Rosler et al., 1992).

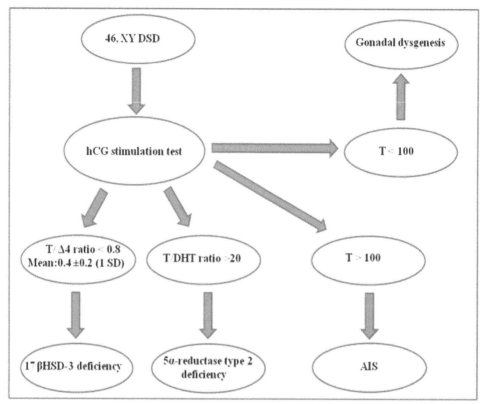

Fig. 2. A diagnostic algorithm to elucidate the various etiologies of 46,XY DSD. The diagram shows the importance of hCG stimulation in the diagnosis of 46,XY DSD. Upon hCG stimulation, if the T/Δ4-A ratio is >0.8, the diagnosis of 17β- HSD3 can be suspected; if the T/DHT ratio is >20, a diagnosis of 5α-reductase deficiency can be suspected. If the response of T is >100 ng/dl, androgen insensitivity syndrome (AIS) is possible. However, if the response is <100 ng/dl, causes of gonadal dysgenesis should be sought. Once a diagnosis is suspected, molecular genetic studies can be used for definitive diagnosis.

### 4.4 Molecular diagnosis

*HSD17B3* gene alterations have been identified in patients showing clinical and biochemical characteristics of 17β-HSD3 deficiency. The disease is genetically heterogeneous and genotype-phenotype correlations have not been found.

To date, 27 mutations in the *HSD17B3* gene have been reported. These include intronic splice junction abnormalities, exonic deletions and missense mutations (Table 2) (Mains et al., 2008). The majority are missense mutations inherited as homozygous or compound heterozygous mutations, occurring most frequent in exons 3,9,10 of the gene; 4 are splice junction abnormalities (Andersson et al., 1996; Boehmer et al., 1999), 1 is a small deletion (Δ777-783), and 1 is a thymidine deletion resulting in a frame shift mutation which alters the amino acid sequence from codon position 187 onward with a premature termination in codon 226 (Boehmer et al., 1999; Twesten et al., 2000).

| Age of diagnosis | Phenotype Clinical presentation | Ethnicity | Mutation | Mutation type Effect | Reference |
|---|---|---|---|---|---|
| 16 years | 46,XY DSD; hirsutism, clitoromegaly, failure to menstruate | Iranian | p.Ser65Leu | missense/ inactivates enzyme | Andersson et al., 1996 |
| 6 months, 11 years | 46,XY DSD; female prepubertal external genitalia, pubertal virilization, severe hair growth, voice changes and clitoral enlargement (6 months, child diagnosed because of family history) | South Asian | p.Ala56Thr | missense/ severe impairment of enzyme | Lee et al., 2007 Moghrabi et al., 1998 |
| 4–16 years | 46,XY DSD; ambiguous genitalia, pubertal virilization | Dutch | p.Asn74Thr | missense | Boehmer et al., 1999 |
| 4–43 years | 46,XY DSD; ambiguous genitalia at birth to mild clitoromegaly, pubertal virilization, male gender role, and many reassigned as males if raised as girls | Arab, Dutch, Brazilian, Portuguese | p.Arg80Gln | missense/ impaired enzyme activity (NADPH binding site) | Mendonca et al., 2000 Geissler et al., 1994 Boehmer et al., 1999 Roesler et al., 1996 Roesler et al., 1992 Mendonca et al., 1999 |
| Newborn– 12 years | 46,XY DSD; female external genitalia, palpable gonads, clitoral enlargement and virilization at puberty | Spanish, Italian, Lebanese | p.Arg80Trp | missense/ complete loss of enzyme activity (NADPH binding site) | McKeever et al., 2002 Faienza et al., 2007 Bilbao et al., 1998 |
| 4 months– 15 years | 46,XY DSD; pubertal virilization, mild clitoromegaly, voice changes | English, German | c.325+4,A-T | splice junction/ disrupts splice acceptor site | Mendonca et al., 2000 Boehmer et al., 1999 Andersson et al., 1996 |
| 8, 23, 34 years 15 years | 46,XY DSD; inguinal hernia, failure of breast development, facial and body hair growth, voice changes, clitoral enlargement | Dutch, Brazilian | c.326–1,G-C | splice junction | Mendonca et al., 2000 Geissler et al., 1994 Boehmer et al., 1999 Andersson et al., 1996 Mendonca et al., 1999 Moghrabi et al., 1998 |
| 14,15 years | 46,XY DSD; pubertal virilization, mild clitoromegaly, voice changes | English, German | p.Asn130Ser | missense/ severe impairment of enzyme activity | Lee et al., 2007 Bertelloni et al., 2009 Moghrabi et al., 1998 |

| Unknown | 46,XY DSD | unknown | c.538–1,G-A | splice junction | Mueller § Coovadia, 2009 |
|---|---|---|---|---|---|
| 13 years | 46,XY DSD; clitoromegaly and coarsening of voice, scrotalization of labia majora and inguinal masses | American (Italian, German, Irish) | p.Gln176Pro | missense | Andersson et al., 1996 Moghrabi et al., 1998 |
| 12 years | 46,XY DSD; female prepubertal development, clitoral enlargement at 12 years of age, testes in inguinal canal | German | c.608delT | downstream premature stop codon | Twesten et al., 2000 |
| 10 years | 46,XY DSD; prepubertal female external genitalia, inguinal mass | Turkish | p.Ala188Val | missense/ inactivates enzyme | Boehmer et al., 1999 |
| 12 years | 46,XY DSD; pubertal virilization, facial hair, 4–8 cm phallus and labioscrotal folds | Afghan | p.Met197Lys | missense/ alters secondary protein structure | Lee et al., 2007 |
| 10,16,17 years | 46,XY DSD; prepubertal female external genitalia, pubertal virilization, male gender rol | Syrian, Turkish, Dutch, Greek-American | c.655–1,G-A | splice junction/ disrupts splice acceptance site | Geissler et al., 1994 Boehmer et al., 1999 Andersson et al., 1996 Moghrabi et al., 1998 Ademola Akesode et al., 1977 |
| 13, 18, 21, 26 years | 46,XY DSD; absence of menses, failure of breast development, facial and chest hair and clitoral enlargement, male and female gender identity in siblings | African-Brazilian, Italian | p.Ala203Val | missense/ inactivates enzyme | Mendonca et al., 2000 Geissler et al., 1994 Mendonca et al., 1999 Moghrabi et al., 1998 |
| Unknown | 46,XY DSD; pubertal virilization | Southern Italian | p.Ala203Glu | missense | Mendonca et al., 2000 Bertelloni et al., 2009 |
| Newborn, 20 years | 46,XY DSD; prepubertal female externalgenitalia to perineoscrotal hypospadias, primary amenorrhea, mild clitoromegaly | White American, English | p.Val205Glu | missense/ inactivates enzyme | Lee et al., 2007 Andersson et al., 1996 |

| Newborn | 46,XY DSD; ambiguous genitalia, clitoromegaly (1.5 cm) and posterior fusion and scrotalization of the labia majora which contained palpable masses | German | p.Phe208Ile | missense/ inactivates enzyme | Andersson et al., 1996 |
|---|---|---|---|---|---|
| 2 years, 3 months | 46,XY DSD; inguinal mass, mild clitoromegaly | Italian | p.Leu212Gln | missense/ inactivates enzyme | Geissler et al., 1994 Bertelloni et al., 2006 |
| 14, 15, 21 years | 46,XY DSD; female or ambiguous genitalia at birth, male behaviors in childhood, pubertal virilization, absence of menses, male gender role | White Brazilian, English | p.Glu215Asp | missense/ inactivates enzyme | Mendonca et al., 2000 Lee et al., 2007 Andersson et al.,1996 |
| 2 months, 2, 6, 17 years | 46,XY DSD; clitoromegaly, primary amenorrhea, absent labia minora, severe hypospadias with undermasculinization– raised as males and females | African-American, South Asian | p.Ser232Leu | missense/ inactivates enzyme | Geissler et al.,1994 Lee et al., 2007 Moghrabi et al., 1998 |
| 17 years | 46,XY DSD; clitoromegaly, primary amenorrhea, inguinal masses | African-American, Italian | p.Met235Val | missense/ inactivates enzyme | Geissler et al.,1994 Bertelloni et al., 2006 Moghrabi et al., 1998 |
| 15 years | 46,XY DSD; testes in herniorrhaphy sac, failure to menstruate | Polish | c.777-783delGAT AACC | deletion/ frame shift truncates protein | Andersson et al.,1996 |
| 5, 18 months, 2–4 years | 46,XY DSD; prominent clitoris, palpable inguinal gonads | Pakistani | p.Cys268YT yr | missense/ inactivates enzyme | Lee et al., 2007 Lindqvist et al., 2001 |
| Unknown | 46,XY DSD | French | p.His271Arg | missense/ inactivates enzyme | Bachelot et al., 2006 |
| 12, 14 years | 46,XY DSD; clitoromegaly, failure of breast development and deepening of voice | White American, Dutch | p.Pro282Leu | missense/ inactivates enzyme | Boehmer et al., 1999 Andersson et al.,1996 |
| 6 months | 46,XY DSD; normal female prepubertal genitalia, bilateral inguinal hernia at sonography | Italian, West Indian | p.Gly289Ser | polymorphism / unknown | Boehmer et al., 1999 Bertelloni et al., 2009 |

Table 2. Mutations reported to date in patients with 17β-HSD3 deficiency phenotype

Two missense mutations, the 239 G to A resulting in an Arg to Gln (R80Q) substitution, which is the most frequent alteration described in the Arab population living in the Gaza Strip (Boehmer et al.,1999; Mains et al., 2008; Rosler et al., 1996), and the 238 C to T resulting in an Arg to Trp (R80W) substitution (Bilbao et al, 1998; Faienza et al., 2007) involve the same arginine residue in exon 3 at position 80. This site has been extensively studied by systematic replacement of the wild-type arginine at position 80 and has been shown to be extremely important for both forming the salt bridge with the terminal phosphate moiety of the NADPH, as well as providing for a hydrophobic pocket for the purine ring of the adenosine portion of the NADPH (McKeever et al., 2002). Thus, this arginin is critical for cofactor binding and the substitution by different amino acids results in alteration of cofactor preference, switching from NADPH to NADH (Payne § Hales, 2004).

One polymorphic substitution (G289S) has been described in a heterozygous form in apparently normal individuals. This polymorphism does not impair the kinetic properties of the normal enzyme (Moghrabi et al., 1998). A possible role of the G289S variation has been demonstrate in prostate cancer (Margiotti et al., 2002).

Most gene alterations severely compromise the enzyme activity, but the R80Q mutation results in a 17β-HSD3 residual enzyme activity (20%), showing a significantly lower reaction velocity as compared to the normal enzyme (Geissler et al., 1994).

### 4.5 Worldwide distribution of ancient and *de novo* mutations

Haplotype analysis of genetic markers flanking the *HSD17B3* gene has been performed to establish the ancient or *de novo* occurrence of mutations described in European, North American, Latin American, Australian and Arab populations (Boehmer et al., 1999). Dutch, German, white Australian and white American patients carrying the 325+4,A –T mutation share the same genetic markers and seem to have a common European ancestor. A founder effect was also demonstrated for the R80Q mutation that is common in Dutch, Arab (in Gaza), white Brazilian, and white Portuguese patients. As this mutation is associated with a specific haplotype, a common ancestor introduced during the Phoenician migration has been hypothesized (Rosler et al., 2006). An additional founder effect has been suggested for 655-1,G-T mutation found in Greeks, Turks and Syrians patients that may have spread to the Mediterranean area during Ottoman Empire (Boehmer et al., 1999). On the contrary, patients harboring the 326-1,G-C and the c.Pro282Leu mutations have a different marker genotype suggesting that these are the novo mutations (Boehmer et al., 1999).

### 4.6 Genotype-phenotype correlation

No phenotype-genotype correlation has been noted in 17β-HSD3 deficiency, as exemplified by members of the same family who have different phenotypes despite the same genotype (Lee et al., 2007). A variable T/Δ4-A ratio after human chorionic gonadotropin (hCG) stimulation was also seen despite the same homozygous mutation in different subjects of the same pedigree. This can be attributed to the extratesticular ability of some subjects to convert Δ4-A to T by other enzymes such as 17β-HSD5 (Qiu et al., 2004).

### 4.7 Imaging studies

Imaging studies that reveal the absence of mullerian structures and persistent wolffian structures also point to the diagnosis of 17β-HSD3 deficiency, but this is not pathognomonic as 5α-reductase type 2 deficiency will also have similar findings. Histological evidence from gonadal tissue may show normal testicular structures, which can help to exclude any structural abnormalities (testicular dysgenesis) as the cause for the 46,XY DSD. Despite an early orchidopexy, an absent spermatogenesis has been seen in patients affected with 17β-HSD3 deficiency raised as males (Dumic et al., 1985). So far, no patient with 17β-HSD3 deficiency was fertile although raised as male, thus infertility appears to be the rule in adulthood (Tab. 3) (Bertelloni et al., 2009a; Rosler et al., 1996).

| Patients | Epididimus | Testes ml[a]  SDS | Spematogonia cells | Sertoli cells | Leydig | Micro-calcifications |
|---|---|---|---|---|---|---|
| 1 | Yes | 1.4  –1.0 | Scarce | Normal | Normal | No |
| 2 | Yes | 1.0  –0.5 | Present (sub-normal) | Normal | Normal | Yes |
| 3 | Yes | 2.0   2.0 | Present | Normal | Normal | No |
| 4 | Yes | 9.0   1.3 | Absent/very scarce | Normal | Hypertrophic | No |

[a] mean of the two gonads; SDS: SD score.
Normal values from Cassorla et al., 1981 for patients 1-3 and from Taranger et al., 1976 for patient 4.

Table 3. Gonadal findings in 4 subjects with 17β-HSD3 deficiency

### 4.8 Gender behavior

In the absence of a correct diagnosis before puberty, most patients with 17β-HSD deficiency are raised as females and undergo virilization during adolescence due to extratesticular conversion of Δ4-A to T, secondary to some residual function of the enzyme and increased substrate availability in Δ4-A at puberty (Andersson et al., 1996). In cases with partial virilization, early post-natal diagnosis and consequence successful androgen treatment may result in a male sex assignment and in a nearly normal male phenotype in adulthood. Gonadectomy is recommended before puberty for those individuals who have been raised as females and wish to remain so. In these subjects, female sex characteristics should be induced or maintained with appropriate hormone replacement therapy (Hiort et al., 2003). Vaginal dilation using the modified Frank's procedure or vaginal reconstruction surgery may be necessary to create a vaginal cavity with adequate capacity for sexual relations (Castro-Magana et al., 1993). The patient and family will need appropriate psychological counseling to accept the diagnosis and the infertility that accompanies it (Gooren, 2002). In patients with a male attitude, it is possible to achieve adequate male development without medical intervention, when corrective surgery has been judged to be warranted (Boehmer et al., 1999; Farkas § Rosler, 1993; Rosler et al., 1996). Exogenous T treatment does not seem to yield additional benefits in adulthood (Mendonca et al., 2000; Farkas § Rosler, 1993), while pre-operative T administration may result in a better cosmetic appearance of the external genitalia (Farkas § Rosler., 1993). Gender role changes have been reported in 39-60% of cases of 17β-HSD3 deficiency who have been raised as girls (Wilson, 1999). Genetic and endocrine evidence indicates that androgens play an important role in male gender behavior and identity. However the fact that many individuals with mutations of the 5α-reductase and 17β-HSD3 encoding genes do not change their gender role behavior implies that other factors (social, psychological or biological) contribute to modulating human sexual behavior. Because gender-appropriate rearing, and not the chromosomal, gonadal or genital factors plays a crucial role in gender identity development, early diagnosis and treatment if patients with the 17β-HSD3 deficiency is very important.

## 4.9 Psychological aspects

Sex assignment of children with DSD is a subject of intense debate. The early pioneers in this field coined the term 'optimal gender policy', which advocated for early corrective surgery to help the affected children and their parents to facilitate stable gender identity and appropriate gender role behavior (Money et al., 1955) . Opponents of early surgery argue for a 'full consent policy', in which surgery is not performed in non-emergency situations before full consent may be obtained from the child (Kipnis § Diamond, 1998). In 17β-HSD3 deficiency, as in all situations characterized by severe undervirilization (Sinnecker stage 5 or 4), is not always feasible to wait the start of the virilization and/or the age for a reliable full consent for major intervention, because in this waiting period the patient could assume a female gender role and identity. According to the recent guidelines regarding ethical principles and recommendations for the medical management of DSD in children and adolescents, the parents take the first-line responsibility in defining what might be best for the child, and this might vary according to their individual experience and lifestyle, cultural expectations and religious beliefs (Wiesemann et al., 2010). The child, according to his or her developmental level, can express own preference. Each case must be weighed on its own merits. When there is a doubt, the psychological and social support of the child and the parent is to be ranked higher than the creation of biological normalcy.

## 4.10 Malignancy risk

The external genitalia are mostly female in 17β-HSD3 deficiency, but the internal structures are derivatives of wolffian structures. The testes are usually positioned in the inguinal canal, sometimes at the labia majora and rarely in the abdominal cavity (Mendonca et al., 2000). The consensus statement for management of DSD puts the risk of germ cell malignancy at 28% in 17β-HSD3 deficiency (Houk et al., 2006; Hughes et al., 2006). This puts it in the intermediate risk group for malignancies and close monitoring is recommended for someone who is raised as a male rather than having gonadectomy at the time of diagnosis.

## 5. Conclusions

Diagnosis and consequently early treatment of the 17β-HSD3 deficiency is frequently difficult because clinical signs are often mild or absent from birth until puberty. Moreover, the 17β-HSD3 deficiency is clinically indistinguishable from other forms of 46,XY DSD such as AIS or 5α-reductase 2 gene deficiency. The correct diagnosis can be arrived at by systematic endocrine evaluation and, most importantly, by the calculation of the T/Δ4-A ratio. The diagnostic power of biochemical parameters is not always specific, because no normal reference range has yet been established in strictly age-matched controls and because of overlapping with other causes of 46,XY DSD due to impaired T biosynthesis. Molecular genetic testing confirms the diagnosis and provides the orientation for genetic counseling. A high index of suspicion should be present for any female who presents with inguinal hernias or mild clitoromegaly in infancy or early childhood. The virilization in the adolescent girl should also arouse suspicion. Since there are unique clinical implications based on the diagnosis of this condition, it is important to be as prompt and accurate as possible. In conclusion, endocrine evaluation is an important tool for the selection of patients with a suspected 17β-HSD3 deficiency. In these patients, mutational analysis of the *HSD17B3* gene, supported by a knowledge of the ethnic distribution of mutations, is irreplaceable in confirming the diagnosis.

# 6. References

Adamski, J., Carstensen, J., Husen, B., Kaufmann, M., de Launoit, Y., Leenders, F., Markus, M. § Jungblut, P.W. (1996). New 17 beta-hydroxysteroid dehydrogenases. Molecular and cell biology of the type IV porcine and human enzymes. *Annals of the New York Academy of Sciences*, 784, pp. 124–136.

Andersson, S., Geissler, W.M., Wu, L., Davis, D.L., Grumbach, M.M., New, M.I., Schwarz, H.P., Blethen, S.L., Mendonca,

B.B., Bloise, W., Witchel, S.F., Cutler, G.B. Jr, Griffin, J.E., Wilson, J.D. § Russel, D.W. (1996). Molecular genetics and pathophysiology of 17 beta-hydroxysteroid dehydrogenase 3 deficiency. *The Journal of Clinical Endocrinology § Metabolism*, 81, pp. 130–136.

Balducci, R., Toscano, V., Wright, F., Bozzolan, F., Di Piero, G., Maroder, M., Panei, P., Sciarra, F. § Boscherini, B. (1985).

Familial male pseudohermaphroditism with gynaecomastia due to 17 beta-hydroxysteroid dehydrogenase deficiency. A report of 3 cases. *Clinical Endocrinology*, 23, pp. 439–444.

Baulieu, E.E. (1991). Neurosteroids: a new function in the brain. *Biology of the Cell*, 71 (1-2), pp. 3-10.

Bertelloni, S., Federico, G. § Hiort, O. (2004). 17β -Hydroxysteroid dehydrogenase-3 deficiency: genetics, clinical findings, diagnosis and molecular biology. *The Italian Journal of Pediatrics*, 30, pp. 32–38.

Bertelloni, S., Maggio, M.C., Federico, G., Baroncelli, G. § Hiort, O. (2006). 17beta-hydroxysteroid dehydrogenase-3 deficiency: a rare endocrine cause of male-to-female sex reversal. *Gynecological Endocrinology*, 22, pp. 488–494.

Bertelloni, S., Dati, E. § Hiort, O. (2009a). Diagnosis of 17β-hydroxysteroid dehydrogenase deficiency: a review. *Expert Review of Endocrinology and Metabolism*, 4, pp. 53-65.

Bertelloni, S., Balsamo, A., Giordani, L., Fischetto, R., Russo, G., Delvecchio, M., Gennari, M., Nicoletti, A., Maggio, M.C., Concolino, D., Cavallo, L., Cicognani, A., Chiumello, G., Hiort, O., Baroncelli, G.I. § Faienza, M.F. (2009b). 17beta-hydroxysteroid dehydrogenase-3 deficiency: from pregnancy to adolescence. *Journal of Endocrinology Investigation*, 32, pp. 666-670.

Bilbao, J.R., Loridan, L., Audì, L., Gonzalo, E.§ Castaño, L. (1998). A novel missense (R80W) mutation in 17β hydroxysteroid dehydrogenase type 3 gene associated with male pseudohermaphroditism. *European Journal of Endocrinology*, 139, pp. 330-333.

Boehmer, A.L., Brinkmann, A.O., Sandkuijl, L.A., Halley, D.J., Niermeijer, M.F., Andersson, S., de Jong, F.H., Kayserili, H., de Vroede, M.A., Otten, B.J., Rouwe, C.W., Mendonca, B.B., Rodrigues, C., Bode, H.H., de Ruiter, P.E., Delemarre-van de Waal, H.A. § Drop, S.L. (1999). 17beta-hydroxysteroid dehydrogenase-3 deficiency: diagnosis, phenotypic variability, population genetics, and worldwide distribution of ancient and de novo mutations. *The Journal of Clinical Endocrinology § Metabolism,* 84, pp. 4713–4721.

Can, S., Zhu, Y.S., Cai, L.Q., Ling, Q., Katz, M.D., Akgun, S., Shackleton, C.H. § Imperato-McGinley, J. (1998). The identification of 5 alpha-reductase-2 and 17 beta-hydroxysteroid dehydrogenase-3 gene defects in male pseudohermaphrodites from a Turkish kindred. *The Journal of Clinical Endocrinology § Metabolism,* 83(2), pp. 560-569.

Casey, M.L., MacDonald, P.C. § Andersson, S. (1994). 17 beta-hydroxysteroid dehydrogenase type 2: chromosomal assignment and progestin regulation of gene expression in human endometrium. *The Journal of Clinical Investigation,* 94, pp. 2135-2141.

Cassorla, F.G., Golden, S.M., Johnsonbaugh, R.E., Heroman, W.M., Loriaux, D.L. § Sherins, R.J. (1981). Testicular volume during early infancy. *Journal of Pediatrics,* 99, pp. 742-743.

Castro-Magana, M., Angulo, M. § Uy, J. (1993). Male hypogonadism with gynecomastia caused by late-onset deficiency of testicular 17-ketosteroid reductase. *The New England Journal of Medicine,* 328, pp. 1297-1301.

Dumic, M., Plavsic, V., Fattorini, I. § Ille, J. (1985). Absent spermatogenesis despite early bilateral orchidopexyin 17-ketoreductase deficiency. *Hormone Research* 1985; 22, pp. 100-106.

Eckstein, B., Cohen, S., Farkas, A. § Rosler, A. (1989). The nature of the defect in familial male pseudohermaphroditismin Arabs of Gaza. *The Journal Clinical Endocrinology § Metabolism,* 68, pp. 477–485.

Faisal, A.S., Iqbal, A. § Hughes, I.A. (2000). The testosterone:rostenedione ratio in male undermasculinization. *Clinical Endocrinology,* 53, pp. 697–702.

Faienza, M.F., Giordani, L., Acquafredda, A., Leggio, S., Todarello, O., Trabucco, S., D'Aniello, M., Zecchino, C., Delvecchio, M.§ Cavallo, L. (2007). 46, XY DSD caused by a rare mutation of the 17β-hydroxysteroid type 3 gene. *The Italian Journal of Pediatrics,* 33, pp.13–16.

Farkas, A. § Rosler, A. (1993). Ten years experience with masculinizing genitoplasty in male pseudohermaphroditism due to 17 beta-hydroxysteroid dehydrogenase deficiency. *European Journal of Pediatrics,* 152(suppl 2), pp. S88–S90.

Faienza, M.F., Giordani, L., Delvecchio, M. § Cavallo, L. (2008). Clinical, endocrine, and molecular findings in 17beta-hydroxysteroid dehydrogenase type 3 deficiency. *The Journal of Endocrinology Investigation,* 31, pp. 85-91.

Fomitcheva, J., Baker, M.E., Anderson, E., Lee, G.Y. § Aziz, N. (1998). Characterization of Ke 6, a new 17beta-hydroxysteroid dehydrogenase, and its expression in gonadal tissues. *The Journal of Biological Chemistry,* 273, pp. 22664–22671.

Geissler, W.M., Davis, D.L., Wu, L., Bradshaw, K.D., Patel, S., Mendonca, B.B., Elliston, K.O., Wilson, J.D., Russell, D.W. § Andersson, S. (1994). Male pseudohermaphroditism caused by mutations of testicular 17 beta-hydroxysteroid dehydrogenase 3. *Nature Genetics,* 7, pp. 34–39.

Gobinet, J., Poujol, N. § Sultan, Ch. (2002). Molecular action of androgens. *Molecular and Cellular Endocrinology,* 30, 198(1-2), pp. 15-24.

Goebelsmann, U., Horton, R., Mestman, J.H., Arce, J.J., Nagata, Y., Nakamura, R.M., Thorneycroft, I.H. § Mishell, D.R. Jr. (1973). Male pseudohermaphroditism due to testicular 17 -hydroxysteroid dehydrogenase deficiency. *The Journal of Clinical Endocrinology § Metabolism*, 36(5), pp. 867-879.

Gooren, L.J. (2002). Psychological consequences. *Seminars in Reproductive* Medicine, 20, pp. 285–296

Hammer, F., Drescher, D.G., Schneider, S.B., Quinkler, M., Stewart, P.M., Allolio, B. § Arlt, W. (2005). Sex steroid metabolism in human peripheral blood mononuclear cells changes with aging. *The Journal of Clinical Endocrinology § Metabolism*, 90, pp. 6283–6289.

Hiort, O., Reinecke, S., Thyen, U., Jurgensen, M., Holterhus, P.M., Schon, D. § Richter-Appelt, H. (2003). Puberty in disorders of somatosexual differentiation. *Journal of Pediatric Endocrinology and Metabolism*, 16(suppl 2), pp. 297–306.

Hannema, S.E. § Hughes, I.A. (2007). Regulation of Wolffian duct development. *Hormone Research*, 67, pp. 142–151.

Hiort, O., Reinecke, S., Thyen, U., Jürgensen, M., Holterhus, P.M., Schön, D. § Richter-Appelt, H. (2003). Puberty in disorders of somatosexual differentiation. *Journal of Pediatric Endocrinology and Metabolism*, 16(suppl.2), pp. 297-306.

Hoppe, U., Holterhus, P.M., Wunsch, L., Jocham, D., Drechsler, T., Thiele, S., Marschke, C. § Hiort, O. (2006). Tissue-specific transcription profiles of sex steroid biosynthesis enzymes and the androgen receptor. *Journal of Molecular Medicine*, 84(8), pp. 651-659.

Houk, C.P., Hughes, I.A., Ahmed, S.F. § Lee, P.A. (2006). Writing Committee for the International Intersex Consensus Conference Participants: Summary of consensus statement on intersex disorders and their management. International Intersex Consensus Conference. *Pediatrics*, 118. pp. 753–757.

Hughes, I.A., Houk, C., Ahmed, S.F. § Lee, P.A. (2006). Lawson Wilkins Pediatric Endocrine Society/European Society for Paediatric Endocrinology Consensus Group: Consensus statement on management of intersex disorders. *Journal of Pediatric Urology*, 2, pp. 148–162.

Hughes, I.A. (2008). Disorders of sex development: a new definition and classification. *Best Practice and Research Clinical Endocrinology and Metabolism*, 22, pp. 119-34.

Johannsen, T.H., Ripa, C.P., Mortensen, E.L. § Main, K.M. (2006). Quality of life in 70 women with disorders of sex development. *European Journal Endocrinology*, 155, pp. 877–885.

Khan, N., Sharma, K.K., Andersson, S. § Auchus, R.J. (2004). Human 17beta-hydroxysteroid dehydrogenases types 1, 2, and 3 catalyze bi-directional equilibrium reactions, rather than unidirectional metabolism, in HEK-293. *Archives of Biochemistry and Biophisycs*, 1, 429(1), pp. 50-59.

Kipnis, K. § Diamond, M. (1998). Pediatric ethics and the surgical assignment of sex. *Journal of Clinical Ethics*, 9, pp. 398–410.

Labrie, F. (1991). Intracrinology. *Molecular and Cellular Endocrinology*, 78 (3), pp. C113-118.

Labrie, F., Bélanger, A., Luu-The, V., Labrie, C., Simard, J., Cusan, L., Gomez, J.L. § Candas, B. (1998). DHEA and the intracrine formation of androgens and estrogens in peripheral target tissues: its role during aging. *Steroids*, 63(5-6), pp. 322-328.

Labrie, F., Luu-The, V., Lin, S.X., Simard, J., Labrie, C., El-Alfy, M., Pelletier, G. § Bélanger, A. (2000). Intracrinology: role of the family of 17 beta-hydroxysteroid dehydrogenases in human physiology and disease. *Journal of Molecular Endocrinology*, 25 (1), pp. 1-16.

Lee, Y.S., Kirk, J.M., Stanhope, R.G., Johnston, D.I., Harland, S., Auchus, R.J., Andersson, S. § Hughes, I.A. (2007). Phenotypic variability in 17beta-hydroxysteroid dehydrogenase-3 deficiency and diagnostic pitfalls. *Clinical Endocrinology*, 67, pp. 20-28.

Lukacik, P., Kavanagh, K.L. § Oppermann U. (2006). Structure and function of human 17beta-hydroxysteroid dehydrogenases. *Molecular and Cellular Endocrinology*,248, pp. 61-71.

Luu The V., Labrie, C., Zhao, H.F., Couët, J., Lachance, Y., Simard, J., Leblanc, G., Côtè, J., Bérubé, D., Gagné, R. § Labrie F. (1989). Characterization of cDNAs for human estradiol 17 beta-dehydrogenase and assignment of the gene to chromosome 17: evidence of two mRNA species with distinct 5'-termini in human placenta. *Molecular Endocrinology*, 3, pp. 1301-1309.

Luu The, V. (2001). Analysis and characteristics of multiple types of human 17beta-hydroxysteroid dehydrogenase. *The Journal of Steroid Biochemistry and Molecular Biology*, 76, pp. 143-151.

Mains, L.M., Vakili, B., Lacassie, Y., Andersson, S., Lindqvist, A. § Rock, J.A. (2008). 17beta-hydroxysteroid dehydrogenase 3 deficiency in a male pseudohermaphrodite. *Fertility and Sterility*, 89, 228, pp. e213-e227.

Margiotti, K., Kim, E., Pearce, C.L., Spera, E., Novelli, G. § Reichardt, J.K. (2002). Association of the G289S single nucleotide polymorphism in the HSD17B3 gene with prostate cancer in Italian men. *Prostate*, 15, 53(1), pp. 65-68.

Martel, C., Rhéaume, E., Takahashi, M., Trudel, C., Couët, J., Luu-The, V., Simard, J §, Labrie, F. (1992). Distribution of 17 beta-hydroxysteroid dehydrogenase gene expression and activity in rat and human tissues. *The Journal of Steroid Biochemistry and Molecular Bioloy*, 41(3-8), pp. 597-603.

Marijanovic, Z., Laubner, D., Moller, G., Gege, C., Husen, B., Adamski, J. § Breitling, R. (2003). Closing the gap: identification of human 3-ketosteroid reductase, the last unknown enzyme of mammalian cholesterol biosynthesis. *Molecular Endocrinology*, 17, pp. 1715-1725.

Markus, M., Husen, B., Leenders, F., Jungblut, P.W., Hall, P.F. § Adamski, J. (1995). The organelles containing porcine 17 beta-estradiol dehydrogenase are peroxisomes. *European Journal of Cell Biology*, 68, pp. 263-267.

McKeever, B.M., Hawkins, B.K., Geissler, W.M.,Wu, L., Sheridan, R.P., Mosley, R.T.§ Andersson. S.(2002). Amino acid substitution of arginine 80 in 17beta-hydroxysteroid dehydrogenase type 3 and its effect on NADPH cofactor binding and oxidation/reduction kinetics. *Biochimica and Biophysica Acta*, 1601, pp. 29-37.

Mendonca, B.B., Inacio, M., Arnhold, I.J., Costa, E.M., Bloise, W., Martin, R.M., Denes, F.T., Silva, F.A., Andersson, S., Lindqvist, A., § Wilson, J.D. (2000). Male pseudohermaphroditism due to 17beta-hydroxysteroid dehydrogenase 3 deficiency. Diagnosis, psychological evaluation, and management. Medicine (Baltimore), 79, pp. 299-309.

Miller, W.L., Huang, N., Pandey, A.V., Flück, C.E. § Agrawal, V. (2005). P450 oxidoreductase deficiency: a new disorder of steroidogenesis. *Annals of the New York Academy Science*, 1061, pp. 100-108.

Moghrabi, N. , Hughes, I.A., Dunaif, A. § Andersson, S. (1998). Deleterious missense mutations and silent polymorphism in the human 17betahydroxysteroid dehydrogenase 3 gene (HSD17B3). *The Journal of Clinical § Endocrinology Metabolism*, 83, pp. 2855–2860.

Moeller, G. § Adamski. (2009). Integrated view on 17beta-hydroxysteroid dehydrogenases. *Molecular and Cellular Endocrinology*, 301, pp. 7–19.

Money, J., Hampson, J.G. § Hampson, .JL. (1955). Hermaphroditism: recommendations concerning assignment of sex, c   hange of sex and psychologic management. *Bulletin of the Johns Hopkins Hospital*, 97, pp. 284–300.

Pang, S.Y., Softness, B., Sweeney, W.J. 3rd § New, M.I. (1987). Hirsutism, polycystic ovarian disease, and ovarian 17- ketosteroid reductase deficiency. *The New England Journal of Medicine*, 316(21), pp. 1295-301.

Parisi, M.A., Ramsdell, L.A., Burns, M.W., Carr, M.C., Grady, R.E., Gunther, D.F., Kletter, G.B., Mc-Cauley, E., Mitchell, M.E., Opheim, K.E., Pihoker, C., Richards, G.E., Soules, M.R. § Pagon, R.A. (2007). A gender assessment team: experience with 250 patients over a period of 25 years. *Genetics in Medicine* 2007; 9: 348–357

Payne, A.H. § Hales, D.B. (2004). Overview of steroidogenic enzymes in the pathway from cholesterol to active steroid hormones. *Endocrine Review*, 25(6), pp. 947-970.

Prehn, C., Moller, G. § Adamski, J. (2009). Recent advances in 17beta-hydroxysteroid dehydrogenases. *The Journal of Steroid Biochemistry and Molecular  Biology*, 114, pp. 72–77.

Qiu, W., Zhou, M., Labrie, F. § Lin, S.X. (2004). Crystal structures of the multispecific 17beta-hydroxysteroid dehydrogenase type 5: critical androgen regulation in human peripheral tissues. *Molecular Endocrinology*, 18, pp. 1798–1807.

Quigley, C.A., De Bellis, A., Marschke, K.B., el-Awady, M.K., Wilson, E.M. § French, F.S. (1995). Androgen receptor defects: historical, clinical, and molecular perspectives. *Endocrine Review*, 16(3), pp. 271-321.

Rogers, D.G., Chasalow, F.I. § Blethen, S.L. (1985). Partial deficiency in 17-ketosteroid reductase presenting as gynecomastia. *Steroids*, 45(2), pp. 195-200.

Rosler, A., Belanger, A. § Labrie, F. (1992). Mechanisms of androgen production in male pseudohermaphroditism due to 17 beta-hydroxysteroid dehydrogenase deficiency. *The Journal of Clinical § Endocrinology Metabolism*, 75(3), pp. 773-778.

Rosler, A., Silverstein, S. § Abeliovich, D. (1996). A (R80Q) mutation in 17 beta-hydroxysteroid dehydrogenase type 3 gene among Arabs of Israel is associated with pseudohermaphroditism in males and normal asymptomatic females. *The Journal of Clinical § Endocrinology Metabolism*, 81, pp. 1827–1831.

Rosler, A. (2006). 17 beta-hydroxysteroid dehydrogenase 3 deficiency in the Mediterranean population. *Pediatric Endocrinology Reviews*, 3(suppl 3), pp. 455–461.

Saez, J.M., De Peretti, E., Morera, A.M., David, M. § Bertrand, J. (1971). Familial male pseudohermaphroditism with gynecomastia due to a testicular 17-ketosteroid reductase defect. I. Studies in vivo. *The Journal of Clinical   Endocrinology § Metabolism*, 32, pp. 604–610.

Sinnecker, G.H., Hiort, O., Dibbelt, L., Albers, N., Dorr, H.G., Hauss, H., Heinrich, U., Hemminghaus, M., Hoepffner, W., Holder, M., Schnabel, D. § Kruse, K. (1996). Phenotypic classification of male pseudohermaphroditism due to steroid 5 alpha-reductase 2 deficiency. *American Journal of Medical Genetics*, 63, pp. 223–230.

Stewart, P.M. § Sheppard, M.C. (1992). Novel aspects of hormone action: intracellular ligand supply and its control by a series of tissue specific enzymes. *Molecular and Cellular Endocrinology*, 83(2-3), pp. C13-18.

Taranger, J., Engström, I., Lichtenstein, H., Svennberg-Redegren, I.VI. (1976). Somatic pubertal development. *Acta Paediatrica Scandiva*, 258, pp. 121-135.

Thyen, U., Lanz, K., Holterhus, P.M. § Hiort, O. (2006). Epidemiology and initial management of ambiguous genitalia at birth in Germany. *Hormone Research*, 66, pp.195–203.

Tong, S.Y., Hutson, J.M. § Watts, L.M. (1996). Does testosterone diffuse down the wolffian duct during sexual differentiation? *Journal of Urology*, 155, pp. 2057–2059.

Twesten, W., Holterhus, P., Sippell, W.G., Morlot, M., Schumacher, H., Schenk, B. § Hiort, O. (2000). Clinical, endocrine, and molecular genetic findings in patients with 17beta-hydroxysteroid dehydrogenase deficiency. *Hormone Research*, 53, pp. 26–31.

Ulloa-Aguirre, A., Bassol, S., Poo, J., Mendez, J.P., Mutchinick, O., Robles, C. § Perez-Palacios, G. (1985). Endocrine and biochemical studies in a 46,XY phenotypically male infant with 17-ketosteroid reductase deficiency. *The Journal of Clinical Endocrinology § Metabolism*, 60, pp. 639–643.

Van Poucke, C., Van De Velde, M. § Van Peteghem, C. (2005). Combination of liquid chromatography/tandemmass spectrometry and gas chromatography/mass spectrometry for the detection of 21 anabolic steroid residues in bovine urine. *Journal of Mass spectrometry*, 40(6), pp. 731-738.

Whitney, A.R., Diehn, M., Popper, S.J., Alizadeh, A.A., Boldrick, J.C., Relman, D.A. § Brown, P.O. (2003). Individuality and variation in gene expression patterns in human blood. *Proceedings of the National Academy of Sciences USA*, 100, pp.1896-1901.

Wilson, J.D. (1978). Sexual differentiation. *Annual Review of Physiology*, 40, pp. 279–306.

Wilson, J.D., Griffin, J.E.§ Russell, D.W. (1993). Steroid 5 alpha-reductase 2 deficiency. *Endocrine Review*, 14(5), pp. 577-93. Wilson, J.D. (1999). The role of androgens in male gender role behavior. *Endocrine Review*, 20(5) pp. 726-737.

Wiesemann, C., Ude-Koeller, S., Sinnecker, G.H. § Thyen, U. (2010). Ethical principles and recommendations for the medical management of differences of sex development (DSD)/intersex in children and adolescents. *European Journal of Pediatrics*, 169, pp. 671–679

Wu, L., Einstein, M., Geissler, W.M., Chan, H.K., Elliston, K.O. § Andersson, S. (1993). Expression cloning and characterization of human 17 betahydroxysteroid dehydrogenase type 2, a microsomal enzyme possessing 20 alphahydroxysteroid dehydrogenase activity. *The Journal of Biological Chemistry*, 268, pp.12964–12969.

Xiaofei, D., Rosenfeld, R.L. § Quin, K. (2006). Molecular mechanisms regulating basal expression of 17–β hydroxysteroid dehydrogenase type 3 (HSD17B3) gene promoter in Leydig cells. In: Endocrine, Boston, P1-372.

# 7

# Dehydroepiandrosterone in Nonalcoholic Fatty Liver Disease

Yoshio Sumida[1] et al.*
*[1]Center for Digestive and Liver Diseases, Nara City Hospital,
Japan*

## 1. Introduction

Nonalcoholic fatty liver disease (NAFLD) is the most common chronic liver disease (CLD) in many developed countries and results in a serious public health problem worldwide. NAFLD includes a wide spectrum of liver diseases, ranging from simple fatty liver, which is usually a benign and nonprogressive condition, to nonalcoholic steatohepatitis (NASH) which may progress to liver cirrhosis (LC), hepatic failure and hepatocellular carcinoma (HCC) in the absence of significant alcohol consumption (Ludwig et al., 1980, Matteoni et al. 1999). About a third of people with NAFLD will develop NASH, and about 20% of people with NASH will go on to liver fibrosis and cirrhosis, with its accompanying risk of liver failure and even HCC (Yasui et al. 2011). In Japan, current best estimates make the prevalence of NAFLD approximately 20% and of NASH 2% to 3% in the general population. Pathophysiology of primary NASH still hasn't been completely clarified. According to the "two-hits" model of NASH pathogenesis proposed by Day and James (Day & James. 1999), excessive triglyceride accumulation is the most likely first step. The second step may relate to an increase in oxidative stress (Sumida et al. 2011a), which, in turn, triggers liver cell necrosis and activation of hepatic stellate cells, both leading to fibrosis and ultimately to the development of LC. Although the number of NASH cases in women is known to be higher than in men over 50 years of age, the mechanisms remain unknown (Hashimoto & Tokushige, 2011). According to our study produced by Japan Study Group of NAFLD (JSG-NAFLD) including nine hepatology centers in Japan (Sumida et al., 2011b), NASH patients with significant or advanced fibrosis (Brunt stage 2-4) was more prevalent in females than in males (Fig.1). Although plausible mechanisms have been proposed, including estrogen deficiency after menopause, iron accumulation generating hydroxylradicals via Fenton reaction (Sumida et al., 2009), and so on, precise mechanisms have not been clarified. Although several factors have been associated with more advanced NAFLD, the biological basis of the histological diversity of severity of NAFLD [i.e., why some patients develop simple fatty liver and others develop NASH with advanced fibrosis] remains unknown. More advanced NAFLD is characterized by insulin resistance, oxidative stress, and advanced fibrosis.

* Kyoko Sakai[1], Tomoyuki Ohno[1], Kazuyuki Kanemasa[1], Yutaka Inada[2], Naohisa Yoshida[2],
Kohichiroh Yasui[2], Yoshito Itoh[2], Yuji Naito[2], Toshikazu Yoshikawa[2]
[1]Center for Digestive and Liver Diseases, Nara City Hospital, Japan
[2]Department of Gastroenterology and Hepatology, Kyoto Prefectural University of Medicine, Kyoto, Japan

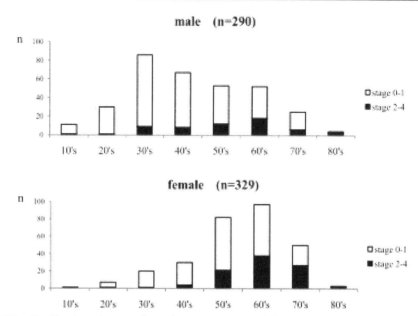

Fig. 1. The distribution of age and gender in patients with biopsy-proven NAFLD (n=619) according to fibrosis stage (stage 0-2 or stage 3-4) in Japan Study Group of NAFLD (JSG-NAFLD), including nine hepatology centers throughout Japan.

Endocrine hormones control cell metabolism and the distribution of body fat and, therefore, may contribute to the development of NAFLD/ NASH. Dehydroepiandrosterone (DHEA), and its interchangeable sulfated form, DHEA sulfate (DHEA-S), is the most abundant circulating steroid hormone and is produced primarily by the zona reticularis of the adrenal cortex in response to adrenocorticotropic hormone. DHEA has been known to have a variety of functions, including anti-oxidative stress, decreasing insulin resistance, anti-atherosclerosis, and anti-osteoporosis (Baulieu et al. 2000). DHEA-S concentration is independently and inversely related to death from any cause and death from cardiovascular disease in men over age 50. It has been postulated that DHEA and DHEA-S may be discriminators of life expectancy and aging (Phillips et al. 2010). In this chapter, we describe here the role of DHEA or DHEA-S in the pathogenesis or treatment of NAFLD.

## 2. NAFLD and dehydroepiandrosterone

### 2.1 What is dehydroepiandrosterone?
DHEA, and its interchangeable sulfated form, DHEA-S (Fig 2.), are the most abundant circulating steroid hormone in healthy individuals. They are produced from cholesterol by the zona reticularis of the adrenal cortex. DHEA is produced from cholesterol through two cytochrome P450 enzymes. Cholesterol is converted to pregnenolone by the enzyme P450 scc (side chain cleavage); then another enzyme, CYP17A1, converts pregnenolone to 17α-Hydroxypregnenolone and then to DHEA. (Fig 3) (Arlt, 2004). DHEA is made primarily in the adrenal glands (which also produce about 150 other hormones) and released into the blood. In different organs it is converted into a variety of more commonly known steroid

hormones, including androstenedione, testosterone, and estrogen. DHEA and DHEA-S levels peak at approximately age 25 years and decrease progressively thereafter, falling to 5% of peak levels by the ninth decade. DHEA is a potential mediator of ROS synthesis (Bednarek-Tupikowska et al., 2000) and has also been reported to augment insulin sensitivity (Lasco et al., 2001, Jakubowicz et al., 1995, Kawano, 2000, Dhatariya et al., 2005) and peroxisome proliferator activation. (Poynter & Daynes, 1998, Peters et al., 1996), a transcription factor that regulates lipid metabolism, and procollagen type I, collagen precursor that has been associated with hepatic fibrosis of NASH. Both cross-sectional and longitudinal data have clearly indicated that serum concentrations of DHES-S decrease with age. Advocates of DHEA recommend it to prevent the effects of aging.

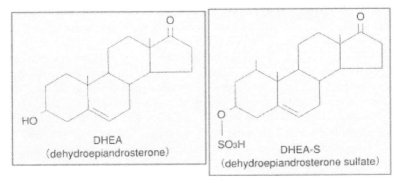

Fig. 2. DHEA and DHEA-S

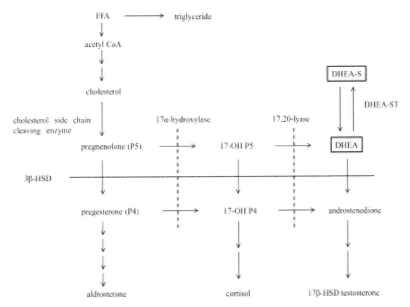

Fig. 3. Synthesis pathway of DHEA and DHEA-S

## 2.2 The significance of serum DHEA-S levels

Whereas DHEA levels naturally reach their peak in the early morning hours, DHEAS levels show no diurnal variation. From a practical point of view, measurement of DHEAS is preferable to DHEA, as levels are more stable. The Baltimore Longitudinal Study of Aging (BLSA) is a multidisciplinary observational study of the physiological and psychological aspects of human aging and diseases and conditions that increase with age. In BLSA, men who had higher DHEAS levels had significantly greater longevity than men with lower levels. (Roth et al., 2002) In Japan, a 27-year study in a community-based cohort (Tanushimaru study) indicated that DHEAS level may be a predictor of longevity in men, independent of age, blood pressure, and plasma glucose (Enomoto et al, 2008). Low serum levels of DHEA(-S) predict death from all causes, cardiovascular disease, and ischemic heart disease in elderly Swedish men. (Ohlsson et al., 2010) On the basis of these results, serum DHEA level is known to be an indicator of longevity at least in men and is often determined in anti-aging checkups (Nishizaki et al., 2009) . Elevated levels of DHEA are found in patients with Cushing syndrome or congenital adrenal hyperplasia, while DHEA levels are reported to be low in some people with anorexia, end-stage kidney disease, type 2 diabetes, AIDS, adrenal insufficiency, and in the critically ill. Some studies suggested that low serum DHEA-S levels were associated with the metabolic syndrome (Muller et al., 2005, Chen et al., 2010). In contrast, several studies found that DHEA levels are not different between subjects with metabolic syndrome and without. (Fukui et al., 2007, Haring et al., 2009, Akishita et al., 2010) It is suggested that age per se is an important correlate of the associations between DHEA-S and metabolic variables. In this way, the previous studies regarding the association between endogenous DHEA-S level and metabolic syndrome are inconsistent. Previous studies have shown that diabetic patients with high serum levels of insulin have lower serum levels of DHEA and DHEA-S. (Yamaguchi et al., 1998). A negative correlation between DHEA and hyperinsulinemia has been repeatedly demonstrated. (Kauffman et al., 2006, Saygili et al., 2005, Vasarhelyi et al., 2003). Fukui and colleagues reported that low levels of DHEA are associated with atherosclerosis and deterioration of urinary albumin excretion in male patients with type 2 diabetes (Fukui et al., 2004, 2005, 2006). Similarly, Serum DHEA-S level seem to be associated with atherosclerosis in diabetic postmenopausal women independent of age, body stature, diabetic status, and other atherosclerotic risk factors (Kanazawa et al., 2008).

## 2.3 DHEA-S levels in NAFLD

Recently, Charlton *et al.* observed that levels of DHEA are significantly lower in patients with histologically advanced NASH, as compared with patients with mild NASH or simple fatty liver. (Charlton M, 2009). DHEA levels exert a good sensitivity and specificity in discriminating patients with more advanced histological disease, as shown by the receiver operating characteristic (ROC) analysis. To validate their results, we also determined circulating DHEA levels in Japanese patients with 133 biopsy-proven NAFLD. Of 133 patients, 90 patients were diagnosed as NASH: 73 patients had stage 0–2, and 17 had stage 3 or 4. In addition, 399 sex- and age-matched healthy people participating in health checkups who had normal levels of alanine aminotransferase (ALT) levels (≤ 30 IU/L) were also enrolled as the control group. Body mass index (BMI), aspartate aminotransferase (AST), ALT, γGT, triglyceride, and HOMA-IR were significantly higher in NAFLD patients than those in the control group, whereas serum DHEA-S levels were similar between both groups. Consistent with our result, in patients with polycystic ovary syndrome (PCOS), DHEA-S levels were similar between those with NAFLD and without. (Kauffman et al., 2010). According to a cross-sectional population-based study derived from data of 1912 men, however, the highest risk of hepatic steatosis was found in subjects with the highest serum DHEA-S levels (Völzke H et al., 2010). DHEA and DHEAS levels of post menopausal women with fatty liver were greater than those of post menopausal women with normal histology. (Saruç et al., 2003) These results are contrast to our study. Discrepancies between these studies and ours might be explained by differences in the selection of subjects, sex, size of the study populations and ethnicity.

Only in our NAFLD patients, NASH patients had lower levels of serum DHEA-S levels compared to non-NASH patients (Fig 4). Serum DHEA levels were negative correlated with age in males and females (Fig 5). A " dose effect " of lower DHEA-S and advanced fibrosis was observed, with a mean DHEA-S of 170.4±129.2, 137.6±110.5, 96.2±79.3, 61.2±46.3, and

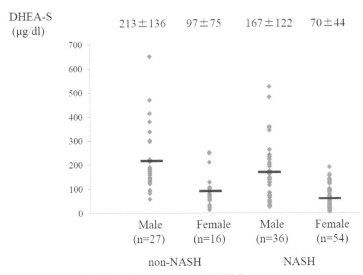

Fig. 4. Serum DHEA levels in biopsy-proven NAFLD.

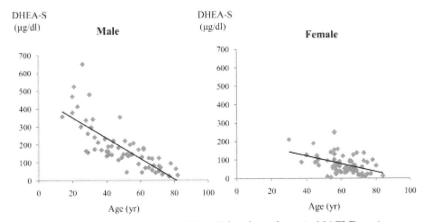

Fig. 5. The relationship between serum DHEA-S levels and age in NAFLD patients

30.0±32.0, for fibrosis stages 0, 1, 2, 3 and 4, respectively. The area under the ROC curve for DHEA in separating patients with and without advanced fibrosis was 0.788. The sensitivity of a DHEA-S-value of 66 mg/dL or less for the presence of more advanced NAFLD was 76.5% and specificity was 73.3% (85/116) (Fig 6)(Sumida et al., 2010a). Our data suggest that patients with DHEA-S levels greater than 66 µg/dL are highly unlikely to have advanced NAFLD (4/89 patients, sensitivity 76% and specificity 73%). Multivariate logistic regression analyses found that serum level of DHEA-S below 66µg/ml was selected as an independent predictor for advanced fibrosis even after adjusting for age, gender and insulin resistance (Table 1). We intended to support the concept that the association between low levels of DHEA and worsening histology is independent of age, sex and insulin resistance. Decreased levels of DHEA can have important roles in the progression hepatic fibrosis in NAFLD. It is expected that determinant of serum DHEA become a predictor of hepatic fibrosis in NAFLD. A 53-year female who had been pointed out her fatty liver without any medications was referred to our hospital because of thrombocytopenia (platelet count $4.6×10^4$/µl). Her BMI was 31.6kg/m² and she had mildly elevated transaminase activities (AST 61IU/l, ALT 59IU/l) and prolonged prothrombin time (66%). Laparoscopic findings revealed nodular liver and her liver histology showed NASH (Brunt grade 3, stage 4) (Fig 7). Her DHEA-S levels was the lowest (5µg/dl) among our NAFLD patients.

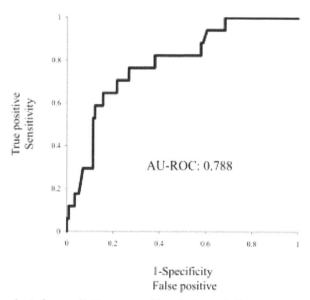

Fig. 6. ROC analysis for predicting severe fibrosis (stage 3-4).

Free fatty acids (FFAs), which lead to oxidative stress in NASH, are the major source of DHEA (Fig 3). The inability to produce appropriate amounts of DHEA in response to FFAs may translate into a more rapid and worsening progression toward NASH (Manco et al., 2008). Serum DHEA-S levels depend on adrenal DHEA production and its hepatic metabolism mediated by DHEA sulfotransferase (DHEA-ST) which catalyzes sulfonation of DHEA to form DHEA-S. It is hypothesized that a low level of DHEA-S was due to a defect in sulfurylation in patients with hepatic cirrhosis, since DHEA-ST is synthesized in the liver

| Variables | Odds ratio | 95% confidence interval | P-value |
|---|---|---|---|
| DHEA-S ≦66 μg/dl | 4.9549 | 1.1691-20.9996 | 0.0229 |
| age≧65 yr | 2.8962 | 0.7843-10.6948 | 0.1106 |
| sex (female) | 1.9494 | 0.3765-10.0935 | 0.4264 |
| HOMA-IR≧5 | 2.3671 | 0.6276-8.9273 | 0.2033 |
| BMI ≧28 kg/m² | 1.0446 | 0.2619-4.1658 | 0.9508 |
| Diabetes | 1.6007 | 0.3904-6.5023 | 0.5107 |
| Dyslipidemia | 0.2500 | 0.0682-0.9162 | 0.0364 |
| Hypertension | 0.4184 | 0.1022-1.7126 | 0.2256 |

HOMA-IR, homeostasis assessment model for insulin resistance; BMI, body mass index

Table 1. Logistic regression models of the association of NAFLD (advanced versus mild) with dehydroepiandrosterone sulfate (DHEA-S) levels and other clinical variables

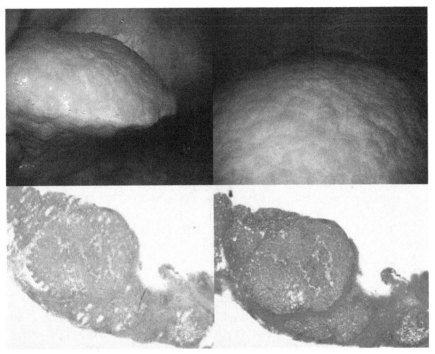

Fig. 7. Laparoscopic findings and liver histology of a case of NASH-LC who was referred to Center for Digestive and Liver Diseases, Nara City Hospital. A: laparoscopy (lt lobe), B: laparoscopy (rt lobe), C: microscopy (HE stain), D: microscopy (Masson-trichrome stain).

(Franz et al., 1979). It was also important to consider whether low levels of DHEA-S might occur as a result of CLD in general versus a specific phenomenon of histologically more advanced NAFLD.

Nakajima T et al revealed that telomere shortening, a marker of senescence, could be associated with hepatic steatosis, insulin resistance, oxidative stress in the liver, and impaired regenerative response in NAFLD patients (Nakajima et al., 2006). The hepatic expression of senescence marker protein-30 (SMP30), which was identified as an antioxidant and anti-apoptotic protein, decreased in the proportion of the hepatic fibrosis in NAFLD patients (Park et al., 2010). These results suggest that the association of aging with NASH pathogenesis is noteworthy.

### 2.4 DHEA as a candidate for the treatment of NASH

There is no specific established treatment for NASH. Management of NASH consists of lifestyle modification including a healthy diet and physical exercise. DHEA has been widely touted as an anti-aging supplement. For years DHEA was promoted as a miracle weight loss drug, based upon some rodent studies that indicated DHEA was effective in controlling obesity in rats and mice. Other rodent studies found similar promising results for DHEA in preventing cancer, arteriosclerosis and diabetes. A randomized, double-blind, placebo-controlled trial showed that DHEA replacement therapy significantly decreases not only in visceral fat area and subcutaneous fat area, but also in insulin resistance. (Villareal & Holloszy, 2004). In contrast, DHEA replacement has no detectable effect on body composition, physical performance, insulin action, or quality of life (Nair et al., 2006). Therapeutic benefits of hormone supplementation for the treatment of aging, insulin resistance and cardiovascular disease remain obscure and controversial. DHEA can cause higher than normal levels of androgens and estrogens in the body, and theoretically may increase the risk of prostate, breast, ovarian, and other hormone-sensitive cancers. A protective effect of DHEA was reported in an orotic acid-induced animal model of fatty liver disease (Goto et al., 1998). Since the clinical usefulness of DHEA for NAFLD patients has never been investigated, there is a great need for prospective, randomized, multicenter and well-designed trials.

## 3. Conclusion

Recent studies have demonstrated that more advanced NAFLD, as indicated by the presence of NASH with advanced fibrosis stage, is strongly associated with low circulating DHEA-S. Although NASH patients with severe fibrosis are frequently observed in aged-female patients, the precise mechanisms of this phenomenon remain to be resolved. Lower levels of serum DHEA in females compared to in males may contribute to the fibrosis progression of NASH. There are thus several potential mechanisms for DHEA deficiency to promote histological progression in NAFLD. DHEA deficiency presents an appealing new therapeutic target for the treatment and prevention of NASH. Since the association of NAFLD with endocrine diseases such as hypothyroidism (Liangpunsakul & Chalasani, 2003), adult growth hormone deficiency (Takahashi et al. 2007), and PCOS (Baranova et al. 2011) has recently been suggested, the pathogenesis of NASH should be explored in the view of anti-aging medicine or endocrinology (Loria et al.,2010).

## 4. Acknowledgment

This study was supported by a Grant from the Chiyoda Mutual Life Foundation.

## 5. References

Akishita, M. & Fukai, S. & Hashimoto, M. & Kameyama, Y. & Nomura, K. & Nakamura, T. & Ogawa, S. & Iijima, K. & Eto, M. & Ouchi ,Y. (2010). Association of low testosterone with metabolic syndrome and its components in middle-aged Japanese men. *Hypertens Res* Vol.33, No.6, pp. 587-591

Arlt W. (2004). Dehydroepiandrosterone and ageing. *Best Pract Resn Clin Endocrinol Metab* Vo.18, No.3, pp. 363-380.

Baranova, A. & Tran TP. & Birerdinc A. & Younossi ZM. (2011). Systematic review: association of polycystic ovary syndrome with metabolic syndrome and non-alcoholic fatty liver disease. Aliment Pharmacol Ther Vol. 33, No.7, pp. 801-814.

Baulieu, EE. &Thomas, G. & Legrain, S . & Lahlou, N. & Roger, M. & Debuire, B. & Faucounau, V. & Girard, L. & Hervy, MP. & Latour, F. & Leaud, MC. & Mokrane, A. & Pitti-Ferrandi, H. & Trivalle, C. & de Lacharrière, O. & Nouveau, S. & Rakoto-Arison, B. & Souberbielle, JC. & Raison, J. & Le Bouc, Y. & Raynaud, A. & Girerd, X. & Forette F. (2000). Dehydroepiandrosterone (DHEA), DHEA sulfate, and aging: contribution of the DHEAge Study to a sociobiomedical issue. *Proc Natl Acad Sci U S A* Vol. 97, No. 8, pp. 4279-4284.

Bednarek-Tupikowska, G. & Gosk, I. & Szuba, A. &Bohdanowicz-Pawlak, A. & Kosowska, B. & Bidzinska B, et al. (2006). Influence of dehydroepiandrosterone on platelet aggregation, superoxide dismutase activity and serum lipid peroxide concentrations in rabbits with induced hypercholesterolemia. *Med SciMonit* Vol. 6, No.1, pp. 40-45.

Charlton M. & Angulo, P. & Chalasani, N. & Merriman, R. & Viker, K. & Charatcharoenwitthaya, P. & Sanderson, S. & Gawrieh, S. & Krishnan, A. & Lindor K (2008). Low circulating levels of dehydroepiandrosterone in histologically advanced nonalcoholic fatty liver disease. *Hepatology* Vo. 47, No.2, pp. 484-492.

Chen, YC. & Chang, HH. & Wen, CJ. & Lin, WY. & Chen, CY. & Hong, BS. & Huang KC. (2010). Elevated serum dehydroepiandrosterone sulphate level correlates with increased risk for metabolic syndrome in the elderly men. *Eur J Clin Invest* Vo. 40, No.3, 220-225.

Day, CP. & James, OF. (1998). Steatohepatitis: a tale of two "hits"? *Gastroenterology* Vol. 114, No.4, pp. 842-845.

Dhatariya, K. & Bigelow, ML. & Nair, KS. (2005). Effect of dehydroepiandrosterone replacement on insulin sensitivity and lipids in hypoadrenal women. *Diabetes* Vol. 54, No.3, pp. 765-769.

Enomoto, M. & Adachi, H. & Fukami, A. & Furuki, K. & Satoh, A. & Otsuka, M. & Kumagae, S. & Nanjo, Y. & Shigetoh, Y. & Imaizumi T. (2008). Serum dehydroepiandrosterone sulfate levels predict longevity in men: 27-year follow-up study in a community-based cohort (Tanushimaru study). *J Am Geriatr Soc* Vol. 56, No.6, pp. 994-998.

Franz, C. & Watson, D. & Longcope, C. (1979). Estrone sulfate and dehydroepiandrosterone sulfate concentrations in normal subjects and men with cirrhosis. *Steroids* Vol, 34, No.5, pp. 563–573.

Fukui, M. & Kitagawa, Y. & Nakamura, N. & Kadono, M. & Hasegawa, G. & Yoshikawa T. (2004). Association between urinary albumin excretion and serum dehydroepiandrosterone sulfate concentration in male patients with type 2 diabetes: a possible link between urinary albumin excretion and cardiovascular disease. *Diabetes Care* Vol. 27, No.12, pp. 2893-2897.

Fukui, M. & Kitagawa, Y. & Nakamura, N. & Kadono, M. & Yoshida, M. & Hirata, C. & Wada, K. & Hasegawa, G. & Yoshikawa T. (2005). Serum dehydroepiandrosterone sulfate concentration and carotid atherosclerosis in men with type 2 diabetes. *Atherosclerosis* Vol. 181, No.2, pp. 339-344

Fukui, M. & Kitagawa, Y. & Kamiuchi, K. & Hasegawa, G. & Yoshikawa, T. & Nakamura, N. (2006). Low serum dehydroepiandrosterone sulfate concentration is a predictor for deterioration of urinary albumin excretion in male patients with type 2 diabetes. *Diabetes Res Clin Pract*, Vol. 73, No.1, pp. 47-50.

Fukui, M. & Ose, H. & Kitagawa, Y. & Kamiuchi, K. & Nakayama, I. & Ohta, M. Obayashi, H. & Yamasaki, M. & Hasegawa, G. & Yoshikawa, T. & Nakamura, N. (2007). Metabolic syndrome is not associated with markers of subclinical atherosclerosis, serum adiponectin and endogenous androgen concentrations in Japanese men with Type 2 diabetes. *Diabet Med* Vo. 24, No. 8, pp. 864-871

Goto, H. & Yamashita, S. & Makita T. (1998). Preventive effects of dehydroepiandrosterone acetate on the fatty liver induced by orotic acid in male rats. *Exp Anim* Vol. 47, No.4, pp. 257-260.

Haring, R. & Völzke, H. & Felix, SB. & Schipf, S. & Dörr, M. & Rosskopf, D. & Nauck, M. & Schöfl, C. &Wallaschofski, H. (2009). Prediction of metabolic syndrome by low serum testosterone levels in men: results from the study of health in Pomerania. *Diabetes* Vol. 58, No. 9, pp. 2027-2031.

Hashimoto, E. &Tokushige, K. (2011). Prevalence, gender, ethnic variations, and prognosis of NASH. *J Gastroenterol* Vo. 46, No. Suppl 1, pp. 63-69.

Jakubowicz, D. & Beer, N. & Rengifo R. (1995). Effect of dehydroepiandrosterone on cyclic-guanosine monophosphate in men of advancing age. *Ann N Y Acad Sci* Vol. 774, pp. 312-315.

Kanazawa, I. & Yamaguchi, T. & Yamamoto, M. & Yamauchi, M. & Kurioka, S. & Yano, S. & Sugimoto T. (2008). Serum DHEA-S level is associated with the presence of atherosclerosis in postmenopausal women with type 2 diabetes mellitus. *Endocr J* Vol. 55, No. 4, pp. 667-675.

Kauffman, RP. & Baker, VM. & DiMarino, P. & Castracane, VD. (2006). Hyperinsulinemia and circulating dehydroepiandrosterone sulfate in white and Mexican American women with polycystic ovary syndrome. *Fertil Steril, Vol.* 85, No.4, pp. 1010-1016.

Kauffman, RP. & Baker, TE. & Baker, V. & Kauffman, MM. & Castracane, VD. (2010). Endocrine factors associated with non-alcoholic fatty liver disease in women with polycystic ovary syndrome: do androgens play a role? *Gynecol Endocrinol* Vo. 26, No. 1, pp. 39-46

Kawano, M. (2000). Complement regulatory proteins and autoimmunity. *Arch Immunol Ther Exp (Warsz)* Vol.48, No.5, pp.367-372.

Lasco, A. & Frisina, N. & Morabito, N. & Gaudio, A. & Morini, E. & Trifiletti A, et al. (2001). Metabolic effects of dehydroepiandrosterone replacement therapy in post-menopausal women. *Eur J Endocrinol* Vol. 145, No.4, pp. 457-461.

Liangpunsakul, S. & Chalasani N.(2003). Is hypothyroidism a risk factor for non-alcoholic steatohepatitis? J Clin Gastroenterol Vol. 37, No.4, pp. 340-343.

Loria, P. & Carulli, L. & Bertolotti, M. & Lonardo, A. (2009). Endocrine and liver interaction: the role of endocrine pathways in NASH. *Nat Rev Gastroenterol Hepatol* Vol. 6, No.4, pp. 236-247.

Ludwig, J. & Viggiano, TR. & McGill, DB. & Oh BJ. (1980). Nonalcoholic steatohepatitis: Mayo Clinic experiences with a hitherto unnamed disease. *Mayo Clin Proc* Vol.55, No. 7, pp. 434-438.

Manco, M. & Bottazzo G. (2008). Does the hormone of eternal youth protect against nonalcoholic steatohepatitis? *Hepatology* Vo. 48, No.4, pp. 1351.

Matteoni, CA. & Younossi, ZM. & Gramlich, T. *et al.* (1999). Nonalcoholic fatty liver diseases: a spectrum of clinical and pathological severity. *Gastroenterology* Vol. 116, No.6, pp. 1413-1419.

Muller, M. & Grobbee, DE. & den Tonkelaar, I. & Lamberts SW. & van der Schouw, YT. (2005) Endogenous sex hormones and metabolic syndrome in aging men. *Journal of Clinical Endocrinology and Metabolism* Vol. 90, No.5, pp. 2618-2623.

Nair, KS. & Rizza, RA. & O'Brien P. & Dhatariya, K. & Short, KR. & Nehra, A. & Vittone, JL. & Klee, GG. & Basu, A. & Basu, R. & Cobelli, C. & Toffolo, G. & Dalla Man, C. & Tindall, DJ. &, Melton, LJ 3rd. & Smith, GE. & Khosla, S. & Jensen, MD. (2006). DHEA in elderly women and DHEA or testosterone in elderly men. *N Engl J Med* Vol. 355, No.16, pp. 1647-1659.

Nakajima, T. & Moriguchi, M. & Katagishi, T. & (2006). Premature telomere shortening and impaired regenerative response in hepatocytes of individuals with NAFLD. *Liver Int* No. 26, No.1, pp. 23-31.

Nishizaki, Y. & Kuwahira, I. & Kawada, H. & Kubo, A. . & Kataoka, K. & Tanaka, S. & Sueno, T. & Isozaki, M. & Kobayashi, H. & Nakamura, Y. & Tanino, R. & Ishii, N. & Inoko H. (2009). Beneficial effects of medical advice provided to elderly persons under the anti-aging health check-up system at Tokai University Tokyo Hospital. *Tokai J Exp Clin Med* Vo. 34, No. 4, pp. 142-151.

Ohlsson, C. & Labrie, F. & Barrett-Connor, E. & Karlsson, MK. & Ljunggren, O. & Vandenput, L. & Mellström, D. & Tivesten, A. (2010). Low serum levels of dehydroepiandrosterone sulfate predict all-cause and cardiovascular mortality in elderly Swedish men. *J Clin Endocrinol Metab* Vo. 95, No. 9, pp. 4406-4414.

Park, H. & Ishigami, A. & Shima, T. & Mizuno, M. & Maruyama, N. & Yamaguchi, K. & Mitsuyoshi, H. & Minami, M. & Yasui, K. & Itoh, Y. & Yoshikawa, T. & Fukui, M. & Hasegawa, G. & Nakamura, N. & Ohta M. & Obayashi, H. & Okanoue T. (2010). Hepatic senescence marker protein-30 is involved in the progression of nonalcoholic fatty liver disease. *J Gastroenterol* Vol. 45, No.4, pp. 426-434.

Peters, JM. & Zhou, YC. & Ram, PA. & Lee, SS. & Gonzalez, FJ. &Waxman DJ. (1996). Peroxisome proliferator-activated receptor alpha required for gene induction by dehydroepiandrosterone-3 beta-sulfate. *Mol Pharmacol* Vol.50, No.1, pp. 67-74.

Phillips, AC. & Carroll, D. & Gale, CR. & Lord, JM. & Arlt, W. & Batty GD.(2010). Cortisol, DHEAS, their ratio and the metabolic syndrome: evidence from the Vietnam Experience Study. *Eur J Endocrinol* Vo. 162, No.5, 919-923.

Poynter, ME. & Daynes, RA. (1998). Peroxisome proliferator-activated receptor alpha activation modulates cellular redox status, represses nuclear factor-kappaB signaling, and reduces inflammatory cytokine production in aging. *J Biol Chem* Vo. 273, No.49, pp. 32833-32841.

Roth, GS. & Lane, MA. . & Ingram, DK. & Mattison, JA. & Elahi, D. & Tobin, JD. & Muller, D. & Metter, EJ. (2002). Biomarkers of caloric restriction may predict longevity in humans. *Science* Vo. 297, No. 5582, pp. 811.

Saruç, M. & Yüceyar, H. & Ayhan, S. & Türkel, N. & Tuzcuoglu, I. & Can M. (2003). The association of dehydroepiandrosterone, obesity, waist-hip ratio and insulin resistance with fatty liver in postmenopausal women--a hyperinsulinemic euglycemic insulin clamp study. *Hepatogastroenterology,* vol.50, No.51, pp. 771-774.

Saygili F, Oge A, Yilmaz C. (2005). Hyperinsulinemia and insulin insensitivity in women with nonclassical congenital adrenal hyperplasia due to 21-hydroxylase deficiency:

the relationship between serum leptin levels and chronic hyperinsulinemia. *Horm Res*, Vol.63, No.6, pp.270-274.

Sumida, Y. & Yoshikawa, T. & Okanoue T. (2009). Role of hepatic iron in non-alcoholic steatohepatitis. *Hepatol Res* Vol. 39, No.3, pp. 213-222.

Sumida, Y. & Yonei, Y. & Kanemasa, K. et al. (2010). Lower circulating levels of dehydroepiandrosterone, independent of insulin resistance, is an important determinant of severity of nonalcoholic steatohepatitis in Japanese patients. *Hepatol Res* Vo. 40, No.9, pp. 901-910.

Sumida, Y. & Eguchi, Y. & Ono, M. (2010). Current status and agenda in the diagnosis of nonalcoholic steatohepatitis in Japan. *World J Hepatol* Vol. 2, No.10, pp. 374-383.

Sumida, Y. & Naito, Y. & Yoshikawa, T. (2011). Free Radicals and nonalcoholic fatty liver disease (NAFLD)/nonalcoholic steatohepatitis (NASH). *Free Radical Biology in Digestive Diseases* Vol. 29, pp. 144-155.

Sumida, Y. & Yoneda, M. & Hyogo, H. & Yamaguchi, K. & Ono, M. & Fujii, H. & Eguchi, Y. & Suzuki Y. & Imai, S. & Kanemasa, K. & Fujita, K. & Chayama, K. & Yasui, K. & Saibara, T. & Kawada, N. & Fujimoto, K. & Kohgo, Y. & Okanoue, T. ; Japan Study Group of Nonalcoholic Fatty Liver Disease (JSG-NAFLD). (2011). A simple clinical scoring system using ferritin, fasting insulin, and type IV collagen 7S for predicting steatohepatitis in nonalcoholic fatty liver disease. *J Gastroenterol.* Vol. 46, No. 2, pp. 257-268.

Takahashi, Y. & Iida, K. & Takahashi, K. & Yoshioka, S. & Fukuoka, H. & Takeno, R. & Imanaka, M. & Nishizawa, H. & Takahashi, M. & Seo, Y. & Hayashi, Y. & Kondo, T. & Okimura, Y. & Kaji, H. & Kitazawa, R. & Kitazawa, S. & Chihara, K.(2007). Growth hormone reverses nonalcoholic steatohepatitis in a patient with adult growth hormone deficiency. Gastroenterology Vol.132, No.3, pp. 938-943.

Vasarhelyi, B. & Bencsik, P. & Treszl, A. & Bardoczy, Z. & Tulassay, T. & Szathmari M. (2003). The effect of physiologic hyperinsulinemia during an oral glucose tolerance test on the levels of dehydroepiandrosterone (DHEA) and its sulfate (DHEAS) in healthy young adults born with low and with normal birth weight. *Endocr J.* Dec Vol. 50, No. 6, pp. 689-695.

Villareal, DT. & Holloszy JO. (2004). Effect of DHEA on abdominal fat and insulin action in elderly women and men: a randomized controlled trial. *JAMA* Vol. 292, No.18, pp. 2243-2248.

Völzke, H. & Aumann, N. & Krebs, A. & Nauck, M. & Steveling, A. & Lerch, MM. & Rosskopf, D. & Wallaschofski H. (2010). Hepatic steatosis is associated with low serum testosterone and high serum DHEAS levels in men. *Int J Androl* Vol. 33, No.1, pp. 45-53.

Yamaguchi, Y. & Tanaka, S. & Yamakawa, T. & Kimura, M. & Ukawa, K. & Yamada, Y. & Ishihara, M. & Sekihara H.(1998). Reduced serum dehydroepiandrosterone levels in diabetic patients with hyperinsulinaemia. *Clin Endocrinol (Oxf)*, Vol. 49, No. 3, pp.377-383.

Yasui, K. & Hashimoto, E. & Komorizono, Y. & Koike, K. & Arii, S. & Imai, Y. & Shima, T. & Kanbara, Y. & Saibara, T. & Mori, T. & Kawata, S. & Uto, H. & Takami, S. & Sumida, Y. & Takamura, T. & Kawanaka, M. & Okanoue T; Japan NASH Study Group, Ministry of Health, Labour, and Welfare of Japan. (2011). Characteristics of patients with nonalcoholic steatohepatitis who develop hepatocellular carcinoma. *Clin Gastroenterol Hepatol* Vol. 9, No. 5, pp. 428-433

# 8

# Steroid Hormones in *Drosophila*: How Ecdysone Coordinates Developmental Signalling with Cell Growth and Division

Leonie Quinn[1], Jane Lin[2], Nicola Cranna[1], Jue Er Amanda Lee[1],
Naomi Mitchell[1] and Ross Hannan[2,3,4]
*[1]Department of Anatomy and Cell Biology, University of Melbourne,*
*[2]Peter MacCallum Cancer Centre, St Andrews Place, East Melbourne,*
*[3]Department of Biochemistry and Molecular Biology, University of Melbourne,*
*[4]Department of Biochemistry and Cell Biology, Monash University,*
*Australia*

## 1. Introduction

### 1.1 The ecdysone pathway directs *Drosophila* development

Ecdysone is the major steroid hormone in all holometabolous insects responsible for driving the metamorphosis of larval tissues into adult structures. During metamorphosis, ecdysone is essential for upregulating the genes required to control apoptosis and differentiation, essential processes for removal of larval structures which have become obsolete and for tissue remodelling. In addition, ecdysone directs cell growth and division in many tissues throughout the larval to pupal transition. This chapter will discuss the many diverse mechanisms reported for connecting the ecdysone pulse to the developmentally regulated cell growth and cycle progression required for tissue growth and for insects to reach their target body size.

Like all other holometabolous insects, the size of *Drosophila* adult flies is set by the size of the larvae prior to metamorphosis, at the time of pupariation when feeding has ceased and growth can no longer occur. The major developmental hormone in *Drosophila*, the steroid hormone 20-hydroxyecdysone (20E), commonly known as ecdysone, is required for all the developmental transitions needed for metamorphosis (Figure 1-3; (Thummel 1995, 1996, 2001)). Ecdysone is produced in and released by the prothoracic gland (PG), a component of the ring gland, which also contains the corpora allata (CA) and corpora cardiaca (CC) (Figure 1; (Zitnan et al. 2007; McBrayer et al. 2007)). Ecdysone release is controlled by a complex combination of upstream factors, including peptide hormones and neuropeptide signals (see section 2.2). For example, Prothoracicotropic hormone (PTTH) from the central nervous system (CNS) is required to regulate the synthesis and release of ecdysone from the PG (McBrayer et al. 2007).

Ecdysone pulses from the PG are required for all aspects of morphogenesis, starting with the formation of the body plan during late embryogenesis, hatching and development of the first larval instar, and for cuticle moulting at the end of the first and second instars. A large

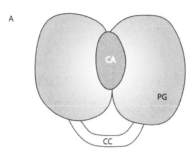

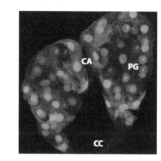

Fig. 1. **The ring gland.** An important organ in *Drosophila* is the ring gland, which is situated in between the two brain lobes in the larvae. (A) Diagram of the components of the ring gland: the prothoracic gland (PG), the corpora allata (CA) and corpora cardiaca (CC). Ecdysone is produced by the PG, whilst the CA is thought to synthesise the Juvenile hormone. (B) A confocal image of a 3rd instar prothoracic gland overexpressing GFP.

titre of ecdysone is released at the end of the third instar, in the wandering larvae in preparation for pupation, which marks the beginning of adult tissue metamorphosis (Figure 3; (Thummel 1995, 1996, 2001)).

Insect metamorphosis is characterized by vast changes in tissue morphology, where larval tissues are replaced by adult structures. In *Drosophila*, the pulse of ecdysone at the end of the third larval instar initiates metamorphosis (Riddiford 1993). During metamorphosis, an extensive range of larval structures respond to the ecdysone pulse, which triggers the complex array of cellular responses required to achieve conversion from the larval tissue to give the adult (Bender et al. 1997). This begins with the secretion of glue proteins for the larvae to attach itself onto a surface for puparium development. Subsequently ecdysone drives the larval body to shorten, and promotes the subsequent cuticle darkening and hardening required to form the pupal case. During the late larval to early pupal stages the ecdysone pulse drives removal of obsolete larval tissues, such as the larval gut and salivary glands (Thummel 2001).

The major morphological changes for metamorphosis involve development of adult structures from the imaginal discs, which are epithelial structures formed from invaginations of the ectoderm during embryogenesis (Gates and Thummel 2000). The imaginal discs include 2 pairs for the eye/antenna, wing, and halteres, 3 pairs for the legs and a single disc for the gonads, which evert, elongate, and differentiate during metamorphosis

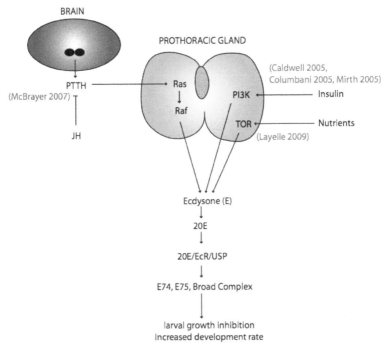

Fig. 2. **The ecdysone pathway.** Abbreviations: Juvenile hormone (JH), prothoracicotropic hormone (PTTH), Target of Rapamycin (TOR), 20-hydroxyecdysone (20E), ecdysone receptor (EcR), Ultraspiracle (USP), prothoracic gland (PG). References are in blue.

(Alberts 2002). Ecdysone triggers the imaginal disc eversion and elongation, which is accomplished through cell shape changes, rather than by additional cell division (Condic, Fristrom, and Fristrom 1991). As the new appendages emerge from the imaginal discs, the larval tissues undergo programmed cell death and are eventually replaced by the adult structures (Ward et al. 2003). About 12 hours after puparium formation, another major ecdysone pulse initiates the prepupal-pupal transition, and forms the basic body plan of the adult fly. This pulse causes the head to evert from the anterior end of the puparium, the final growth of leg and wings, as well as the removal of most of the remaining larval tissues (Ward et al. 2003). The following 4 days of pupal development involves terminal differentiation of the remaining tissues to form the adult fly (Figure 3; reviewed in (Thummel 2001)).

## 1.2 Ecdysone, EcR and USP structure and function
Insect metamorphosis is achieved by the cascade of gene transcription triggered by ecdysone, which activates the ecdysone receptor (EcR), a member of the nuclear receptor family, and its receptor binding partner Ultraspiricle (USP) (Thummel 1996, 1990, 1995; Koelle et al. 1991) (Figure 2). The *EcR* gene spans 77kb in length, and through the use of two promoters and as a result of alternate splicing, encodes three major protein isoforms EcR-A, EcR-B1, EcR-B2. All three isoforms have conserved DNA binding domains and ligand binding domains but differ in their N-terminal regions, with variable N terminal domains of 197, 226 and 17 amino acid residues, respectively (Koelle et al. 1991; Talbot, Swyryd, and Hogness 1993).

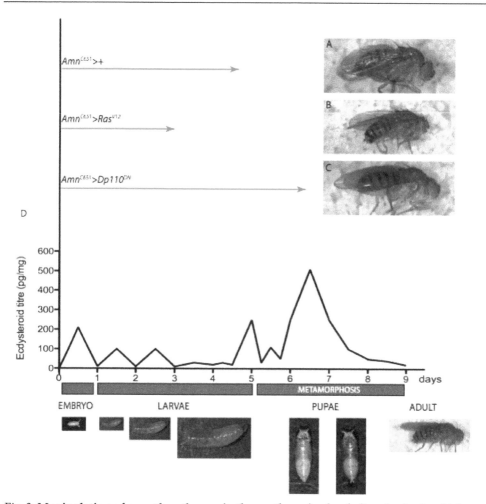

Fig. 3. **Manipulation of growth pathways in the prothoracic gland alters body size.** Light micrographs of female adult flies raised at 25°C bearing the genotypes: (A) control ($Amn^{C651}$>+) (B) overexpressing activated $Ras$ ($Amn^{C651}$>$Ras^{V12}$) in the PG (C) overexpressing dominant negative $PI3K$ ($AmnC651$>$Dp110^{DN}$) in the PG. Red arrows indicate length of larval growth period. (D) Graph of ecdysone titres during *Drosophila* development (modified from (Thummel, 2001)).

Although EcR can bind ecdysone alone, optimal binding to the ecdysone response elements (*EcRE*) and activation of transcriptional targets requires the addition of USP (Grad et al. 2001; Grebe, Fauth, and Spindler-Barth 2004). USP exhibits a strong structural and functional similarity to the orthologous vertebrate retinoid X receptor (RXR) (Yao et al. 1992; Oro, McKeown, and Evans 1990). Like RXR, which forms heterodimers with non-steroid receptors for thyroid hormone, retinoic acid and vitamin D, and thereby activates them for DNA-binding (Mangelsdorf and Evans 1995), USP interacts with each of the EcR isoforms to form DNA-binding heterodimers (Yao et al. 1992; Bender et al. 1997). In this respect

*Drosophila* EcRs are, therefore, analogous to the vertebrate family of RXR heterodimeric receptors rather than the vertebrate family of steroid hormone receptors, which bind DNA as homodimers (Beato and Klug 2000). Therefore, similar to vertebrate nuclear receptors, the EcR/USP heterodimer functions as a ligand-dependent transcription factor. In the presence of the ecdysone ligand, the appropriate EcR nuclear receptor isoform dimerizes with USP, and the complex is stabilised by the active form of ecdysone, 20-hydroxyecdysone (20E) to allow efficient binding to the ecdysone response element (*EcRE*) (Hall and Thummel 1998; Yao et al. 1993) and transcriptional activation of ecdysone-responsive genes (D'Avino and Thummel 1998; Kozlova and Thummel 2002; Thummel 2002; Thummel, Burtis, and Hogness 1990; Urness and Thummel 1995). Genes that are directly activated by the 20E/EcR/USP complex include three "early" ecdysone pathway genes; *E74*, *E75* and the *Broad-Complex* (*BR-C*), which all encode transcription factors. The E74, E75 and BR-C transcription factors control the late genes in order to elicit the biological changes associated with each ecdysone pulse. This hierarchy of gene activation is required for modulating expression of the many cell death, cell cycle and differentiation genes required for metamorphosis (Thummel 1996, 2001). *E74* encodes two proteins with an identical ETS DNA binding domain, designated E74A and E74B (Burtis et al. 1990; Thummel, Burtis, and Hogness 1990). *E75* encodes three members of the nuclear receptor superfamily (designated E75A, E75B, and E75C), which are often referred to as orphan nuclear receptors due to their unidentified ligand (Segraves and Hogness 1990). The *BR-C* is a multigene locus, which encodes several zinc finger proteins (DiBello et al. 1991). To increase the output of the ecdysone pulse, EcR provides an autoregulatory loop to activate its own transcription and further increase receptor levels in response to the ecdysone ligand (Koelle et al. 1991).

### 1.3 Ecdysone signalling coordinates proliferation, death and differentiation
Metamorphosis of *Drosophila* requires co-ordination of proliferation (cell growth and division), differentiation and death in order to form an adult fly of the appropriate size and with correctly differentiated structures. An essential process driven by the ecdysone pulse is the removal of larval tissues no longer required in the adult (Baehrecke 2000). The process of steroid hormone driven apoptosis is an important part of tissue remodelling, whereby selective death removes unwanted cells towards generating the mature structure (Rusconi, Hays, and Cagan 2000; Thummel 2001). For example, the histolysis of the larval salivary gland and midgut at the end of metamorphosis is stage-specific, ecdysone triggered, programmed cell death, which results in the removal of the component of these larval structures no longer required in the adult fly. In line with an apoptotic mechanism, previous studies have shown that cell death activators are upregulated in the third instar larval tissues, including the salivary glands and midgut in response to ecdysone (reviewed in (Jiang, Baehrecke, and Thummel 1997; Baehrecke 2000; Yin and Thummel 2005)).

The ecdysone pulse is also essential for differentiation and patterning of the larval imaginal tissues required for development of adult structures (Hall and Thummel 1998; D'Avino and Thummel 2000, 1998; Zheng et al. 2003). As cell division and patterning are tightly linked in *Drosophila* imaginal tissues, the process of metamorphosis controlled by ecdysone involves coordination of the developmental signals that regulate proliferation and differentiation. Although much work has focused on the downstream targets linking the ecdysone pathway to programmed cell death and cell differentiation (Baehrecke 2000; Jiang, Baehrecke, and

Thummel 1997; Yin and Thummel 2005), the relationship between ecdysone and cell cycle is a relatively unexplored field. Here we review the evidence that the ecdysone pulse is critical for controlling cell growth and division in *Drosophila*.

### 1.4 Linking the Ecdysone pulse to cell cycle

In *Drosophila*, cell growth and cell cycle progression are regulated by a number of key genes, which have been shown to control the cell cycle in an analogous manner in all multicellular organisms. These include the *Drosophila* orthologue of the mammalian *c-myc* transcription factor and oncogene, dMyc, which drives growth and progression through G1 to S-phase (Johnston et al. 1999), the essential G1 to S-phase Cyclin complex, Cyclin E (CycE) and its Cyclin-dependent-kinase (Cdk) partner Cdk2, which triggers S-phase by promoting DNA replication (Knoblich et al. 1994; Neufeld et al. 1998; Richardson et al. 1995), and the *Drosophila* orthologue of the Cdc25 phosphatase, String (Stg), which is required for G2/M progression and promotes mitotic entry by activating the Cdk1/Cyclin B complex (Edgar and Datar 1996). CycE and Stg are the rate limiting factors for S-phase and mitosis, respectively, and both are activated by the *Drosophila* orthologue of human E2F1 protein, dE2F1 (Neufeld et al. 1998). dE2F1 responds to the relevant Cdk-Cyclin complex (CycE/Cdk2 for S-phase and CycB/Cdk1 for mitosis) to coordinate cell cycle progression from G1 to S-phase and G2 into mitosis (Reis and Edgar 2004).

During metamorphosis, following removal of the obsolete larval structures, proliferation of the remaining tissue occurs in an ecdysone-dependent manner to produce adult structures. For example, during pupal development the larval midgut is removed by apoptosis and is replaced through proliferation of the remaining tissue to form the adult midgut (Jiang, Baehrecke, and Thummel 1997). Microarray analysis has revealed that the ecdysone signal is associated with the activation of key cell cycle genes, including *Cyclin B, Cdc2* and *Cyclin D*, during the initiation of midgut metamorphosis (Li and White 2003). Analysis of *EcR* null mutants also revealed that EcR function was necessary for the cell cycle and growth genes to be activated in the larval midgut, suggesting that the ecdysone pathway is required for cell division control. The body of this chapter will discuss how the ecdysone pulse achieves changes to cell growth and cell cycle progression. First we will describe how ecdysone levels dictate body size cell extrinsically by controlling developmental timing. Then we will discuss how ecdysone works with its receptors, in a tissue autonomous manner to control transcription of cell cycle genes, which most likely occurs indirectly by modifying the activity of developmental signalling pathways.

## 2. Cell extrinsic effects of ecdysone on larval growth and body size

The ecdysone pulse can act indirectly to affect larval growth as a consequence of the link between the ecdysone titre and developmental timing. Here we will discuss how cell extrinsic effects of the ecdysone pathway control *Drosophila* larval growth and final body size non-autonomously, at least in part, through interactions between the ecdysone and insulin pathways (King-Jones and Thummel 2005; Shingleton 2005; Mirth and Riddiford 2007; Nijhout 2008).

### 2.1 The prothoracic gland directs body size

The prothoracic gland (PG) is tightly associated with the developmental timing of all holometabolous insects, including *Drosophila*, as it produces the ecdysone pulse that dictates the timing of the larval-pupal transition and metamorphosis. As the adult fly size is determined by the size of the larvae at the pupal molt, the timing of ecdysone release plays a vital role in the growth of the fly (reviewed in (King-Jones and Thummel 2005)). Studies in 2005 demonstrated the importance of the size of the PG and its effect on ecdysone production and, therefore, determination of the final adult fly size (Caldwell, Walkiewicz, and Stern 2005; Colombani et al. 2005; Mirth, Truman, and Riddiford 2005). Specifically, these groups reported a role for insulin signalling in the PG, and also characterised a size-assessing feature of the PG (Figure 3). As a size-assessment tissue, inhibiting the growth of the PG causes an underestimation of body size and results in pupation at a larger size, whereas promoting this tissue's growth results in smaller flies (Mirth, Truman, and Riddiford 2005). Consistent with this, overexpression of activated *PI3K* or *Ras* (*Ras^V12*), both key components of growth control pathways in flies and mammals, specifically in the PG resulted in a larger PG but reduced the pupal and adult size (Caldwell, Walkiewicz, and Stern 2005; Colombani et al. 2005; Mirth, Truman, and Riddiford 2005), which we have recapitulated as shown in Figure 3 (compare 3B with 3A). Conversely, overexpression of a dominant negative isoform of *PI3K* (*Dp110^DN*) reduced the PG size but resulted in larger pupae and adults, due to an extended larval growth period (Figure 3, compare C with A). Furthermore, through measurements of the ecdysone target *E74B* or through an enzyme immunoassay for ecdysteroid titres, it was shown that the extended larval growth period was due to reduced ecdysone levels, which was most likely a result of a smaller PG (Caldwell, Walkiewicz, and Stern 2005; Colombani et al. 2005; Mirth, Truman, and Riddiford 2005).

## 2.2 PTTH regulates of ecdysone levels

In insects, the production and release of ecdysone is responsive to the prothoracicotropic hormone (PTTH), a small, secreted peptide. PTTH is thought to induce the transcription of ecdysone biosynthetic genes that encode enzymes driving the series of dehydrogenation and hydroxylation reactions required to synthesise the active metabolite 20E from the cholesterol precursor (Marchal et al. 2010). In *Drosophila* PTTH is produced by a pair of bilateral neurosecretory cells in the brain, which innervate the prothoracic gland (PG) ((Figure 2; (McBrayer et al. 2007)). PTTH is expressed throughout 3rd instar in an 8 hour cyclic pattern, with upregulation noticed around 12 hours before pupariation (McBrayer et al. 2007). Ablation of the neurons that produce PTTH results in a 5-day developmental delay in the onset of pupariation, larger 3rd instar larvae and pupae, and adults with larger wings due to increased cell number. In line with the predicted role for PTTH in modulating ecdysone synthesis and release, larvae lacking PTTH producing neurons have reduced ecdysone titres. This suggests PTTH normally modulates ecdysone levels to coordinate larval growth with the onset of metamorphosis. However, as the ecdysone levels still eventually peak in larvae with ablated neurons, PTTH may not be the sole factor required for increasing ecdysone titres (McBrayer et al. 2007). Thus PTTH might be required in addition to the insulin-dependent growth pathways discussed above, to coordinate larval growth with ecdysone-induced moulting and metamorphosis (Figure 2-3).

## 2.3 Juvenile hormone controls PTTH release and ecdysone production

The signals required for metamorphosis have been extensively studied in the tobacco hornworm *Manduca sexta*. In this insect, the pulse of ecdysone in the last larval instar is inhibited by another hormone, the Juvenile Hormone (JH). In the case of JH, levels need to drop below a threshold for metamorphosis to begin (Nijhout and Williams 1974, 1974; Dominick and Truman 1985). Whether the drop in JH abundance signals the attainment of critical weight, which defines the larval size response to starvation (Davidowitz, D'Amico, and Nijhout 2003), or reaching critical weight initiates the drop in JH levels is unclear. However, at least in *Manduca*, a drop of JH levels below a critical threshold is required for PTTH to be released and activate the production of ecdysone to start metamorphosis. As pupae do not receive any additional nutrition, the transition into pupation marks the termination of larval growth and establishes the final adult size.

For *Drosophila*, the role of JH in regulating PTTH is not as well defined. Studies suggests PTTH may operate upstream to set the critical weight as loss of PTTH results in an increase in critical weight and an extended developmental delay (Figure 3; (McBrayer et al. 2007)). Control of developmental timing is likely achieved by minor pulses of PTTH and subsequent ecdysone pulses, which occur prior to the major ecdysone peak. This is consistent with the observation that loss of PTTH impairs ecdysone release and leads to developmental delays and larger adult flies (McBrayer et al. 2007). As ecdysone levels determine the transition from each developmental stage the PG, therefore, plays a critical role in regulating *Drosophila* organ and tissue growth.

### 2.4 Ecdysone controls animal growth rate via the fat body

In holometabolous insects, growth is mainly restricted to the larval period and maturation occurs during metamorphosis or pupal development. In all multicellular animals, tissue growth relies on the insulin-signalling pathway, which couples nutrition with growth (Edgar 2006; Britton et al. 2002). A recent study suggests an ecdysone-dependent control mechanism for restricting growth to the juvenile period, where ecdysone controls growth rate via effects on the growth regulator Myc in the fat body (Delanoue, Slaidina, and Leopold 2010). The fat body, which is functionally homologous to the vertebrate liver, appears to act as a relay tissue for the control of larval growth by circulating ecdysone. Loss of Ecdysone receptor (EcR) function in fat body increases dMyc expression and its ability to upregulate growth by increasing ribosome biogenesis and protein translation. Together with RNA profiling of dissected fat bodies, this suggests that EcR signalling represses dMyc and its downstream targets. Importantly, manipulation of dMyc levels in the fat body is sufficient to affect animal growth-rate. In addition, the downregulation of dMyc in fat cells is required for growth inhibition by ecdysone as the growth increase induced by silencing EcR in the fat body is suppressed by cosilencing dMyc. This work suggests a model where the rise of ecdysone levels at the end of the juvenile period represses dMyc expression in the fat body. This steroid hormone-dependent inhibition restricts ribosome biosynthesis and translation efficiency in fat cells via dMyc and, therefore, induces a general pause in the growth program that precedes entry into metamorphosis.

The ability of circulating ecdysone to control dMyc expression during the pupal stage was found to be specific to the fat body. For example, *dmyc* mRNA levels were elevated in fat body after reducing the level of circulating ecdysone via inhibition of PI3K pathway in the prothoracic gland, but at this stage *dmyc* levels are not altered in wing imaginal discs (Delanoue, Slaidina, and Leopold 2010). Interestingly, inhibition of ecdysone gene activation at the earlier 3rd larval instar stage revealed that EcR function is actually required for normal levels of *dmyc* transcription in some tissues. In these studies, blocking the ecdysone pathway in wing imaginal disc cells using EcR dominant negative (dN) transgenes results in reduced levels of *dmyc* promoter activity (Cranna and Quinn 2009). Thus the effect of ecdysone on this key growth regulator appears to be both 1) developmental-stage specific; being required for *dmyc* activation in the wing at the earlier growth phase but not after pupariation and 2) tissue specific; resulting in downregulation of *dmyc* expression in the fat body, but not in the wing disc during pupariation.

The lack of consensus binding sites for EcR/Usp (EcREs) in the *dmyc* promoter region suggests that *dmyc* is not a direct target of EcR-mediated gene repression in the fat body or activation in the wing, but rather that EcR signalling indirectly controls *dmyc* transcription. Although the fat-specific target of EcR leading to altered *dmyc* expression is unknown, in the wing imaginal disc EcR has been shown to modulate levels of the Wingless morphogen (Mitchell et al. 2008), which in turn can lead to downregulation of *dmyc* transcription (Herranz et al. 2008; Johnston et al. 1999).

### 2.5 Interplay between insulin pathway and ecdysone determines final body size

Taken together the above findings suggest that the insulin-signalling pathway acts in the prothoracic gland (PG) to regulate the release of ecdysone and determine the length of the larval growth period (Caldwell, Walkiewicz, and Stern 2005; Colombani et al. 2005; King-Jones et al. 2005; Mirth, Truman, and Riddiford 2005; Shingleton 2005; Prober and Edgar 2002). For instance, increased PG growth occurs when PI3-kinase (PI3K, a downstream regulator of the insulin pathway) is upregulated in the PG (Caldwell, Walkiewicz, and Stern 2005; Mirth, Truman, and Riddiford 2005). The PG overgrowth causes accelerated metamorphosis, which results in reduced adult size due to the rapid progression through the larval growth stage. Precocious ecdysone release, as measured by premature increase in levels of the early response ecdysone genes, correlates with this disruption to larval growth. Conversely, reducing growth of the PG, using a dominant negative form of PI3K, results in longer larval growth periods and larger adults due to slower ecdysone release and delayed onset of pupariation. More recently it has been shown that Target of Rapamycin (TOR) may link the ecdysone-regulated development to the PI3K mediated growth pathways (Layalle, Arquier, and Leopold 2008; reviewed in (Nijhout 2008)).

The levels of ecdysone release are therefore inversely proportional to larval growth and adult body size; with early onset of the ecdysone peak giving small flies and reduced ecdysone prolonging the growth period to give larger adults. Thus the time spent in the larval growth phase is a critical determinant of body size, with longer growth periods resulting in more cell division cycles and delayed onset of differentiation. In the next section we address the question of how the ecdysone pulse works to affect rates of cell growth and cell cycle progression within specific larval tissues. In particular we discuss the developmental signalling pathways implicated in linking cell cycle patterning of larval imaginal tissues to the ecdysone titre.

### 3. Cell intrinsic roles for ecdysone, EcR and USP in cell growth and division

The *Drosophila* imaginal discs (see also Introduction 1.1), which form the adult head structures (eyes and antenna), appendages (wings and legs) and genitalia, have provided an excellent model for studying developmental signals controlling cell proliferation. The imaginal disc precursor cells arise early in embryonic development from invaginations of the embryonic epithelium (Alberts 2002). By the early larval stage each disc consists of a ball of around 10-50 undifferentiated stem cells, which undergo extensive growth and proliferation to comprise up to 100,000 cells by the end of the third larval instar. The imaginal discs start differentiation at the end of third instar and complete the process by the end of pupariation, when all adult structures such as the wings, legs and eyes have developed (Fristrom and Fristrom 1993). The third instar larval stage is a critical stage of *Drosophila* development, containing the major growth and proliferation of all tissues required to form the adult fly (Church and Robertson 1966). Indeed the size of the adult fly is determined at the time when the pupal case is formed, as after this the animal cannot feed again until eclosion. Here we will discuss the developmental signals (including Wingless, Dpp, Hedgehog, Notch) controlling growth of the eye and wing imaginal discs, and how ecdysone impacts on these signalling pathways to control cell division.

### 3.1 Ecdysone mediates morphogenetic Furrow progression in the eye imaginal disc

The *Drosophila* eye is composed of an ordered array of photoreceptor clusters or ommatidia, which develop from an epithelial monolayer known as the eye imaginal disc, via an organised pattern of proliferation and differentiation (Figure 4; (Ready, Hanson, and Benzer 1976; Wolff and Ready 1991)). Differentiation of the ommatidia occurs in a wave that moves from the posterior toward the anterior (Thomas and Zipursky 1994). The margin between the asynchronously dividing anterior cells and the differentiated posterior cells is marked by the morphogenetic furrow (MF) (Ready, Hanson, and Benzer 1976). Mitotic division cycles become synchronized in the MF where cells are delayed in G1 and a subset of photoreceptor cells are specified. The remaining retinal cells synchronously re-enter the cell cycle in the "Second Mitotic Wave" (SMW), which is composed of a tight band of DNA synthesis and mitosis (Figure 4). These final cell divisions provide the cells required for differentiation of the ommatidial structures that form the adult eye (Ready, Hanson, and Benzer 1976; Wolff and Ready 1991).

Studies in the eye primordium of the tobacco hornworm moth, *Manduca sexta*, suggest that progression of the MF, including proliferation and differentiation of ommatidial clusters, requires ecdysone. Eye primordia proliferation responds to a critical concentration of ecdysone and below this threshold cells arrest in the G2 phase of the cell cycle (Champlin and Truman 1998). Premature exposure to high levels of ecdysone will also result in MF arrest and precocious maturation of ommatida (Champlin and Truman 1998). These cell cycle responses to ecdysone are consistent with the moderate ecdysone pulse during the larval stage first stimulating eye proliferation and the high levels of ecdysone released after pupariation driving cell cycle exit and eye maturation.

The ecdysone pathway has also been implicated in regulation of MF progression in the *Drosophila* larval eye imaginal disc. The *ecdysoneless* mutation (*ecd-ts*) is a hypomorphic temperature-sensitive allele, which reduces ecdysone secretion from the ring gland (Henrich et al. 1987). Homozygous *ecd-ts* flies show eye defects when shifted to the restrictive temperature during the third instar larval stage (Brennan, Ashburner, and Moses 1998). Consistent with the MF moving much more slowly than normal in the *ecd-ts* mutant, delayed eye differentiation was shown using the neuronal marker Elav.

Microarray analysis has linked the ecdysone pulse during metamorphosis to transcriptional changes in mitogenic signalling molecules, which are essential for coordinating cell cycle and patterning of imaginal tissues. The observation that ecdysone signalling was essential for the activation of factors involved in regulatory signalling pathways such as Wg, Notch

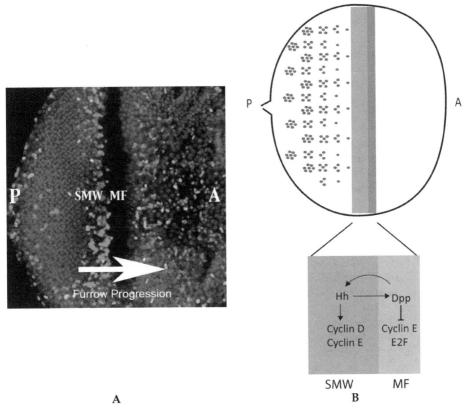

Fig. 4. **A - Eye imaginal disc differentiation occurs in a wave that moves from posterior (P) to anterior (A).** The margin between the asynchronously dividing anterior cells and the differentiated posterior cells is marked by the morphogenetic furrow (MF), where cells are delayed in G1. Mitotic division cycles become synchronized in the "Second Mitotic Wave" (SMW), which is composed of a tight band of DNA synthesis (Marked by BrdU in red) and mitosis (marked by PH3 in green). **B - The Hedgehog (Hh) and Dpp pathways control cell division in the larval eye.** *Drosophila* eye development is dependent on *hedgehog* (*hh*) expression posterior to the MF and *decapentaplegic* (*dpp*) expression within the MF. Hh and Dpp regulate key cell cycle genes to coordinate cell cycle and differentiation. Dpp and Hh act redundantly to ensure G1 arrest, thus cells unable to respond to Dpp will arrest later in response to Hh. Dpp and Hh inhibit Cyclin E and dE2F1 in the cells comprising the MF. In the anterior of the MF, Hh acts to promote cell division in the SMW by upregulating Cyclin D to promote cell growth and Cyclin E to drive S-phase entry.

and Dpp, suggests there might be many connections between ecdysone, developmental pathways and cell cycle regulation during metamorphosis in *Drosophila* (Li and White 2003). The first evidence for these connections in the *Drosophila* larval eye imaginal disc came from studies implicating the ecdysone pathway in regulation of MF progression via effects on Hh and Dpp (Brennan, Ashburner, and Moses 1998; Brennan et al. 2001). In *Drosophila*, eye development is dependent on *hedgehog* (*hh*) expression posterior to the MF (Heberlein,

Wolff, and Rubin 1993; Heberlein et al. 1995) and *decapentaplegic* (*dpp*) expression within the MF (Figure 4; (Blackman et al. 1991)). *Drosophila* Dpp is a member of the mammalian transforming growth factor-beta (TGF-beta) family of secreted proteins. TGF-beta can behave as a tumour-suppressor or oncogene depending on the tissue microenvironment, thus pathway inhibition or activation can result in cancer progression (Serra and Moses 1996; Derynck, Akhurst, and Balmain 2001; Wakefield and Roberts 2002; Bachman and Park 2005; Elliott and Blobe 2005; Jakowlew 2006; Massague 2008). Aberrant Hh signalling has also been associated with human cancer, with much literature linking activation of the pathway with increased tumour progression (Toftgard 2000; Vestergaard, Bak, and Larsen 2005; Evangelista, Tian, and de Sauvage 2006; Epstein 2008; Varjosalo and Taipale 2008). In the eye disc, Dpp and Hedgehog (Hh) act redundantly to ensure G1 arrest within the MF (Penton, Selleck, and Hoffmann 1997; Horsfield et al. 1998; Firth and Baker 2005) where both pathways can inhibit Cyclin E and dE2F1 (Escudero and Freeman 2007). In addition to this cell cycle inhibitory role of Hh in the MF, Hh promotes cell division in the SMW by upregulating Cyclin D to promote cell growth and Cyclin E to drive S-phase entry (Figure 4; (Duman-Scheel et al. 2002)).

In line with ecdysone regulating eye development via Hh, the phenotype observed in *ecdysoneless* (*ecd-ts*) mutant is similar to phenotypes resulting from *hh* loss of function (Heberlein et al. 1995). In addition, the decreased levels of Hh protein posterior to the MF in *ecd-ts* larval eye discs are consistent with *hh* being a downstream target of the ecdysone signal (Brennan, Ashburner, and Moses 1998). The delayed MF progression may be, therefore, a consequence of the requirement for Hh in activation of the S-phase genes *cyclin D* and *cyclin E* and, therefore, cell cycle re-entry in the SMW (Duman-Scheel et al. 2002). Indeed, the failure of MF movement in *ecd-ts* mutants is likely a result of impaired cell cycle progression as S-phase numbers were dramatically decreased in the SMW (Brennan, Ashburner, and Moses 1998). Consistent with reduced cell division within the SMW, levels of the mitotic cyclin, Cyclin B, were also reduced posterior to the MF (Brennan, Ashburner, and Moses 1998).

The USP receptor has also been implicated in regulation of cell cycle progression and differentiation in the developing eye imaginal disc. Loss-of-function *usp* clones spanning the morphogenetic furrow show an anterior shift in expression of the MF-specific marker Dpp, consistent with premature progression of the MF and a role for USP in repressing morphogenetic furrow movement (Zelhof et al. 1997). In addition, loss of USP results in ectopic activation of many genes involved in cell fate specification in the eye, including the differentiation markers Spalt and Atonal (Zelhof et al. 1997). Although expression of these differentiation markers occurs prematurely, specification of cells contributing to the ommatidia occurs normally. The cell cycle analysis of *usp* mutant clones suggested that although the MF was advanced, cell cycle progression was disrupted in the SMW. First staining for Cyclin A, as a marker for cells in either S or G2 phase, revealed fewer Cyclin A-positive cells in *usp-* clones posterior to the morphogenetic furrow (Ghbeish et al. 2001). Similarly, although the Cyclin B band was not shifted in *usp-* clones posterior to the MF, the numbers of cells expressing Cyclin B were reduced (Ghbeish and McKeown 2002). The reduction in cell cycle markers posterior of the MF suggests that USP is required for cell cycle progression in the SMW. In support of cell cycle induction in the SMW depending on the presence of USP protein, *usp* overexpression using the *GMR*-promoter, which is only expressed posterior of the furrow, can rescue the loss of Cyclin B in the *usp* mutant clone. As progression through the SMW and differentiation are tightly coupled, the reduced cell cycles in *usp-/-* clones may be the underlying cause of the premature differentiation observed (Zelhof et al. 1997).

Together these data show that reduction in either ecdysone or USP results in reduced cell cycles. Paradoxically, however, *usp* mutations increase the rate of MF movement (Zelhof et al. 1997; Ghbeish et al. 2001; Ghbeish and McKeown 2002) while loss of ecdysone stops the MF (Brennan, Ashburner, and Moses 1998; Brennan et al. 2001). One explanation for these observations is that in the absence of ligand, the EcR/USP heterodimer normally acts as a repressor at certain *EcRE*s. For these target genes ecdysone would be required to relieve the transcriptional repression caused by unliganded binding of the EcR/USP complex. This idea emerged from the finding that the *Broad-complex* (*BR-C*), which encodes the family of zinc-finger transcription factors upregulated early in response to high ecdysone titres (Karim, Guild, and Thummel 1993), becomes ectopically expressed in loss-of-function wing imaginal disc cells for either *usp* (Schubiger and Truman 2000) or *EcR* (Schubiger et al. 2005). Although concrete evidence is lacking, the idea is that the early (pre-ecdysone pulse) repressive effect of the EcR/USP heterodimer at the *BR-C* promoter will be lost in either *EcR* or *usp* mutants.

The apparently contradictory effects of USP and ecdysone in the eye might actually be a consequence of the differential effects of the pathway on *BR-C* transcription. The Z1 isoform of the *BR-C* (*BrC-Z1*) is normally expressed posterior to the MF but not anterior to the MF (Emery, Bedian, and Guild 1994; Bayer, Holley, and Fristrom 1996) and reduced induction of *BrC-Z1* occurs in *ecd-ts* eye discs (Brennan, Ashburner, and Moses 1998). Loss of USP function has the opposite effect, leading to high level BrC-Z1 protein expression both anterior and posterior to the MF, which might occur as a consequence of de-repression of *BR-C* transcription (Brennan et al. 2001). This high level of BrC-Z1 protein in *usp* mutant clones may explain the MF advancement phenotypes, as ectopic BrC-Z1 protein has been shown to induce premature differentiation of photoreceptor cells (Zelhof et al. 1997; Ghbeish et al. 2001; Ghbeish and McKeown 2002).

Yet even though *BrC-Z1* expression is downregulated in *ecd-ts* mutants (Brennan, Ashburner, and Moses 1998), *BrC-Z1* loss of function eye imaginal discs are phenotypically different (Ghbeish et al. 2001), suggesting that other downstream targets of ecdysone pathway transcription mediate the reported effects on eye development. Like *ecd-ts*, impaired *BrC-Z1* function results in decreased levels of Hh, defective MF progression and photoreceptor recruitment. However, unlike the findings for *ecd-ts*, reduced levels of Cyclin B were not detected in *BrC-Z1* loss of function clones (Ghbeish et al. 2001). Rather loss of *BrC-Z1* function results in defects in ommatidial assembly, suggesting a role for *BR-C* in post-MF differentiation rather than cell cycle regulation in the SMW (Brennan et al. 2001). This suggests that some ecdysone regulation in the eye is mediated by BrC-Z1, but that an alternate target(s) of the ecdysone pathway regulates the cell cycle activity required for SMW cell cycles and MF progression.

The *ecd-ts* and USP studies suggest a role for the ecdysone pathway and the USP receptor in furrow progression, however, analysis of *EcR* mutant clones led to the conclusion that EcR was not required for furrow progression (Brennan et al. 2001). This was surprising given the EcR isoforms are the major mediators of the ecdysone signal, combined with the *Manduca Sexta* (Champlin and Truman 1998, 1998) and *Drosophila* studies (Brennan, Ashburner, and Moses 1998) that have demonstrated a requirement for ecdysone in MF progression. This led the authors of this study to propose a novel hormone transduction pathway involving an uncharacterized receptor to explain USP functioning independent of EcR in the eye, which could occur via heterodimerisation of USP with one of the 16 orphan nuclear receptors identified in *Drosophila* (Sullivan and Thummel 2003). For example USP has been found to heterodimerize with the orphan nuclear receptor, DHR38, to regulate cuticle formation (Kozlova et al. 1998; Sutherland et al. 1995). The USP/DHR38 complex responds to a different class of ecdysteroids in larval fat body and epidermis in an EcR independent manner, which does not involve direct binding of the ecdysone ligand to either DHR38 or USP (Baker et al. 2003). However, as *DHR38* expression does not appear to be induced by ecdysteroids in the larval eye (Baker et al. 2003), it is unlikely that DHR38 partners USP during eye development. We believe it is premature to rule out a function for EcR in MF progression as the absence of a furrow progression phenotype reported (Brennan et al. 2001) may be a consequence of perdurance of EcR protein after clone induction. As studies using dominant negative EcR transgenes have shown that EcR is required for normal signalling and cell cycle progression in the wing (discussed in section 3.2; (Mitchell et al. 2008; Cranna and Quinn 2009)), similar methods should be used to inhibit EcR activity before any definitive conclusions about whether EcR is required for eye proliferation can be made.

Together the evidence suggests that larval ecdysone signalling is essential for cell cycle progression in the eye imaginal disc. The effect of ecdysone on cell division may, in part, be mediated by increasing Hedgehog (Hh) signalling (Brennan, Ashburner, and Moses 1998) posterior to the MF to drive S-phase gene activity and cell cycle progression in the second mitotic wave (SMW) (Duman-Scheel et al. 2002). In addition to this cell cycle promoting role of ecdysone via Hh activity in the SMW, the shift in the Dpp band of expression in *usp*-clones suggests the ecdysone pathway might also act on Dpp to coordinate G1 arrest in the furrow with division in the SMW (Escudero and Freeman 2007; Firth and Baker 2005). Further work is required to understand how ecdysone might coordinate these developmental signals with the G1 arrest/MF formation and stimulation of the SMW required for eye development (Figure 4).

### 3.2 The ecdysone pathway regulates cell cycle progression in the larval wing disc

Like the eye disc, the larval wing disc is also comprised of an epithelial sheet, which can be divided into distinct domains based on cell fate in the adult wing; the notum, hinge and pouch (Figure 5). The wing pouch, which ultimately forms the adult wing blade, has been a focus for studying signals impacting upon cell cycle, as wing morphogenesis involves patterned cell cycles that are tightly linked with developmental signalling (Johnson, Grenier, and Scott 1995; Johnston and Edgar 1998; Johnston et al. 1999; Johnston and Sanders 2003; Baker 2007).

Early studies demonstrated that Crol, which is a zinc finger transcription factor, is activated in late larval imaginal discs by the steroid hormone ecdysone (D'Avino and Thummel 1998). Pupal lethal, hypomorphic *crol* mutants (*crol⁴⁴¹⁸*) have defects in ecdysone-induced gene expression (D'Avino and Thummel 1998). Crol is both necessary and sufficient for cell cycle progression in the wing imaginal disc as *crol* mutant clones in the wing pouch fail to proliferate, whilst overexpression of *crol* results in ectopic proliferation (Mitchell et al. 2008). Crol is also required to downregulate the Wingless (Wg) pathway, which normally acts to drive cell cycle exit and differentiation (Figure 5). Therefore, by inhibiting the Wg pathway, *crol* drives wing disc cell division and potentially provides a link between the ecdysone pathway and the developmental signals that regulate cell cycle patterning (discussed in more detail section 3.3; Figure 6).

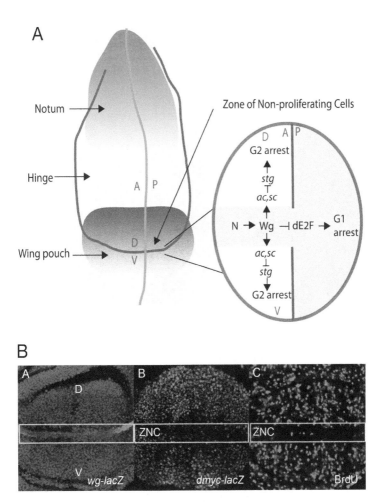

Fig. 5. **(A) - *Drosophila* wing imaginal disc patterning.** (A) The orange domain forms the notum, the blue region gives the hinge and the purple region (the pouch) forms the wing blade. The green line marks the anterior-posterior (A/P) boundary while the red line defines the dorsal-ventral (D/V) boundary. (B) Within D/V boundary of the pouch, Notch (N) expression activates Wingless (Wg) in the central domain. In the anterior compartment, *Wg* induces G2 arrest via *string* (*stg*) through *Achaete* (*ac*) and *Scute* (*sc*). In the posterior compartment, *Wg* induces G1 arrest via repression of dE2F. **(B) - Wg protein, *dmyc* expression and cell cycle patterning in the *Drosophila* wing pouch.** (A) Wg protein (red) is strongly expressed along the dorsal-ventral boundary of the wing pouch. (B) β-gal antibody staining (pink) of *dmyc-lacZ* discs shows a pattern consistent with *dmyc* transcription throughout the cycling cells of the pouch and downregulation of *dmyc* within the G1 arrested cells of the zone of non-proliferating cells (ZNC). (C) The ZNC can be seen by the reduced BrdU staining (red) for S-phase.

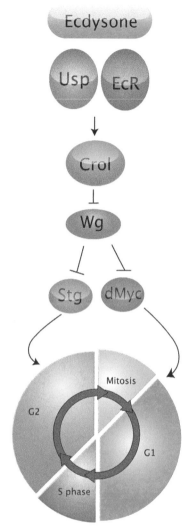

Fig. 6. **Working model connecting Crol to steroid hormone signalling and cell cycle progression in the wing pouch.** Crol is up-regulated in response to ecdysone signalling and increased Crol results in decreased *wg* mRNA expression. Reduced Wg signalling leads to increased *dmyc* expression to drive S-phase and mitosis via increased Stg.

In addition, EcR function is required for wing imaginal disc cell cycles as inactivation of signalling through the EcR/USP/ecdysone complex results in reduced cell division (Cranna and Quinn 2009; Mitchell et al. 2008). In this work the pathway was inhibited using either of 2 dominant negative EcR isoforms; 1) the *EcRA* dominant negative (dN) receptor (EcRAdN), which still binds ecdysone, USP and the *EcRE*, but is defective in the activation of target-gene transcription due to a mutation in the ligand binding domain (LBD) (Cherbas et al. 2003); or 2) the EcR-B2 dominant negative receptor, which dimerizes with USP and binds the *EcRE*, but cannot bind ecdysone, thus preventing optimal activation of ecdysone responsive genes (Cherbas et al. 2003; Hu, Cherbas, and Cherbas 2003). Blocking the EcR signal via overexpression of either *EcRAdN* or *EcRB2dN* in third instar wing imaginal disc flip-out clones (Pignoni and Zipursky 1997) results in a significant decrease in S-phase progression and mitosis, as measured by BrdU incorporation (Figure 7) and staining for anti-phosphohistone-H3, respectively (Cranna and Quinn 2009; Mitchell et al. 2008). Consistent with ecdysone signalling through EcR/USP normally being required for *dmyc* transcription, reduced *dmyc* promoter activity was observed in *EcRAdN* clones generated in the *dmyc-lacZ* enhancer trap background (Cranna and Quinn 2009). Thus ecdysone signalling through EcR/USP might normally control cell cycle progression in the wing imaginal disc by upregulating dMyc to drive growth by increasing ribosome biogenesis and protein translation (Johnston et al. 1999) and S phase via increased activity of the G1 cyclins (Duman-Scheel, Johnston, and Du 2004). Together this suggests EcR signalling might modulate cell growth and division of the wing imaginal disc by modulating *dmyc* levels (Cranna and Quinn 2009).

In support of the reduced cell division in loss-of-function EcR cells being mediated by Crol, EcRAdN clones generated in the heterozygous *crol* mutant background show a further, significant reduction in cell cycle progression, when compared with either EcRdN cells alone or *crol* heterozygotes (Figure 7). This suggests that the reduction in cell cycle resulting from loss of EcR is sensitive to the level of Crol and that the ecdysone pathway normally regulates cell cycle in a Crol-dependent manner.

### 3.3 EcR is required for *Wingless* repression

A key signalling molecule in the morphogenesis of the wing is the Wingless (Wg) protein, a member of the Wnt family of secreted morphogens. Wg is secreted in a band across the dorsal-ventral (D/V) boundary in the wing pouch (Figure 5; (Williams, Paddock, and Carroll 1993)) and is essential for cell cycle arrest in a region of the wing disc called the "Zone of Non-Proliferating Cells", or ZNC, at the end of larval development. The Wg pathway acts to downregulate key cell cycle genes (eg. *dmyc*, *cycE*, *dE2F1* and *stg*) to link the Wg patterning signal to the cell cycle delay preceding the onset of differentiation at the wing margin (Johnston and Edgar 1998; Johnston et al. 1999; Johnston and Sanders 2003; Duman-Scheel, Johnston, and Du 2004). Indeed, the cell cycle arrest in the ZNC mediated by Wg is required for these cells to differentiate and develop into the adult wing blade (Figure 5; (Johnston and Edgar 1998; Johnston et al. 1999)).

In the wing pouch EcR signalling is required for repression of *wg* transcription (Mitchell et al. 2008; Cranna and Quinn 2009), which together with the data above showing EcR is required for cell division, suggests the ecdysone signal might normally control cell cycle via Wg (Figure 6). Consistent with EcR normally being required to repress *wg* transcription, expansion of the *wg* expression domain occurs in *UAS-EcRAdN* (Mitchell et al. 2008) and *UAS-EcRBdN* (Cranna and Quinn 2009) "flip-out" clones generated in a *wg-lacZ* enhancer trap background (Kassis et al. 1992). These results suggest repression of *wg* transcription in the wing pouch is dependent on the ecdysone pathway. Given that increased Wg protein causes reduction of cell cycle regulators such as *dmyc* and *stg*, leading to decreased cells in S-phase and mitosis in the pouch (Figure 5; (Johnston and Edgar 1998; Johnston et al. 1999)), this finding is consistent with the reduced cell cycles observed in *EcR* loss-of-function clones.

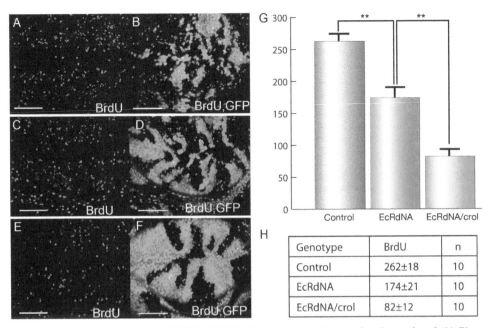

Fig. 7. **S phase progression in UAS-EcRAdN clones is sensitive to the dose of crol.** (A,B) Representative images of the wing pouch with control clones in heterozygous crol mutant (crolk05205) background; (C,D) UAS-EcRdN-A clones and (E,F) UAS-EcRdN-A clones in heterozygous crol mutant background, (A, C, E) S-phase is shown using BrdU (red), (B, D, F) GFP (green) marks clonal tissue. Scale bars indicate 50μm. (G) Quantification of S-phases for each of the genotypes; heterozygous *crol* mutant, UAS-EcRAdN alone and EcRAdN in the heterozygous *crol* mutant background. A significant reduction in the number of S-phase cells was found for the UAS-EcRdN-A alone compared to the control (p=0.0055) and for the UAS-EcRdN-A in the *crol* mutant background compared to UAS-EcRdN-A alone (p=0.0011). (H) Mean number of BrdU (S-phase) cells + SEM in control (clones in tissue heterozygous for the crol mutant); UAS-EcRdN-A alone and UAS-EcRdN-A in the *crol* mutant background. n=sample size.

Together this data suggests that EcR activity and the ecdysone-responsive transcription factor Crol are required for cell cycle progression in the wing imaginal disc (Mitchell et al. 2008). First Crol affects the Wg pathway by downregulating *wg* transcription and driving cells through the Wg-mediated cell cycle arrest (Mitchell et al. 2008). In support of ecdysone acting upstream of Crol to regulate the Wg pathway, blocking EcR activity in the wing results in increased *wg* transcription and reduced cell cycle progression, which is further impaired by halving the dose of *crol* (Figure 7). As Wg is one of the key developmental signals required for inhibition of cell cycle progression in the wing pouch (Duman-Scheel, Johnston, and Du 2004; Johnston and Edgar 1998; Johnston et al. 1999; Johnston and Sanders 2003; Milan 1998), this would be consistent with EcR regulating cell cycle by acting to increase levels of *crol* transcription, which will in turn decrease levels of Wg signalling. Thus we would predict that ecdysone/EcR/USP would normally act to upregulate Crol and drive cell cycle progression in the wing pouch via inhibition of Wg (Figure 6).

Cross-talk between the Wg pathway and other signalling pathways is required to coordinate proliferation and patterning of the wing imaginal disc. Dpp is expressed in a band of cells in the anterior compartment along the anterior-posterior boundary (Lecuit et al. 1996) and is required for cell cycle progression and tissue growth (Martin-Castellanos and Edgar 2002). Proliferation is dependent on careful regulation of the relative levels of the Dpp and Wg signalling pathways (Edgar and Lehner 1996). The Hedgehog (Hh) (Strigini and Cohen 2000) and Notch (N) (de Celis, Garcia-Bellido, and Bray 1996) pathways are key upstream regulators of Wg in the wing disc. Notch activity also plays a role in cell cycle arrest during wing development (Herranz et al. 2008; Johnston and Edgar 1998). Notch is activated in cells along the dorso-ventral (D/V) boundary (ZNC) of the wing disc, where it is required for Wg expression (de Celis, Garcia-Bellido, and Bray 1996). The activation of Wg target genes *achaete* (*ac*) and *scute* (*sc*) specifically within the anterior compartment of the cells flanking the D/V boundary results in downregulation of the mitotic inducer, Cdc25c/Stg, to arrest these cells in G2 (Johnston and Edgar 1998). The expression of Notch within the D/V boundary prevents the G2 arrest, allowing Wg to mediate G1 arrest within the anterior cells comprising the D/V boundary and all cells comprising the posterior compartment ZNC (Figure 5); (Johnston and Edgar 1998; Johnston et al. 1999). More recent reports have demonstrated that Notch also acts downstream of Wg to control G1 to S phase progression in the ZNC (Herranz et al. 2008). Together these studies suggest that a Wg and N "double-repression mechanism" controls cell cycle exit in the ZNC through controlling levels of *dmyc* expression, which drives growth and regulates the S phase transcription factor, E2F1 (Johnston and Edgar 1998; Johnston et al. 1999; Herranz et al. 2008). Thus, interplay between these signalling pathways is essential for cell cycle patterning and differentiation of the wing pouch, which is required to form the adult wing.

The Hh pathway is critical for regulating *wg* transcription during wing development (Murone, Rosenthal, and de Sauvage 1999), but as ectopic levels of the Hh pathway activator, Ci, were not detected in *crol* mutant clones, Crol is unlikely to affect *wg* transcription indirectly via the Hh pathway (Mitchell et al. 2008). Notch is required for Wg expression (de Celis, Garcia-Bellido, and Bray 1996) and plays a critical role in cell cycle arrest during wing development (Herranz et al. 2008; Johnston and Edgar 1998). The Notch target, En(spl)m7 was not however decreased in *crol* over-expressing cells, suggesting Notch signalling is not downregulated by Crol (Mitchell et al. 2008). The effects of Crol on cell cycle in the wing via downregulation of *wg* transcription are therefore unlikely to be due to indirect effects on either the Notch or Hh pathways. Future studies are therefore aimed to determine whether Crol mediates ecdysone signalling via repression of Wg by directly binding the *wg* promoter to down-regulate *wg* transcription.

### 3.4 Ecdysone couples growth and division in larval histoblasts

Another *Drosophila* tissue where ecdysone has been connected with control of growth and/or cell division is the developing histoblast, which gives rise to the abdominal epithelium (Ninov, Chiarelli, and Martin-Blanco 2007). In the canonical cell division cycles of the eye and wing imaginal discs DNA synthesis is coupled with cell division; cells grow in G1, initiate DNA replication and enter S phase, which is separated from mitosis by the G2 phase. In these cells G1 progression is stimulated by growth factors, which trigger cell growth and activate the G1-S cell cycle machinery (see Introduction 1.4), including the cyclin/Cdk complexes and E2F activity. The progression from G2 to mitosis is coupled to S phase and is controlled by mitotic cyclin/Cdk complexes, which are activated by removal of the inhibitory phosphates from Cdk1 by the Cdc25 phosphatases (eg. String in *Drosophila*) (Edgar and O'Farrell 1990). For cells to maintain their size, cell cycle progression must be accompanied by cell growth. However, during morphogenesis of the *Drosophila* abdominal epidermis from histoblasts, growth and division are uncoupled. The progenitor abdominal histoblasts are quiescent during the larval stages, but undergo rapid proliferation after pupation and eventually form the adult abdominal epidermis. Neither cell size nor division rate is constant for the developmentally regulated divisions that histoblast cells undergo during the larval and pupal stages. The onset of histoblast proliferation occurs 1–2 h after pupal formation (Ninov, Chiarelli, and Martin-Blanco 2007), which follows the ecdysone maximum at 0 h APF (Thummel 2001) and recent work has revealed that ecdysone is important for coupling growth and proliferation in abdominal histoblasts (Ninov, Manjon, and Martin-Blanco 2009).

In contrast to the wing and eye epithelium, during larval stages histoblasts grow in a G2 arrested state prior to entering a proliferative stage during pupal metamorphosis (Hayashi 1996; Lawrence, Casal, and Struhl 1999, 1999). During larval stages the arrested histoblasts accumulate cellular mass in a process dependent on the insulin receptor/PI3K pathway and the transition to a proliferative state is initiated by ecdysone-dependent string/Cdc25 phosphatase transcription (Ninov, Manjon, and Martin-Blanco 2009). The latter can occur because the larval histoblasts have preaccumulated stores of the G1 cyclin, Cyclin E, which is sufficient to trigger S phase after mitosis. These cells show a progressive reduction of cell size as a consequence of the lack of a growth phase. After depletion of the stored Cyclin E, histoblasts proliferate more slowly and G1 is restored and cell proliferation again depends on growth factor signalling, requiring epidermal growth factor receptor (EGFR) signalling during the G2/M transition and the insulin receptor/PI3K-pathway for growth.

Initiation of histoblast division by ecdysone/EcR occurs via transcriptional control of the cell cycle regulator String (Ninov, Manjon, and Martin-Blanco 2009). Previous work has shown that *string* overexpression triggers cell-cycle progression in embryonic and imaginal cells previously arrested in G2 (Edgar and O'Farrell 1990; Edgar, Lehman, and O'Farrell 1994; Milan, Campuzano, and Garcia-Bellido 1996), but not in G1-arrested cells (Kylsten and Saint 1997). Accordingly, the overexpression of String, but not Cyclin A, Cyclin B, or Cdk1, in histoblasts triggered their premature hyperproliferation in larval stages (Ninov, Manjon, and Martin-Blanco 2009). Although ecdysone is necessary to trigger histoblast proliferation (Ninov, Chiarelli, and Martin-Blanco 2007), upregulation of *string* transcription in larval stages bypasses the requirement for ecdysone pathway activity. As the block to histoblast proliferation following EcR knockdown with RNAi (Ninov, Chiarelli, and Martin-Blanco 2007) can be overcome by overexpression of *string*, which can still promote ectopic histoblast proliferation in the EcR loss of function cells (Ninov, Manjon, and Martin-Blanco 2009). As an indirect measure of *string* transcription a *string*-enhancer trap element was used, which revealed that EcR knockdown reduces *string* promoter activity. The authors also demonstrated reduced *string* mRNA levels by in situ hybridization. Further experiments are, however, required to determine whether these changes in *string* transcription are due to direct effects of EcR or mediated by another transcriptional regulator. Together this work revealed that the ecdysone pulse at the larval–pupal transition is required for the *string* transcription triggering histoblast proliferation at the onset of abdomen metamorphosis.

## 4. Summary and conclusions

At the level of the whole animal, ecdysone controls larval growth and final body size through interactions with the insulin pathway (King-Jones and Thummel 2005; Shingleton 2005; Mirth and Riddiford 2007; Nijhout 2008). The insulin-signalling pathway acts in the prothoracic gland (PG) to regulate the release of ecdysone, therefore influencing the rate and duration of larval growth. For instance, PG overgrowth causes accelerated metamorphosis, which results in reduced adult size due to the rapid progression through the larval growth stage. Conversely, reducing growth of the PG results in longer larval growth periods and larger adults due to slower ecdysone release and delayed onset of pupariation. Correct timing of the critical peak in ecdysone is therefore essential for controlling larval growth and adult body size.

In the imaginal tissues and larval histoblasts ecdysone most likely regulates cell cycle genes indirectly by modulating upstream developmental signalling pathways. The effect of ecdysone on promoting SMW division in the eye may, in part, be mediated by Hedgehog (Hh) signalling (Brennan, Ashburner, and Moses 1998), and might coordinate this division with the G1 arrest in the furrow via the Dpp signal (Escudero and Freeman 2007; Firth and Baker 2005). In the wing imaginal disc, cell cycle progression requires EcR activity, which is associated with changes to the levels of *wingless* transcription. These changes in Wg may be mediated by the ecdysone-responsive transcription factor Crol (Mitchell et al. 2008) since EcR regulates cell cycle progression in a Crol dependent manner (Figure 7). Thus, by regulating the Wg pathway, which is known to control cell cycle in the wing (Johnston and Edgar 1998; Johnston and Sanders 2003; Herranz et al. 2008), the Crol transcription factor may provide a link between the ecdysone pulse and developmental cell cycle regulation in the wing (Figure 6; (Mitchell et al. 2008)). At the larval–pupal transition ecdysone activates *string* transcription in the histoblasts, triggering exit from G2 phase and histoblast proliferation. It will be of interest to determine whether these changes in *string* transcription are due to direct effects of EcR or, like the cell cycle changes occurring in imaginal tissues, are mediated by changes to developmental signalling.

Together the studies discussed here highlight the diverse mechanisms by which the ecdysone signal can impact on cell division in a range of tissues at different developmental time points. Further work is required to elucidate the molecular mechanisms underlying the ability of ecdysone to modify levels of the complex array of signals required for development.

## 5. References

Alberts, Bruce. 2002. *Molecular biology of the cell*. 4th ed. New York: Garland Science.

Bachman, K. E., and B. H. Park. 2005. Duel nature of TGF-beta signalling: tumor suppressor vs. tumor promoter. *Curr Opin Oncol* 17 (1):49-54.

Baehrecke, E. H. 2000. Steroid regulation of programmed cell death during Drosophila development. *Cell Death Differ* 7 (11):1057-62.

Baker, K. D., L. M. Shewchuk, T. Kozlova, M. Makishima, A. Hassell, B. Wisely, J. A. Caravella, M. H. Lambert, J. L. Reinking, H. Krause, C. S. Thummel, T. M. Willson, and D. J. Mangelsdorf. 2003. The Drosophila orphan nuclear receptor DHR38 mediates an atypical ecdysteroid signalling pathway. *Cell* 113 (6):731-42.

Baker, N. E. 2007. Patterning signals and proliferation in Drosophila imaginal discs. *Curr Opin Genet Dev*.

Bayer, C. A., B. Holley, and J. W. Fristrom. 1996. A switch in broad-complex zinc-finger isoform expression is regulated posttranscriptionally during the metamorphosis of Drosophila imaginal discs. *Dev Biol* 177 (1):1-14.

Beato, M., and J. Klug. 2000. Steroid hormone receptors: an update. *Hum Reprod Update* 6 (3):225-36.

Bender, M., F. B. Imam, W. S. Talbot, B. Ganetzky, and D. S. Hogness. 1997. Drosophila ecdysone receptor mutations reveal functional differences among receptor isoforms. *Cell* 91 (6):777-88.

Blackman, R. K., M. Sanicola, L. A. Raftery, T. Gillevet, and W. M. Gelbart. 1991. An extensive 3' cis-regulatory region directs the imaginal disk expression of decapentaplegic, a member of the TGF-beta family in Drosophila. *Development* 111 (3):657-66.

Brennan, C. A., M. Ashburner, and K. Moses. 1998. Ecdysone pathway is required for furrow progression in the developing Drosophila eye. *Development* 125 (14):2653-64.

Brennan, C. A., T. R. Li, M. Bender, F. Hsiung, and K. Moses. 2001. Broad-complex, but not ecdysone receptor, is required for progression of the morphogenetic furrow in the Drosophila eye. *Development* 128 (1):1-11.

Britton, J. S., W. K. Lockwood, L. Li, S. M. Cohen, and B. A. Edgar. 2002. Drosophila's insulin/PI3-kinase pathway coordinates cellular metabolism with nutritional conditions. *Dev Cell* 2 (2):239-49.

Burtis, K. C., C. S. Thummel, C. W. Jones, F. D. Karim, and D. S. Hogness. 1990. The Drosophila 74EF early puff contains E74, a complex ecdysone-inducible gene that encodes two ets-related proteins. *Cell* 61 (1):85-99.

Caldwell, P. E., M. Walkiewicz, and M. Stern. 2005. Ras activity in the Drosophila prothoracic gland regulates body size and developmental rate via ecdysone release. *Curr Biol* 15 (20):1785-95.

Champlin, D. T., and J. W. Truman. 1998. Ecdysteroid control of cell proliferation during optic lobe neurogenesis in the moth Manduca sexta. *Development* 125 (2):269-77.

― ― ―. 1998. Ecdysteroids govern two phases of eye development during metamorphosis of the moth, Manduca sexta. *Development* 125 (11):2009-18.

Cherbas, L., X. Hu, I. Zhimulev, E. Belyaeva, and P. Cherbas. 2003. EcR isoforms in Drosophila: testing tissue-specific requirements by targeted blockade and rescue. *Development* 130 (2):271-84.

Church, R. B., and F. W. Robertson. 1966. Biochemical analysis of genetic differences in the growth of Drosophila. *Genet Res* 7 (3):383-407.

Colombani, J., L. Bianchini, S. Layalle, E. Pondeville, C. Dauphin-Villemant, C. Antoniewski, C. Carre, S. Noselli, and P. Leopold. 2005. Antagonistic actions of ecdysone and insulins determine final size in Drosophila. *Science* 310 (5748):667-70.

Condic, M. L., D. Fristrom, and J. W. Fristrom. 1991. Apical cell shape changes during Drosophila imaginal leg disc elongation: a novel morphogenetic mechanism. *Development* 111 (1):23-33.

Cranna, N., and L. Quinn. 2009. Impact of steroid hormone signals on Drosophila cell cycle during development. *Cell Div* 4:3.

D'Avino, P. P., and C. S. Thummel. 1998. crooked legs encodes a family of zinc finger proteins required for leg morphogenesis and ecdysone-regulated gene expression during Drosophila metamorphosis. *Development* 125 (9):1733-45.

— — —. 2000. The ecdysone regulatory pathway controls wing morphogenesis and integrin expression during Drosophila metamorphosis. *Dev Biol* 220 (2):211-24.

Davidowitz, G., L. J. D'Amico, and H. F. Nijhout. 2003. Critical weight in the development of insect body size. *Evol Dev* 5 (2):188-97.

de Celis, J. F., A. Garcia-Bellido, and S. J. Bray. 1996. Activation and function of Notch at the dorsal-ventral boundary of the wing imaginal disc. *Development* 122 (1):359-69.

Delanoue, R., M. Slaidina, and P. Leopold. 2010. The steroid hormone ecdysone controls systemic growth by repressing dMyc function in Drosophila fat cells. *Dev Cell* 18 (6):1012-21.

Derynck, R., R. J. Akhurst, and A. Balmain. 2001. TGF-beta signalling in tumor suppression and cancer progression. *Nat Genet* 29 (2):117-29.

DiBello, P. R., D. A. Withers, C. A. Bayer, J. W. Fristrom, and G. M. Guild. 1991. The Drosophila Broad-Complex encodes a family of related proteins containing zinc fingers. *Genetics* 129 (2):385-97.

Dominick, O. S., and J. W. Truman. 1985. The physiology of wandering behaviour in Manduca sexta. II. The endocrine control of wandering behaviour. *J Exp Biol* 117:45-68.

Duman-Scheel, M., L. A. Johnston, and W. Du. 2004. Repression of dMyc expression by Wingless promotes Rbf-induced G1 arrest in the presumptive Drosophila wing margin. *Proc Natl Acad Sci U S A* 101 (11):3857-62.

Duman-Scheel, M., L. Weng, S. Xin, and W. Du. 2002. Hedgehog regulates cell growth and proliferation by inducing Cyclin D and Cyclin E. *Nature* 417 (6886):299-304.

Edgar, B. A. 2006. How flies get their size: genetics meets physiology. *Nat Rev Genet* 7 (12):907-16.

Edgar, B. A., and S. A. Datar. 1996. Zygotic degradation of two maternal Cdc25 mRNAs terminates Drosophila's early cell cycle program. *Genes Dev* 10 (15):1966-77.

Edgar, B. A., D. A. Lehman, and P. H. O'Farrell. 1994. Transcriptional regulation of string (cdc25): a link between developmental programming and the cell cycle. *Development* 120 (11):3131-43.

Edgar, B. A., and C. F. Lehner. 1996. Developmental control of cell cycle regulators: a fly's perspective. *Science* 274 (5293):1646-52.

Edgar, B. A., and P. H. O'Farrell. 1990. The three postblastoderm cell cycles of Drosophila embryogenesis are regulated in G2 by string. *Cell* 62 (3):469-80.

Elliott, R. L., and G. C. Blobe. 2005. Role of transforming growth factor Beta in human cancer. *J Clin Oncol* 23 (9):2078-93.

Emery, I. F., V. Bedian, and G. M. Guild. 1994. Differential expression of Broad-Complex transcription factors may forecast tissue-specific developmental fates during Drosophila metamorphosis. *Development* 120 (11):3275-87.

Epstein, E. H. 2008. Basal cell carcinomas: attack of the hedgehog. *Nat Rev Cancer* 8 (10):743-54.

Escudero, L. M., and M. Freeman. 2007. Mechanism of G1 arrest in the Drosophila eye imaginal disc. *BMC Dev Biol* 7:13.

Evangelista, M., H. Tian, and F. J. de Sauvage. 2006. The hedgehog signalling pathway in cancer. *Clin Cancer Res* 12 (20 Pt 1):5924-8.

Firth, L. C., and N. E. Baker. 2005. Extracellular signals responsible for spatially regulated proliferation in the differentiating Drosophila eye. *Dev Cell* 8 (4):541-51.

Fristrom, J. W., and D. Fristrom. 1993. *The Metamorphic Development of the Adult Epidermis.* Edited by M. Bates. Vol. 2, *The Development of Drosophila melanogaster*: Cold Spring Harbour Laboratory Press.

Gates, J., and C. S. Thummel. 2000. An enhancer trap screen for ecdysone-inducible genes required for Drosophila adult leg morphogenesis. *Genetics* 156 (4):1765-76.

Ghbeish, N., and M. McKeown. 2002. Analyzing the repressive function of ultraspiracle, the Drosophila RXR, in Drosophila eye development. *Mech Dev* 111 (1-2):89-98.

Ghbeish, N., C. C. Tsai, M. Schubiger, J. Y. Zhou, R. M. Evans, and M. McKeown. 2001. The dual role of ultraspiracle, the Drosophila retinoid X receptor, in the ecdysone response. *Proc Natl Acad Sci U S A* 98 (7):3867-72.

Grad, I., A. Niedziela-Majka, M. Kochman, and A. Ozyhar. 2001. Analysis of Usp DNA binding domain targeting reveals critical determinants of the ecdysone receptor complex interaction with the response element. *Eur J Biochem* 268 (13):3751-8.

Grebe, M., T. Fauth, and M. Spindler-Barth. 2004. Dynamic of ligand binding to Drosophila melanogaster ecdysteroid receptor. *Insect Biochem Mol Biol* 34 (9):981-9.

Hall, B. L., and C. S. Thummel. 1998. The RXR homolog ultraspiracle is an essential component of the Drosophila ecdysone receptor. *Development* 125 (23):4709-17.

Hayashi, S. 1996. A Cdc2 dependent checkpoint maintains diploidy in Drosophila. *Development* 122 (4):1051-8.

Heberlein, U., C. M. Singh, A. Y. Luk, and T. J. Donohoe. 1995. Growth and differentiation in the Drosophila eye coordinated by hedgehog. *Nature* 373 (6516):709-11.

Heberlein, U., T. Wolff, and G. M. Rubin. 1993. The TGF beta homolog dpp and the segment polarity gene hedgehog are required for propagation of a morphogenetic wave in the Drosophila retina. *Cell* 75 (5):913-26.

Henrich, V. C., R. L. Tucker, G. Maroni, and L. I. Gilbert. 1987. The ecdysoneless (ecd1ts) mutation disrupts ecdysteroid synthesis autonomously in the ring gland of Drosophila melanogaster. *Dev Biol* 120 (1):50-5.

Herranz, H., L. Perez, F. A. Martin, and M. Milan. 2008. A Wingless and Notch double-repression mechanism regulates G1-S transition in the Drosophila wing. *Embo J* 27 (11):1633-45.

Horsfield, J., A. Penton, J. Secombe, F. M. Hoffman, and H. Richardson. 1998. decapentaplegic is required for arrest in G1 phase during Drosophila eye development. *Development* 125 (24):5069-78.

Hu, X., L. Cherbas, and P. Cherbas. 2003. Transcription activation by the ecdysone receptor (EcR/USP): identification of activation functions. *Mol Endocrinol* 17 (4):716-31.

Jakowlew, S. B. 2006. Transforming growth factor-beta in cancer and metastasis. *Cancer Metastasis Rev* 25 (3):435-57.

Jiang, C., E. H. Baehrecke, and C. S. Thummel. 1997. Steroid regulated programmed cell death during Drosophila metamorphosis. *Development* 124 (22):4673-83.

Johnson, R. L., J. K. Grenier, and M. P. Scott. 1995. patched overexpression alters wing disc size and pattern: transcriptional and post-transcriptional effects on hedgehog targets. *Development* 121 (12):4161-70.

Johnston, L. A., and B. A. Edgar. 1998. Wingless and Notch regulate cell-cycle arrest in the developing Drosophila wing. *Nature* 394 (6688):82-4.

Johnston, L. A., D. A. Prober, B. A. Edgar, R. N. Eisenman, and P. Gallant. 1999. Drosophila myc regulates cellular growth during development. *Cell* 98 (6):779-90.

Johnston, L. A., and A. L. Sanders. 2003. Wingless promotes cell survival but constrains growth during Drosophila wing development. *Nat Cell Biol* 5 (9):827-33.

Karim, F. D., G. M. Guild, and C. S. Thummel. 1993. The Drosophila Broad-Complex plays a key role in controlling ecdysone-regulated gene expression at the onset of metamorphosis. *Development* 118 (3):977-88.

Kassis, J. A., E. Noll, E. P. VanSickle, W. F. Odenwald, and N. Perrimon. 1992. Altering the insertional specificity of a Drosophila transposable element. *Proc Natl Acad Sci U S A* 89 (5):1919-23.

King-Jones, K., J. P. Charles, G. Lam, and C. S. Thummel. 2005. The ecdysone-induced DHR4 orphan nuclear receptor coordinates growth and maturation in Drosophila. *Cell* 121 (5):773-84.

King-Jones, K., and C. S. Thummel. 2005. Developmental biology. Less steroids make bigger flies. *Science* 310 (5748):630-1.

Knoblich, J. A., K. Sauer, L. Jones, H. Richardson, R. Saint, and C. F. Lehner. 1994. Cyclin E controls S phase progression and its down-regulation during Drosophila embryogenesis is required for the arrest of cell proliferation. *Cell* 77 (1):107-20.

Koelle, M. R., W. S. Talbot, W. A. Segraves, M. T. Bender, P. Cherbas, and D. S. Hogness. 1991. The Drosophila EcR gene encodes an ecdysone receptor, a new member of the steroid receptor superfamily. *Cell* 67 (1):59-77.

Kozlova, T., G. V. Pokholkova, G. Tzertzinis, J. D. Sutherland, I. F. Zhimulev, and F. C. Kafatos. 1998. Drosophila hormone receptor 38 functions in metamorphosis: a role in adult cuticle formation. *Genetics* 149 (3):1465-75.

Kozlova, T., and C. S. Thummel. 2002. Spatial patterns of ecdysteroid receptor activation during the onset of Drosophila metamorphosis. *Development* 129 (7):1739-50.

Kylsten, P., and R. Saint. 1997. Imaginal tissues of Drosophila melanogaster exhibit different modes of cell proliferation control. *Dev Biol* 192 (2):509-22.

Lawrence, P. A., J. Casal, and G. Struhl. 1999. hedgehog and engrailed: pattern formation and polarity in the Drosophila abdomen. *Development* 126 (11):2431-9.

– – –. 1999. The hedgehog morphogen and gradients of cell affinity in the abdomen of Drosophila. *Development* 126 (11):2441-9.

Layalle, S., N. Arquier, and P. Leopold. 2008. The TOR pathway couples nutrition and developmental timing in Drosophila. *Dev Cell* 15 (4):568-77.

Lecuit, T., W. J. Brook, M. Ng, M. Calleja, H. Sun, and S. M. Cohen. 1996. Two distinct mechanisms for long-range patterning by Decapentaplegic in the Drosophila wing. *Nature* 381 (6581):387-93.

Li, T. R., and K. P. White. 2003. Tissue-specific gene expression and ecdysone-regulated genomic networks in Drosophila. *Dev Cell* 5 (1):59-72.

Madhavan, M. M., and K. Madhavan. 1980. Morphogenesis of the epidermis of adult abdomen of Drosophila. *J Embryol Exp Morphol* 60:1-31.

– – –. 1984. Do larval epidermal cells possess the blueprint for adult pattern in Drosophila? *J Embryol Exp Morphol* 82:1-8.

Mangelsdorf, D. J., and R. M. Evans. 1995. The RXR heterodimers and orphan receptors. *Cell* 83 (6):841-50.

Marchal, E., H. P. Vandersmissen, L. Badisco, S. Van de Velde, H. Verlinden, M. Iga, P. Van Wielendaele, R. Huybrechts, G. Simonet, G. Smagghe, and J. Vanden Broeck. 2010. Control of ecdysteroidogenesis in prothoracic glands of insects: a review. *Peptides* 31 (3):506-19.

Martin-Castellanos, C., and B. A. Edgar. 2002. A characterization of the effects of Dpp signalling on cell growth and proliferation in the Drosophila wing. *Development* 129 (4):1003-13.

Massague, J. 2008. TGFbeta in Cancer. *Cell* 134 (2):215-30.

McBrayer, Z., H. Ono, M. Shimell, J. P. Parvy, R. B. Beckstead, J. T. Warren, C. S. Thummel, C. Dauphin-Villemant, L. I. Gilbert, and M. B. O'Connor. 2007. Prothoracicotropic hormone regulates developmental timing and body size in Drosophila. *Dev Cell* 13 (6):857-71.

Milan, M. 1998. Cell cycle control in the Drosophila wing. *Bioessays* 20 (12):969-71.

Milan, M., S. Campuzano, and A. Garcia-Bellido. 1996. Cell cycling and patterned cell proliferation in the wing primordium of Drosophila. *Proc Natl Acad Sci U S A* 93 (2):640-5.

Mirth, C. K., and L. M. Riddiford. 2007. Size assessment and growth control: how adult size is determined in insects. *Bioessays* 29 (4):344-55.

Mirth, C., J. W. Truman, and L. M. Riddiford. 2005. The role of the prothoracic gland in determining critical weight for metamorphosis in Drosophila melanogaster. *Curr Biol* 15 (20):1796-807.

Mitchell, N., N. Cranna, H. Richardson, and L. Quinn. 2008. The Ecdysone-inducible zinc-finger transcription factor Crol regulates Wg transcription and cell cycle progression in Drosophila. *Development* 135 (16):2707-16.

Murone, M., A. Rosenthal, and F. J. de Sauvage. 1999. Hedgehog signal transduction: from flies to vertebrates. *Exp Cell Res* 253 (1):25-33.

Neufeld, T. P., A. F. de la Cruz, L. A. Johnston, and B. A. Edgar. 1998. Coordination of growth and cell division in the Drosophila wing. *Cell* 93 (7):1183-93.

Nijhout, H. F. 2008. Size matters (but so does time), and it's OK to be different. *Dev Cell* 15 (4):491-2.

Nijhout, H. F., and C. M. Williams. 1974. Control of moulting and metamorphosis in the tobacco hornworm, Manduca sexta (L.): cessation of juvenile hormone secretion as a trigger for pupation. *J Exp Biol* 61 (2):493-501.

— — —. 1974. Control of moulting and metamorphosis in the tobacco hornworm, Manduca sexta (L.): growth of the last-instar larva and the decision to pupate. *J Exp Biol* 61 (2):481-91.

Ninov, N., D. A. Chiarelli, and E. Martin-Blanco. 2007. Extrinsic and intrinsic mechanisms directing epithelial cell sheet replacement during Drosophila metamorphosis. *Development* 134 (2):367-79.

Ninov, N., C. Manjon, and E. Martin-Blanco. 2009. Dynamic control of cell cycle and growth coupling by ecdysone, EGFR, and PI3K signalling in Drosophila histoblasts. *PLoS Biol* 7 (4):e1000079.

Oro, A. E., M. McKeown, and R. M. Evans. 1990. Relationship between the product of the Drosophila ultraspiracle locus and the vertebrate retinoid X receptor. *Nature* 347 (6290):298-301.

Penton, A., S. B. Selleck, and F. M. Hoffmann. 1997. Regulation of cell cycle synchronization by decapentaplegic during Drosophila eye development. *Science* 275 (5297):203-6.

Peter, A., P. Schottler, M. Werner, N. Beinert, G. Dowe, P. Burkert, F. Mourkioti, L. Dentzer, Y. He, P. Deak, P. V. Benos, M. K. Gatt, L. Murphy, D. Harris, B. Barrell, C. Ferraz, S. Vidal, C. Brun, J. Demaille, E. Cadieu, S. Dreano, S. Gloux, V. Lelaure, S. Mottier, F. Galibert, D. Borkova, B. Minana, F. C. Kafatos, S. Bolshakov, I. Siden-Kiamos, G. Papagiannakis, L. Spanos, C. Louis, E. Madueno, B. de Pablos, J. Modolell, A.

Bucheton, D. Callister, L. Campbell, N. S. Henderson, P. J. McMillan, C. Salles, E. Tait, P. Valenti, R. D. Saunders, A. Billaud, L. Pachter, R. Klapper, W. Janning, D. M. Glover, M. Ashburner, H. J. Bellen, H. Jackle, and U. Schafer. 2002. Mapping and identification of essential gene functions on the X chromosome of Drosophila. *EMBO Rep* 3 (1):34-8.

Pignoni, F., and S. L. Zipursky. 1997. Induction of Drosophila eye development by decapentaplegic. *Development* 124 (2):271-8.

Prober, D. A., and B. A. Edgar. 2002. Interactions between Ras1, dMyc, and dPI3K signalling in the developing Drosophila wing. *Genes Dev* 16 (17):2286-99.

Ready, D. F., T. E. Hanson, and S. Benzer. 1976. Development of the Drosophila retina, a neurocrystalline lattice. *Dev Biol* 53 (2):217-40.

Reis, T., and B. A. Edgar. 2004. Negative regulation of dE2F1 by cyclin-dependent kinases controls cell cycle timing. *Cell* 117 (2):253-64.

Richardson, H., L. V. O'Keefe, T. Marty, and R. Saint. 1995. Ectopic cyclin E expression induces premature entry into S phase and disrupts pattern formation in the Drosophila eye imaginal disc. *Development* 121 (10):3371-9.

Riddiford, L. M. 1993. Hormone receptors and the regulation of insect metamorphosis. *Receptor* 3 (3):203-9.

Rusconi, J. C., R. Hays, and R. L. Cagan. 2000. Programmed cell death and patterning in Drosophila. *Cell Death Differ* 7 (11):1063-70.

Schubiger, M., C. Carre, C. Antoniewski, and J. W. Truman. 2005. Ligand-dependent derepression via EcR/USP acts as a gate to coordinate the differentiation of sensory neurons in the Drosophila wing. *Development* 132 (23):5239-48.

Schubiger, M., and J. W. Truman. 2000. The RXR ortholog USP suppresses early metamorphic processes in Drosophila in the absence of ecdysteroids. *Development* 127 (6):1151-9.

Segraves, W. A., and D. S. Hogness. 1990. The E75 ecdysone-inducible gene responsible for the 75B early puff in Drosophila encodes two new members of the steroid receptor superfamily. *Genes Dev* 4 (2):204-19.

Serra, R., and H. L. Moses. 1996. Tumor suppressor genes in the TGF-beta signalling pathway? *Nat Med* 2 (4):390-1.

Shingleton, A. W. 2005. Body-size regulation: combining genetics and physiology. *Curr Biol* 15 (20):R825-7.

Strigini, M., and S. M. Cohen. 2000. Wingless gradient formation in the Drosophila wing. *Curr Biol* 10 (6):293-300.

Sullivan, A. A., and C. S. Thummel. 2003. Temporal profiles of nuclear receptor gene expression reveal coordinate transcriptional responses during Drosophila development. *Mol Endocrinol* 17 (11):2125-37.

Sutherland, J. D., T. Kozlova, G. Tzertzinis, and F. C. Kafatos. 1995. Drosophila hormone receptor 38: a second partner for Drosophila USP suggests an unexpected role for nuclear receptors of the nerve growth factor-induced protein B type. *Proc Natl Acad Sci U S A* 92 (17):7966-70.

Talbot, W. S., E. A. Swyryd, and D. S. Hogness. 1993. Drosophila tissues with different metamorphic responses to ecdysone express different ecdysone receptor isoforms. *Cell* 73 (7):1323-37.

Thomas, B. J., and S. L. Zipursky. 1994. Early pattern formation in the developing Drosophila eye. *Trends Cell Biol* 4 (11):389-94.

Thummel, C. S. 1990. Puffs and gene regulation--molecular insights into the Drosophila ecdysone regulatory hierarchy. *Bioessays* 12 (12):561-8.

— — —. 1995. From embryogenesis to metamorphosis: the regulation and function of Drosophila nuclear receptor superfamily members. *Cell* 83 (6):871-7.

— — —. 1996. Files on steroids--Drosophila metamorphosis and the mechanisms of steroid hormone action. *Trends Genet* 12 (8):306-10.

— — —. 2001. Molecular mechanisms of developmental timing in C. elegans and Drosophila. *Dev Cell* 1 (4):453-65.

— — —. 2001. Steroid-triggered death by autophagy. *Bioessays* 23 (8):677-82.

— — —. 2002. Ecdysone-regulated puff genes 2000. *Insect Biochem Mol Biol* 32 (2):113-20.

Thummel, C. S., K. C. Burtis, and D. S. Hogness. 1990. Spatial and temporal patterns of E74 transcription during Drosophila development. *Cell* 61 (1):101-11.

Toftgard, R. 2000. Hedgehog signalling in cancer. *Cell Mol Life Sci* 57 (12):1720-31.

Urness, L. D., and C. S. Thummel. 1995. Molecular analysis of a steroid-induced regulatory hierarchy: the Drosophila E74A protein directly regulates L71-6 transcription. *Embo J* 14 (24):6239-46.

Varjosalo, M., and J. Taipale. 2008. Hedgehog: functions and mechanisms. *Genes Dev* 22 (18):2454-72.

Vestergaard, J., M. Bak, and L. A. Larsen. 2005. The hedgehog signalling pathway in cancer. *Prog Mol Subcell Biol* 40:1-28.

Wakefield, L. M., and A. B. Roberts. 2002. TGF-beta signalling: positive and negative effects on tumorigenesis. *Curr Opin Genet Dev* 12 (1):22-9.

Ward, R. E., P. Reid, A. Bashirullah, P. P. D'Avino, and C. S. Thummel. 2003. GFP in living animals reveals dynamic developmental responses to ecdysone during Drosophila metamorphosis. *Dev Biol* 256 (2):389-402.

Williams, J. A., S. W. Paddock, and S. B. Carroll. 1993. Pattern formation in a secondary field: a hierarchy of regulatory genes subdivides the developing Drosophila wing disc into discrete subregions. *Development* 117 (2):571-84.

Wolff, T., and D. F. Ready. 1991. The beginning of pattern formation in the Drosophila compound eye: the morphogenetic furrow and the second mitotic wave. *Development* 113 (3):841-50.

Yao, T. P., B. M. Forman, Z. Jiang, L. Cherbas, J. D. Chen, M. McKeown, P. Cherbas, and R. M. Evans. 1993. Functional ecdysone receptor is the product of EcR and Ultraspiracle genes. *Nature* 366 (6454):476-9.

Yao, T. P., W. A. Segraves, A. E. Oro, M. McKeown, and R. M. Evans. 1992. Drosophila ultraspiracle modulates ecdysone receptor function via heterodimer formation. *Cell* 71 (1):63-72.

Yin, V. P., and C. S. Thummel. 2005. Mechanisms of steroid-triggered programmed cell death in Drosophila. *Semin Cell Dev Biol* 16 (2):237-43.

Zelhof, A. C., N. Ghbeish, C. Tsai, R. M. Evans, and M. McKeown. 1997. A role for ultraspiracle, the Drosophila RXR, in morphogenetic furrow movement and photoreceptor cluster formation. *Development* 124 (13):2499-506.

Zheng, X., J. Wang, T. E. Haerry, A. Y. Wu, J. Martin, M. B. O'Connor, C. H. Lee, and T. Lee. 2003. TGF-beta signalling activates steroid hormone receptor expression during neuronal remodeling in the Drosophila brain. *Cell* 112 (3):303-15.

Zitnan, D., Y. J. Kim, I. Zitnanova, L. Roller, and M. E. Adams. 2007. Complex steroid-peptide-receptor cascade controls insect ecdysis. *Gen Comp Endocrinol* 153 (1-3):88-96.

# Part 3

## Pharmacology

# 9

# Drug Design Approaches to Manipulate the Agonist-Antagonist Equilibrium in Steroid Receptors

Scott J. Lusher[1,6], Paolo Conti[2], Wim Dokter[3],
Pedro H. Hermkens[2,4] and Jacob de Vlieg[1,5,6]
*Departments of*
*[1]Molecular Design & Informatics,*
*[2]Medicinal Chemistry*
*[3]Immune Therapeutics, MSD, Oss*
*[4]Institute of Molecules & Materials*
*[5]Computational Drug Discovery Group,*
*Radboud University, Nijmegen,*
*[6]Netherlands eScience Center,*
*The Netherlands*

## 1. Introduction

The steroid hormone receptors, the Androgen Receptor (AR), Estrogen Receptors (ERα and ERβ), Glucocorticoid Receptor (GR), Mineralocorticoid Receptor and Progesterone Receptor (PR), have been crucial targets for drug discovery even before their existence was known or understood. The drugs on the market for this sub-class of the nuclear hormone receptors constitute a significant pharmacopeia for the treatment of a vast array of conditions and ailments. Despite the breadth of drugs targeted toward this family, they remain an important target for the pharmaceutical industry.

Key considerations when designing drugs for any family, beyond the on-target pharmaceutical action and safety, is to ensure specificity against related targets, exploration of the most appropriate routes of administration and desirable pharmacokinetic (PK) profiles. Developing non-steroidal modulators for the steroid receptor family has been a key strategy employed to achieve these goals, although there appears to be growing consensus that not being steroidal is insufficient to justify new drugs on its own (Hermkens et al, 2006). Unlike targeting many families, steroid hormone receptor drug discovery also has to balance the need to elicit either agonistic or antagonistic responses depending on the desired indication.

The history of drug discovery for the steroid hormone receptors has tended to follow a common path, beginning with the application of purified endogenous hormone and followed by the application of the first synthetic analogs with improved PK properties or selectivity. For some of the receptors this period was followed by the design of antagonists, including non-steroidal structures. More recently, steroid hormone drug discovery has been dominated by the search for ligands characterized by partial agonistic or partial antagonistic responses, the so called selective modulators. It is hoped and expected that partial agonists and antagonists for the various receptors will provide improved therapeutic profiles. For example, selective GR modulators (SGRMs) could provide their anti-inflammatory action without the undesirable side-effects, including osteoporosis and diabetes, currently associated with oral glucocorticoids (Hudson, Roach, and Higuchi, 2008). Selective ER modulators (SERMs) hold the promise of being active on bone but not breast or endometrial tissue (Shelly et al, 2008;Silverman, 2010), whereas a desirable profile for a selective AR modulator (SARM) would likely have a greater action in bone and muscle compared to the prostate (Gao and Dalton, 2007).

## 2. Molecular basis for partial agonism

The shared domain structure of steroid receptors includes a variable N-terminal domain, a highly conserved DNA-binding domain and a moderately conserved ligand-binding domain (LBD). The LBD domain tends to be the primary target for drug-design. The LBD combines a number of functions, including hormone binding, receptor dimerization and binding to other co-modulating proteins that play a role in the control of transcription. These functions have the ability to influence each other, with ligand-binding, as an example; influencing the pattern of co-modulator recruitment. Specifically, gene activation requires the recruitment of co-modulating proteins to a region of the surface of the LBD formed by helices 3/4, 5 and 12. The position of helix-12, as we will discuss, can be influenced by the nature of the ligand bound to the receptor allowing drugs to influence the binding of co-modulators and consequently gene activation and the resulting biological effects (Bourguet, Germain, and Gronemeyer, 2000;Egea, Klaholz, and Moras, 2000;Kumar and Thompson, 1999;Weatherman, Fletterick, and Scanlan, 1999).

Understanding the molecular basis for partial agonism is hampered by the difficulty in solving the X-ray structures of steroid-receptors in general and specifically complexes including partial active ligands (Nettles et al, 2008). Full agonists stabilize the receptor, and specifically helix-12, in a conformation suited to binding co-activating proteins and full antagonists stabilize the receptor in a conformation suited to binding co-repressing proteins. The apparent reason for the difficulty in co-crystallizing partial agonists is that they do not fully stabilize the receptor in either conformation, adopting some degree of equilibrium between the two (Nettles et al, 2008;Raaijmakers, Versteegh, and Uitdehaag, 2009). This equilibrium allows partially active compounds to bind unique patterns of co-modulators compared to full agonists and antagonists, resulting in their potentially interesting biological effects. Unfortunately as a result it also renders them poorly suited to co-crystallization studies.

The degree of partial activity (how far from either a full agonist or antagonist response) will go some way to determining the profile of co-modulators which will bind. Additionally, the ratio of co-activators compared to co-repressors in each cell type will influence the biological effect of a partial compound. In cells with a high co-activator concentration we would expect partial compounds to show a greater degree of agonistic activity compared to the same ligand in a cell with a high co-repressor concentration. The limitless combination of ligand partiality and co-modulator distribution appears to be a major contributor to the tissue selective responses of partial compounds.

# 3. Mechanisms for ligand-induced partial agonist design

In the absence of a complete record of X-ray structures of steroid receptors bound to agonists, antagonists and partially active compounds, we have to fill in the knowledge gaps with mutation studies and ligand-based structure-activity relationships (SAR). Even with this extra information, our understanding of the mechanisms underpinning the repositioning of helix-12 and the resulting spectrum of partial responses remains relatively naive, but there do appear to be a small number of approaches available to the drug designer who wishes to rationally influence the degree of agonism elicited by their compound series.

1.  Sterically impede the agonistic orientation of Helix-12
2.  Disrupt the function of other indirect stabilizing interactions.
3.  Influence the position of Helix-12 by modulating the end of Helix-11 and the loop between Helices 11 & 12.
4.  Reduce the stabilizing interactions between the ligand and Helix-12.
5.  Straighten Helix-3, and/or disrupt interactions between Helices 3 & 5.

Incorporating these approaches into the optimization of steroid receptor ligands allows the drug-designer to modulate the degree of agonistic and antagonistic response their compounds induce. Pharmacologically it remains difficult to define *a priori* the precise agonistic or antagonistic efficacy (percentage effect or intrinsic activity) required for any desired indication, but it is now possible to generate a series of ligands with tuned efficacies to cover a broad range and then utilize molecular profiling approaches to select the most desirable.

The five basic approaches for generating partially active compounds have been deduced by numerous studies from all members of the steroid receptors and nuclear receptor family in total. For the purposes of this review we present a single receptor case study to demonstrate each of the five mechanisms, but wish to stress that to a greater and lesser degree all mechanisms should be applicable to all steroid receptors.

## 3.1 Sterically impede the agonistic orientation of helix-12
### 3.1.1 Case study: the progesterone receptor

Steroidal anti-progestins are typically differentiated structurally from progestins by the presence of a bulky attachment at their position 11 (Madauss, Stewart, and Williams, 2007). Recent publications of the anti-progestin Mifepristone (Raaijmakers, Versteegh, and Uitdehaag, 2009) and the SPRM Asoprisnil (Madauss et al, 2007) clearly demonstrate that the role of this bulky attachment is to clash with helix-12 and preclude it from adopting its required agonistic position. Both studies also demonstrate an important role specifically for Met909 in the agonism/antagonism balance. Met909 sits within helix-12 at the C-terminal end of the ligand binding domain (LBD), and in the classic agonist conformation of the receptor, is oriented toward the ligand binding pocket. Met909 is typically the only helix-12 residue directly in contact with ligands. The nature of the ligand-Met909 interactions appears to be a key determinant of the receptors function (Petit-Topin et al, 2009). Clashes between Met909 and ligands are likely to destabilize helix-12 (Raaijmakers, Versteegh, and Uitdehaag, 2009), which results in a reduced agonistic response. It has even been suggested that the degree of clash with Met909 might correspond directly to the reduction in agonism (Madauss, Stewart, and Williams, 2007), but this has yet to be shown categorically.

Introducing bulky groups onto PR modulating non-steroidal scaffolds has also been demonstrated to result in partial agonists on a number of occasions (Jones et al, 2005;Kallander et al, 2010;Thompson et al, 2009;Washburn et al, 2009).

### 3.1.2 Additional examples

The existence of a clash between antagonists and helix-12 was first demonstrated for ER by studies comparing the X-ray structures of Estradiol to Raloxifene (Brzozowski et al, 1997) and Diethylstilbestrol to Tamoxifen (Shiau et al, 1998). Numerous reviews of these two studies have been published (Hubbard et al, 2000;Kong, Pike, and Hubbard, 2003;Mueller-Fahrnow and Egner, 1999;Pike et al, 2000;Pike, Brzozowski, and Hubbard, 2000) as have many further studies on the X-ray structures of SERMs, full antagonists and full agonists bound to the ERs (Blizzard et al, 2005;Dykstra et al, 2007;Heldring et al, 2007;Kim et al, 2004;Renaud et al, 2003;Renaud et al, 2005;Tan et al, 2005;Vajdos et al, 2007).

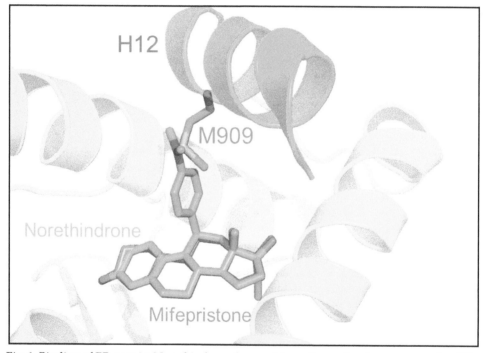

Fig. 1. Binding of PR agonist Norethindrone (orange) from X-ray structure compared to PR antagonist Mifepristone (green) demonstrating clash between antagonists and Met909 in helix-12.

The same helix-12 clash has also been demonstrated for AR (Cantin et al, 2007) and GR (Schoch et al, 2010) in recent X-ray structure determination studies. It was also suggested for GR by a mutagenesis study (Hillmann et al, 2002) that showed that mutating Leu753 (equivalent to Met909 in PR) to a phenylalanine results in a receptor defective in transactivation. We can conclude that the reason for this loss of activation is that an increase in the size of the residue at this position prevents helix-12 from adopting its agonistic conformation due to a clash with the ligand.

## 3.2 Disrupt the function of direct stabilizing interactions
### 3.2.1 Case study: the androgen receptor

The binding of testosterone and dihydrotestosterone to AR demonstrate the existence of crucial receptor stabilizing interactions mediated by agonistic ligands. As we will discuss later, the loop between helix-11 and helix-12 is a key region for mediating partial agonism. As shown in figure 2, AR is stabilized by a ligand mediated hydrogen-bond network from Thr877 in helix-11 to the 17β-OH group in the endogenous steroidal agonists to Asn705 in helix-3 and finally to the backbone of Asp890 in the loop itself (Matias et al, 2000).

Hydroxyflutamide is the active metabolite of the androgen receptor antagonist flutamide. Its antagonism appears to be a result of its inability to complete the entire network of stabilizing hydrogen-bonds (Bohl et al, 2005) also shown in figure 2. The result is that Thr877 is left buried in a predominately hydrophobic pocket, destabilizing the receptor and shifting the agonist-antagonist equilibrium.

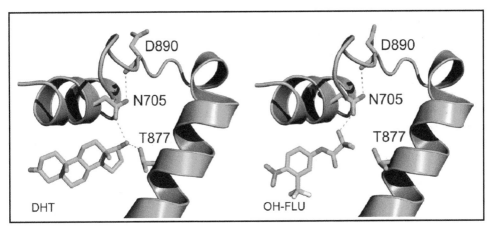

Fig. 2. Left shows the X-ray structure of DHT bound to AR including full hydrogen-bond network. Right shows a model of hydroxyflutamide bound to AR based on the X-ray structure of hydroxyflutamide bound to an AR-T877A mutant.

### 3.2.2 Additional examples

The residue equivalent to AR residue Asn705 in MR is Asn770. Extensive X-ray, SAR and mutation studies have been conducted on Asn770 which demonstrate clearly the existence of a ligand-mediated hydrogen bonding network which is critical for the activation of MR in a similar fashion to the one described for AR (Bledsoe et al, 2005;Hellal-Levy et al, 2000).

Agonistic steroidal ligands for GR and MR are typified by 11β-hydroxyl groups which hydrogen bond to Asn564 in GR and Asn770 in MR respectively. Despite the similarity between MR and PR, the endogenous PR agonist progesterone behaves as an antagonist of PR. This appears to at least in part be due to a lack of an 11β-hydroxyl group on progesterone. It is interesting how the lack of the hydroxyl group doesn't disturb the agonistic activity of PR but does MR.

Another important example of disrupting the function of stabilizing interactions can be seen in the estrogen receptors. In addition to their role in sterically precluding helix-12, SERM side-chains also contain an important basic amine function which is almost ubiquitous amongst this drug class. The role of this nitrogen is to form a salt-bridge to Asp351 in helix-3 of ERα (Asp303 in ERβ). The importance of this salt-bridge is that it requires Asp351 to adopt a new conformation and prevents it from undertaking is usual function of stabilizing the agonistic position of helix-12 by hydrogen-bonding to backbone residues in the helix. It also appears that the exact nature of the interaction between the basic amine and Asp351, including angle, distance and perhaps pKa can influence the biological effect of the ligands.

## 3.3 Modulate the end of helix-11 & the loop between helices-11 & 12
### 3.3.1 Case study: the glucocorticoid receptor

Due to the difficulty in crystallizing partial agonists in complex with steroid-receptors much of the evidence to support these mechanisms has to be inferred from other indirect sources. Some of the most valuable evidence comes from mutagenesis studies including those that indicate that the loop between helix-11 and helix-12 is a hotspot that is crucial to the agonism/antagonism balance in GR.

Mutation of **Ile747**, which sits in the middle of the helix-11 to helix-12 loop, to methionine results in GR having a reduced transactivation potential without affecting the binding of classic glucocorticoids (Vottero et al, 2002). Presumably, the increased size of the residue prevents the correct packing of the loop and therefore destabilizes helix-12.

**Tyr735** at the end of helix-11 is a surface residue whose role is poorly understood, but it has been shown that various mutations (W735F, W735V and W735S) result in a receptor with significant reduction in transactivation activity without affecting ligand binding (Ray et al, 1999;Stevens et al, 2003).

**Thr739** is the last residue in helix-11 whose mutation to alanine has no effect on the binding of triamcinolone acetonide, but does result in a 16-fold reduction in transactivation (Lind et al, 2000).

In addition to these mutation studies, as discussed already, there is also overwhelming evidence across the family to support the hypothesis that **Asn564** is crucial for the agonistic activity of GR and related receptors (Bledsoe et al, 2005;Bledsoe, Stewart, and Pearce, 2004;Fagart et al, 1998;Hellal-Levy et al, 2000;Necela and Cidlowski, 2003;Rafestin-Oblin et al, 2002). The role of Asn564 (Asn705 in AR, Asn770 in MR) was previously discussed.

Tyr735, Thr739 and Ile747, as shown in Fig 3, are all located at the end of helix-11 or in the following loop. Asn564 has an important role in stabilizing the loop. The studies associated with each of these residues indicate how sensitive this region to influencing the agonism/ antagonism balance and therefore the potential to modify its function by ligand design.

The helix-11 to helix-12 loop in steroid-receptors is well suited to drug-design intervention as it forms around the 17β group of steroids and is therefore likely to be in close proximity to most ligands.

Bledsoe and colleagues recognized the importance of this region when solving the first GR-Dexamethasone structure (Bledsoe et al, 2002;Bledsoe, Stewart, and Pearce,2004) as did the group of Kauppi when solving GR complexed with Dexamethasone and RU486, including noting the flexibility of this loop (Kauppi et al, 2003).

### 3.3.2 Additional examples

The importance of the loop region between helix-11 and helix-12 has also been demonstrated by X-ray structure studies for ERα (Pike et al, 1999;Shiau et al, 1998), and mutagenesis studies on MR also support the conclusion that this region of the steroid-receptors is crucial for the agonism/antagonism balance (Fagart et al, 2005).

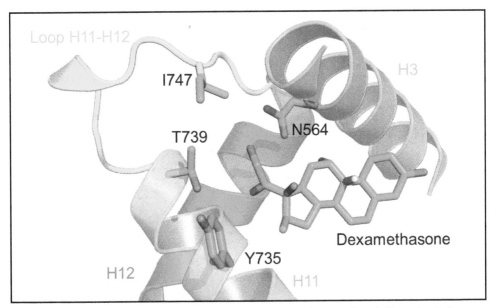

Fig. 3. The loop between helix-11 and helix-12 illustrating key residues believed to influence GR function

### 3.4 Reduce the stabilizing interactions between the ligand and helix-12
### 3.4.1 Case study: the estrogen receptors alpha & beta
Methods for antagonizing or reducing the agonism of steroid receptors that do not involve direct steric clashes with the receptor are often referred to as "passive antagonism". This term was coined by the group of Geoffrey Greene to explain their observations when studying the binding of tetrahydrochyrsene (THC) and its interactions with ERα and ERβ (Shiau et al, 2002).

THC is an ERα agonist and an ERβ antagonist. The group of Greene was able to conclude, after generating X-ray structures of both complexes that THC stabilizes ERα in its agonist conformation but ERβ is in an antagonist conformation. This difference on its own is of significant interest, but the study also demonstrated that the reason for ERβ not adopting an agonist conformation was due to missing stabilizing interactions between the receptor and the ligand. They observe that in ERβ residues Leu476 and Met479 are not positioned correctly by the ligand to form interactions with relevant residues in helix-12 to stabilize its agonist conformation. The result is a failure of THC to stabilize the agonist conformation of helix-12 and therefore a shift in the agonist-antagonist equilibrium. The fact that THC has such differing effects on two such similar receptors illustrates the challenge when following this or any of the five described approaches in drug-design.

### 3.5 Straighten helix-3, and/or disrupt interactions between helices-3 & 5
### 3.5.1 Case study: the mineralocorticoid receptor
It is generally accepted that steroid-receptor activation is facilitated by interactions between helix-3 and helix-5. The correct positioning of the basic component of the charge clamp (Lys579 in GR and Lys785 in MR) and the formation of the hydrophobic pocket in which co-

activators bind is dependent on a bend forming in the middle of helix-3. That bend in helix-3 is induced by a ligand mediated hydrogen bond to helix-5 via the 3-keto group of steroidal ligands. It was initially believed that the importance of the classic interactions between the 3-keto group of steroids and the Glutamine (Glutamate in ERα and ERβ) and Arginine residues in steroid hormones was purely to ensure potent binding of the steroids, but the work of Bledsoe (Bledsoe et al, 2005) and Huyet (Huyet et al, 2007) have demonstrated that is also has a role in the agonism-antagonism balance. Huyet *et al* demonstrated that mutation of either Gln776 or Arg817 in MR to alanine results in previously ligand-mediated agonistic responses being lost.

Bledsoe *et al* have further demonstrated the importance of this bend in helix-3 by characterizing the S810L mutation in MR. This mutation has the effect of stabilizing the agonist conformation of MR, rendering some antagonistic ligands to have an increased agonistic response. Their analysis shows that the role of the S810L mutation is to increase the hydrophobic stabilization between helix-3 and helix-5.

### 3.5.2 Additional example
A recent X-ray structure publication from our group suggests that PR antagonism seen in a compound series can in part be explained by a loss of these same interactions (Lusher et al, 2011).

## 4. Pictorial summary of five drug design approaches

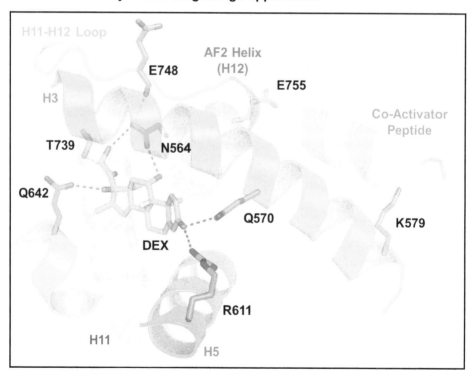

Fig. 4. Binding of Dexamethasone (DEX) to GR

## 4.1 Binding mode of DEX to GR illustrates each of the five design approaches

The binding of Dexamethasone to the Glucocorticoid Receptor (GR) is shown to illustrate the five major routes for reducing agonist efficacy in steroid receptors via the destabilisation of the binding of co-activating proteins. Co-activating proteins bind in a hydrophobic pocket on the surface of the ligand-binding domain (LBD) stabilised by a charge-clamp formed by residues Lys579 in helix-3 and Glu755 in helix-12. [1] Direct clashes between ligands and helix-12 prevent Glu755 from adopting its necessary position and thus prevent the formation of the charge clamp. It has been shown for some receptors that clashes with helix-12 result in the helix adopting a new orientation actually precluding the binding of co-activators by binding in the required hydrophobic pocket. [2] It is probably therefore not a surprise that the positioning of helix-12 can be influenced by the residues that directly precede it. The loop before helix-12 influences its position and is clearly a hotspot that can influence degree of agonism by modifying the ligand. [3] Other interactions also help stabilise helix-12 in its agonist position. For example, in GR, there is a hydrogen-bond network from the ligand to Asn564 in helix-3 to Glu748 in the loop before helix-12. Disruption of this network, by perhaps removing the hydrogen-bonding function in the ligand, can influence the stabilisation of helix-12. [4] In a number of nuclear receptors Helix-12 also makes direct hydrophobic interactions to the ligand. Loss of these interactions, by changing the properties of the ligand, can decrease the stabilisation of helix-12 and therefore alter the agonistic capability of the complex. [5] Finally, the first four approaches are directly or indirectly related to ensuring Glu755, as half of the charge-clamp, is correctly positioned. The second residue in the charge-clamp, Lys579, should not be overlooked. Lys579 is part of helix-3 which itself bends midway along its length. This bend is crucial for ensuring that Lys579 is in the correct position to form the charge-clamp. The bend in helix-3 is partly as a result of its interaction with helix-5. For GR this is largely mediated by a hydrogen-bond network between Gln570 in helix-3, the ligand and Arg611 in helix-5. Disrupting this network by modifying the ligand may influence the distortion in helix-3 and therefore the correct formation of the charge-clamp and therefore co-activator binding.

## 5. Other structure-based design considerations

In addition to exploring the development of partial agonists, structure-based approaches continue to play an important role in the identification of new ligands via virtual screening approaches and other compound optimization tasks. An important lesson in this regard has been our change in understanding the dynamic nature of the steroid-receptor binding pocket. We have seen examples of extensive induced fits for amongst others the glucocorticoid receptor which is able to bind ligands beyond the conventional confines of its binding pocket whilst remaining in an agonistic conformation (Biggadike et al, 2009;Madauss et al, 2008;Suino-Powell et al, 2008). The pocket, behind the crucial helix-3 and helix-5 binding residues, Gln570 and Arg611, is normally water filled. It has already been demonstrated to be a viable ligand-binding region with the potential to improve ligand potency. An interesting note regarding the exploration of the pocket is that GSK report difficulty in combining the use of this pocket with the maintenance of partial agonism (Biggadike et al, 2009). PR has been shown to adapt to steroids baring bulky 17α groups (Madauss et al, 2004) and Trp741 in AR adapts to different ligands, adopting a new position to open an additional channel in the receptor (Bohl et al, 2005).

## 6. Conclusion

As we look to the future of rational and structure-based drug design for the steroid receptors there remain key areas and questions that will dominate research in the short to medium term:

1.  Is each of the five described methods for generating partial compounds equally applicable for each of the receptors? It is generally considered true that ERβ is easier to antagonize than ERα. This is most likely due to the agonist conformation of ERβ being less intrinsically stable than ERα and therefore ensuring that ERβ is more sensitive than ERα in this respect (Pike et al, 1999).
2.  Does the choice of the mechanism for instilling partiality affect the eventual biological activity? Does a compound with a 40% reduction in agonistic activity due to a clash with helix-12 have the same biological effect as a compound with a 40% reduction in agonism due to the loss of other stabilizing interactions?
3.  As described earlier, partial agonists and antagonists are often poor candidates for co-crystallization Recently we have seen the first publications describing methods to circumvent this problem, either by introducing stabilizing mutations into the receptor (Bohl et al, 2007;Fagart et al, 2005;Nettles et al, 2008;Sack et al, 2001) or by generating stable crystals of the receptor using a receptor stabilizing ligand and then exchanging this compound with other compounds of interest via soaking (Raaijmakers, Versteegh, and Uitdehaag, 2009). Both approaches have the potential to dramatically increase our understanding of the biological mechanisms underpinning partial agonism.

## 7. References

Biggadike K, Bledsoe RK, Coe DM, Cooper TW, House D, Iannone MA, Macdonald SJ, Madauss KP, McLay IM, Shipley TJ, Taylor SJ, Tran TB, Uings IJ, Weller V, and Williams SP. 2009. Design and x-ray crystal structures of high-potency nonsteroidal glucocorticoid agonists exploiting a novel binding site on the receptor. *Proc. Natl. Acad. Sci. U. S. A* 106 (43): 18114-18119.

Bledsoe RK, Madauss KP, Holt JA, Apolito CJ, Lambert MH, Pearce KH, Stanley TB, Stewart EL, Trump RP, Willson TM, and Williams SP. 2005. A ligand-mediated hydrogen bond network required for the activation of the mineralocorticoid receptor. *J. Biol. Chem.* 280 (35): 31283-31293.

Bledsoe RK, Montana VG, Stanley TB, Delves CJ, Apolito CJ, McKee DD, Consler TG, Parks DJ, Stewart EL, Willson TM, Lambert MH, Moore JT, Pearce KH, and Xu HE. 2002. Crystal structure of the glucocorticoid receptor ligand binding domain reveals a novel mode of receptor dimerization and coactivator recognition. *Cell* 110 (1): 93-105.

Bledsoe RK, Stewart EL, and Pearce KH. 2004. Structure and function of the glucocorticoid receptor ligand binding domain. *Vitam. Horm.* 68: 49-91.

Blizzard TA, Dininno F, Morgan JD, Chen HY, Wu JY, Kim S, Chan W, Birzin ET, Yang YT, Pai LY, Fitzgerald PM, Sharma N, Li Y, Zhang Z, Hayes EC, DaSilva CA, Tang W, Rohrer SP, Schaeffer JM, and Hammond ML. 2005. Estrogen receptor ligands. Part 9: Dihydrobenzoxathiin SERAMs with alkyl substituted pyrrolidine side chains and linkers. *Bioorg. Med. Chem. Lett.* 15 (1): 107-113.

Bohl CE, Gao W, Miller DD, Bell CE, and Dalton JT. 2005. Structural basis for antagonism and resistance of bicalutamide in prostate cancer. *Proc. Natl. Acad. Sci. U. S. A* 102 (17): 6201-6206.

Bohl CE, Miller DD, Chen J, Bell CE, and Dalton JT. 2005. Structural basis for accommodation of nonsteroidal ligands in the androgen receptor. *J. Biol. Chem.* 280 (45): 37747-37754.

Bohl CE, Wu Z, Miller DD, Bell CE, and Dalton JT. 2007. Crystal structure of the T877A human androgen receptor ligand-binding domain complexed to cyproterone acetate provides insight for ligand-induced conformational changes and structure-based drug design. *J. Biol. Chem.* 282 (18): 13648-13655.

Bourguet W, Germain P, and Gronemeyer H. 2000. Nuclear receptor ligand-binding domains: three-dimensional structures, molecular interactions and pharmacological implications. *Trends Pharmacol. Sci.* 21 (10): 381-388.

Brzozowski AM, Pike AC, Dauter Z, Hubbard RE, Bonn T, Engstrom O, Ohman L, Greene GL, Gustafsson JA, and Carlquist M. 1997. Molecular basis of agonism and antagonism in the oestrogen receptor. *Nature* 389 (6652): 753-758.

Cantin L, Faucher F, Couture JF, de Jesus-Tran KP, Legrand P, Ciobanu LC, Frechette Y, Labrecque R, Singh SM, Labrie F, and Breton R. 2007. Structural characterization of the human androgen receptor ligand-binding domain complexed with EM5744, a rationally designed steroidal ligand bearing a bulky chain directed toward helix 12. *J. Biol. Chem.* 282 (42): 30910-30919.

Dykstra KD, Guo L, Birzin ET, Chan W, Yang YT, Hayes EC, DaSilva CA, Pai LY, Mosley RT, Kraker B, Fitzgerald PM, Dininno F, Rohrer SP, Schaeffer JM, and Hammond ML. 2007. Estrogen receptor ligands. Part 16: 2-Aryl indoles as highly subtype selective ligands for ERalpha. *Bioorg. Med. Chem. Lett.* 17 (8): 2322-2328.

Egea PF, Klaholz BP, and Moras D. 2000. Ligand-protein interactions in nuclear receptors of hormones. *FEBS Lett.* 476 (1-2): 62-67.

Fagart J, Huyet J, Pinon GM, Rochel M, Mayer C, and Rafestin-Oblin ME. 2005. Crystal structure of a mutant mineralocorticoid receptor responsible for hypertension. *Nat. Struct. Mol. Biol.* 12 (6): 554-555.

Fagart J, Wurtz JM, Souque A, Hellal-Levy C, Moras D, and Rafestin-Oblin ME. 1998. Antagonism in the human mineralocorticoid receptor. *EMBO J.* 17 (12): 3317-3325.

Gao W, and Dalton JT. 2007. Expanding the therapeutic use of androgens via selective androgen receptor modulators (SARMs). *Drug Discov. Today* 12 (5-6): 241-248.

Heldring N, Pawson T, McDonnell D, Treuter E, Gustafsson JA, and Pike AC. 2007. Structural insights into corepressor recognition by antagonist-bound estrogen receptors. *J. Biol. Chem.* 282 (14): 10449-10455.

Hellal-Levy C, Fagart J, Souque A, Wurtz JM, Moras D, and Rafestin-Oblin ME. 2000. Crucial role of the H11-H12 loop in stabilizing the active conformation of the human mineralocorticoid receptor. *Mol. Endocrinol.* 14 (8): 1210-1221.

Hermkens PH, Kamp S, Lusher S, and Veeneman GH. 2006. Non-steroidal steroid receptor modulators. *IDrugs.* 9 (7): 488-494.

Hillmann AG, Ramdas J, Multanen K, Norman MR, and Harmon JM. 2000. Glucocorticoid receptor gene mutations in leukemic cells acquired in vitro and in vivo. *Cancer Res.* 60 (7): 2056-2062.

Hubbard RE, Pike AC, Brzozowski AM, Walton J, Bonn T, Gustafsson JA, and Carlquist M. 2000. Structural insights into the mechanisms of agonism and antagonism in oestrogen receptor isoforms. *Eur. J. Cancer* 36 Suppl 4: S17-S18.

Hudson AR, Roach SL, and Higuchi RI. 2008. Recent developments in the discovery of selective glucocorticoid receptor modulators (SGRMs). *Curr. Top. Med. Chem.* 8 (9): 750-765.

Huyet J, Pinon GM, Fay MR, Fagart J, and Rafestin-Oblin ME. 2007. Structural basis of spirolactone recognition by the mineralocorticoid receptor. *Mol. Pharmacol.* 72 (3): 563-571.

Jones DG, Liang X, Stewart EL, Noe RA, Kallander LS, Madauss KP, Williams SP, Thompson SK, Gray DW, and Hoekstra WJ. 2005. Discovery of non-steroidal mifepristone mimetics: pyrazoline-based PR antagonists. *Bioorg. Med. Chem. Lett.* 15 (13): 3203-3206.

Kallander LS, Washburn DG, Hoang TH, Frazee JS, Stoy P, Johnson L, Lu Q, Hammond M, Barton LS, Patterson JR, Azzarano LM, Nagilla R, Madauss KP, Williams SP, Stewart EL, Duraiswami C, Grygielko ET, Xu X, Laping NJ, Bray JD, and Thompson SK. 2010. Improving the developability profile of pyrrolidine progesterone receptor partial agonists. *Bioorg. Med. Chem. Lett.* 20 (1): 371-374.

Kauppi B, Jakob C, Farnegardh M, Yang J, Ahola H, Alarcon M, Calles K, Engstrom O, Harlan J, Muchmore S, Ramqvist AK, Thorell S, Ohman L, Greer J, Gustafsson JA, Carlstedt-Duke J, and Carlquist M. 2003. The three-dimensional structures of antagonistic and agonistic forms of the glucocorticoid receptor ligand-binding domain: RU-486 induces a transconformation that leads to active antagonism. *J. Biol. Chem.* 278 (25): 22748-22754.

Kim S, Wu JY, Birzin ET, Frisch K, Chan W, Pai LY, Yang YT, Mosley RT, Fitzgerald PM, Sharma N, Dahllund J, Thorsell AG, Dininno F, Rohrer SP, Schaeffer JM, and Hammond ML. 2004. Estrogen receptor ligands. II. Discovery of benzoxathiins as potent, selective estrogen receptor alpha modulators. *J. Med. Chem.* 47 (9): 2171-2175.

Kong EH, Pike AC, and Hubbard RE. 2003. Structure and mechanism of the oestrogen receptor. *Biochem. Soc. Trans.* 31 (Pt 1): 56-59.

Kumar R, and Thompson EB. 1999. The structure of the nuclear hormone receptors. *Steroids* 64 (5): 310-319.

Lind U, Greenidge P, Gillner M, Koehler KF, Wright A, and Carlstedt-Duke J. 2000. Functional probing of the human glucocorticoid receptor steroid-interacting surface by site-directed mutagenesis. Gln-642 plays an important role in steroid recognition and binding. *J. Biol. Chem.* 275 (25): 19041-19049.

Lusher SJ. 2011. Structural basis for agonism and antagonism for a set of chemically related progesterone receptor modulators *J.Biol. Chem.* Publication in Press.

Madauss KP, Bledsoe RK, Mclay I, Stewart EL, Uings IJ, Weingarten G, and Williams SP. 2008. The first X-ray crystal structure of the glucocorticoid receptor bound to a non-steroidal agonist. *Bioorg. Med. Chem. Lett.* 18 (23): 6097-6099.

Madauss KP, Deng SJ, Austin RJ, Lambert MH, Mclay I, Pritchard J, Short SA, Stewart EL, Uings IJ, and Williams SP. 2004. Progesterone receptor ligand binding pocket flexibility: crystal structures of the norethindrone and mometasone furoate complexes. *J. Med. Chem.* 47 (13): 3381-3387.

Madauss KP, Grygielko ET, Deng SJ, Sulpizio AC, Stanley TB, Wu C, Short SA, Thompson SK, Stewart EL, Laping NJ, Williams SP, and Bray JD. 2007. A structural and in vitro characterization of asoprisnil: a selective progesterone receptor modulator. *Mol. Endocrinol.* 21 (5): 1066-1081.

Madauss KP, Stewart EL, and Williams SP. 2007. The evolution of progesterone receptor ligands. *Med. Res. Rev.* 27 (3): 374-400.

Matias PM, Donner P, Coelho R, Thomaz M, Peixoto C, Macedo S, Otto N, Joschko S, Scholz P, Wegg A, Basler S, Schafer M, Egner U, and Carrondo MA. 2000. Structural evidence for ligand specificity in the binding domain of the human androgen receptor. Implications for pathogenic gene mutations. *J. Biol. Chem.* 275 (34): 26164-26171.

Mueller-Fahrnow A, and Egner U. 1999. Ligand-binding domain of estrogen receptors. *Curr. Opin. Biotechnol.* 10 (6): 550-556.

Necela BM, and Cidlowski JA. 2003. Crystallization of the human glucocorticoid receptor ligand binding domain: a step towards selective glucocorticoids. *Trends Pharmacol. Sci.* 24 (2): 58-61.

Nettles KW, Bruning JB, Gil G, Nowak J, Sharma SK, Hahm JB, Kulp K, Hochberg RB, Zhou H, Katzenellenbogen JA, Katzenellenbogen BS, Kim Y, Joachmiak A, and Greene GL. 2008. NFkappaB selectivity of estrogen receptor ligands revealed by comparative crystallographic analyses. *Nat. Chem. Biol.* 4 (4): 241-247.

Petit-Topin I, Turque N, Fagart J, Fay M, Ulmann A, Gainer E, and Rafestin-Oblin ME. 2009. Met909 plays a key role in the activation of the progesterone receptor and also in the high potency of 13-ethyl progestins. *Mol. Pharmacol.* 75 (6): 1317-1324.

Pike AC, Brzozowski AM, and Hubbard RE. 2000. A structural biologist's view of the oestrogen receptor. *J. Steroid Biochem. Mol. Biol.* 74 (5): 261-268.

Pike AC, Brzozowski AM, Hubbard RE, Bonn T, Thorsell AG, Engstrom O, Ljunggren J, Gustafsson JA, and Carlquist M. 1999. Structure of the ligand-binding domain of oestrogen receptor beta in the presence of a partial agonist and a full antagonist. *EMBO J.* 18 (17): 4608-4618.

Pike AC, Brzozowski AM, Walton J, Hubbard RE, Bonn T, Gustafsson JA, and Carlquist M. 2000. Structural aspects of agonism and antagonism in the oestrogen receptor. *Biochem. Soc. Trans.* 28 (4): 396-400.

Raaijmakers HC, Versteegh JE, and Uitdehaag JC. 2009. The X-ray structure of RU486 bound to the progesterone receptor in a destabilized agonistic conformation. *J. Biol. Chem.* 284 (29): 19572-19579.

Rafestin-Oblin ME, Fagart J, Souque A, Seguin C, Bens M, and Vandewalle A. 2002. 11beta-hydroxyprogesterone acts as a mineralocorticoid agonist in stimulating Na+ absorption in mammalian principal cortical collecting duct cells. *Mol. Pharmacol.* 62 (6): 1306-1313.

Ray DW, Suen CS, Brass A, Soden J, and White A. 1999. Structure/function of the human glucocorticoid receptor: tyrosine 735 is important for transactivation. *Mol. Endocrinol.* 13 (11): 1855-1863.

Renaud J, Bischoff SF, Buhl T, Floersheim P, Fournier B, Geiser M, Halleux C, Kallen J, Keller H, and Ramage P. 2005. Selective estrogen receptor modulators with conformationally restricted side chains. Synthesis and structure-activity relationship of ERalpha-selective tetrahydroisoquinoline ligands. *J. Med. Chem.* 48 (2): 364-379.

Renaud J, Bischoff SF, Buhl T, Floersheim P, Fournier B, Halleux C, Kallen J, Keller H, Schlaeppi JM, and Stark W. 2003. Estrogen receptor modulators: identification and structure-activity relationships of potent ERalpha-selective tetrahydroisoquinoline ligands. *J. Med. Chem.* 46 (14): 2945-2957.

Sack JS, Kish KF, Wang C, Attar RM, Kiefer SE, An Y, Wu GY, Scheffler JE, Salvati ME, Krystek SR, Jr., Weinmann R, and Einspahr HM. 2001. Crystallographic structures of the ligand-binding domains of the androgen receptor and its T877A mutant complexed with the natural agonist dihydrotestosterone. *Proc. Natl. Acad. Sci. U. S. A* 98 (9): 4904-4909.

Schoch GA, D'Arcy B, Stihle M, Burger D, Bar D, Benz J, Thoma R, and Ruf A. 2010. Molecular switch in the glucocorticoid receptor: active and passive antagonist conformations. *J. Mol. Biol.* 395 (3): 568-577.

Shelly W, Draper MW, Krishnan V, Wong M, and Jaffe RB. 2008. Selective estrogen receptor modulators: an update on recent clinical findings. *Obstet. Gynecol. Surv.* 63 (3): 163-181.

Shiau AK, Barstad D, Loria PM, Cheng L, Kushner PJ, Agard DA, and Greene GL. 1998. The structural basis of estrogen receptor/coactivator recognition and the antagonism of this interaction by tamoxifen. *Cell* 95 (7): 927-937.

Shiau AK, Barstad D, Radek JT, Meyers MJ, Nettles KW, Katzenellenbogen BS, Katzenellenbogen JA, Agard DA, and Greene GL. 2002. Structural characterization of a subtype-selective ligand reveals a novel mode of estrogen receptor antagonism. *Nat. Struct. Biol.* 9 (5): 359-364.

Silverman SL. 2010. New selective estrogen receptor modulators (SERMs) in development. *Curr. Osteoporos. Rep.* 8 (3): 151-153.

Stevens A, Garside H, Berry A, Waters C, White A, and Ray D. 2003. Dissociation of steroid receptor coactivator 1 and nuclear receptor corepressor recruitment to the human glucocorticoid receptor by modification of the ligand-receptor interface: the role of tyrosine 735. *Mol. Endocrinol.* 17 (5): 845-859.

Suino-Powell K, Xu Y, Zhang C, Tao YG, Tolbert WD, Simons SS, Jr., and Xu HE. 2008. Doubling the size of the glucocorticoid receptor ligand binding pocket by deacylcortivazol. *Mol. Cell Biol.* 28 (6): 1915-1923.

Tan Q, Blizzard TA, Morgan JD, Birzin ET, Chan W, Yang YT, Pai LY, Hayes EC, DaSilva CA, Warrier S, Yudkovitz J, Wilkinson HA, Sharma N, Fitzgerald PM, Li S, Colwell L, Fisher JE, Adamski S, Reszka AA, Kimmel D, Dininno F, Rohrer SP, Freedman LP, Schaeffer JM, and Hammond ML. 2005. Estrogen receptor ligands. Part 10: Chromanes: old scaffolds for new SERAMs. *Bioorg. Med. Chem. Lett.* 15 (6): 1675-1681.

Thompson SK, Washburn DG, Frazee JS, Madauss KP, Hoang TH, Lapinski L, Grygielko ET, Glace LE, Trizna W, Williams SP, Duraiswami C, Bray JD, and Laping NJ. 2009. Rational design of orally-active, pyrrolidine-based progesterone receptor partial agonists. *Bioorg. Med. Chem. Lett.* 19 (16): 4777-4780.

Vajdos FF, Hoth LR, Geoghegan KF, Simons SP, LeMotte PK, Danley DE, Ammirati MJ, and Pandit J. 2007. The 2.0 A crystal structure of the ERalpha ligand-binding domain complexed with lasofoxifene. *Protein Sci.* 16 (5): 897-905.

Vottero A, Kino T, Combe H, Lecomte P, and Chrousos GP. 2002. A novel, C-terminal dominant negative mutation of the GR causes familial glucocorticoid resistance through abnormal interactions with p160 steroid receptor coactivators. *J. Clin. Endocrinol. Metab* 87 (6): 2658-2667.

Washburn DG, Hoang TH, Frazee JS, Johnson L, Hammond M, Manns S, Madauss KP, Williams SP, Duraiswami C, Tran TB, Stewart EL, Grygielko ET, Glace LE, Trizna W, Nagilla R, Bray JD, and Thompson SK. 2009. Discovery of orally active, pyrrolidinone-based progesterone receptor partial agonists. *Bioorg. Med. Chem. Lett.* 19 (16): 4664-4668.

Weatherman RV, Fletterick RJ, and Scanlan TS. 1999. Nuclear-receptor ligands and ligand-binding domains. *Annu. Rev. Biochem.* 68: 559-581.

# 10

# Approaches for Searching of Modified Steroid Estrogen Analogues with Improved Biological Properties

Alexander Shavva, Svetlana Morozkina and Olga Galkina
*Saint-Petersburg State University, Chemistry Faculty,*
*Department of Natural Products Chemistry*
*Russia*

## 1. Introduction

Estrogens play a key role in multiple physiological functions in women. They have important actions on bone and lipid metabolism, cardiovascular function, and diffuse effects on other target organs. Estrogens have important roles in cognitive function and influence psychological well-being in women, in development and maintenance of the reproductive system in the female (**Gustafsson, 2003**). The most potent estrogens are 17β-estradiol **1**, estrone **2** and estriol **3** may have tissue-specific roles (**Gruber & Huber, 1999**).

1         2         3

In female body estrogens are formed in ovaries, and as result the menopause is associated with an increased risk of the development of cardiovascular diseases, osteoporosis and many other diseases. In postmenopausal women, many of these functions (positive effect on prevention of osteoporosis and improved serum profile enhanced by the use of estrogen replacement therapy) are achievement. The positive action of estrogens on prophylactic and treatment of osteoporosis has been proved undoubtedly, however other clinical data are considered as contradictory (**Davison & Davis, 2003**). Moreover, during the use of estrogens for HRT the number of strokes is increasing (**Bushnell, 2005**). It was absolutely unexpected because the adverse effect has been observed in experiments on animals. It was also found that during long-term using of estrogens the risk of some oncological diseases is increasing (**Beral, 2003; Beral et al., 2005**). Other side effects, which we discuss later, also indicate the necessity for the search of new safe estrogen analogues with the improved biological properties.

Firstly we consider the results in these directions, and then we discuss the main advantages of the creation of agents with directed biological action, which are perspective for HRT, for the treatment of oncological estrogen-sensitive diseases, cardio-vascular system, osteoporosis, neuroendocrinal diseases. The division of agents on such groups has relative character, because the activity of steroid estrogens has multifunctional character and one compound may be effectively used in various fields. This is a main reason why modified steroid estrogens have the advantage in comparison with huge number of heterocyclic compounds, having more selective action.

Obviously that most perspective search of such compounds is done on the basis of knowledge about estrogen action mechanism, particularity of its structure and metabolism.

Several authors consider that main fast non genomic effects of estrogens are mediated by their membrane receptors (**Levin, 2002; Sak & Evaraus, 2004**). Experimental data about the identity of nuclear and membrane ERα in MCF7 cell are presented in the publication (**Pedram et al., 2009**). Obviously, ligand specificity may be significantly different. Mechanisms of membrane receptors action are still unclear, very often it is not proved that one or another effect is mediated by namely this group of receptors (**Warner & Gustafsson, 2006**). The absence of data about ligand specificity to membrane receptors does not allow to plan the synthesis of modified steroids with selective action, especially taking into account that their activity is realizing on many ways. During the consideration of osteoprotective action of estrogens and its influence on processes of cardio-vascular system we restrict ourselves to state the facts, because the decision concerning the synthesis of potential agents is usually reached on the analogy with known compounds.

## 2. Genomic actions of estrogens

The genomic effects of steroid estrogens are mediated through two subtypes of nuclear α- and β-receptors (ERα and ERβ). In mid 1980s. studies on the cloning of DNA encoding the steroid estrogen receptors were initiated (**Walter et al., 1986; Green, G.L. et al., 1986; Koike et al., 1987**). These studies led to the determination of their primary structure. Later they were assigned to ERα. In 1996, a number researchers discovered new members of the superfamily of nuclear estrogen receptors in rat prostate and ovaries (**Kuipper et al, 1996**) in human and mouse (**Mosselman et al., 1996; Tremblay et al., 1997**) and named it ERβ. Very soon the complete amino acid sequence of human ERβ (hERβ) was determinated (**Ogawa et al., 1998**). It was established that ERβ is significantly shorter than ERα. The comparison of amino acid sequences of these receptors and the investigation of affinity of various ligands to mutant forms of receptors allowed to establish that these receptors have 6 domains.

The N-terminal domains (A/B) have variable length and amino acid sequences. Usually, they exhibit a hormone-independent transactivation function (AF-1) that interacts with the elements of the transcription machinery and activate genes in target organs (**Tzukerman et al., 1994**). Domain C is responsible for the DNA recognition and receptor dimerization. This is a DNA-binding region, consisting approximately 50 amino acids. Domain E (HBD) contains approximately 250 amino acids and ensures the binding of hormones. This domain is the «hinge» - after the binding of ligand with receptors the following conformational rearrangement takes place with the participation of domain D. Clone 29 protein is highly homologous to rat ERα, particularly in DNA-binding domain (95%) and ligand-binding domain (55%) (**Kuipper et al., 1996**). High degree of conservation of DNA-binding domain (96%) and ligand-binding domain (58%) was registered by other authors (**Mosselman et al., 1996**).

Ligand-independent transactivational function AF1 is in zone A/B of both sub-types of receptors, zone E/F of α-receptor of estrogens has additional ligand-independent activation function (**Tora et al., 1989**). ERα has ligand-dependent trans-activation function AF-2.

Without ligand estrogen receptors are in complexes with heat shock proteins (Hsp90, Hsp70, Hsp56, Hsp60, Hsp48, Hsp23), this binding takes place in domain C. Probably, being in complexes with heat shock proteins estrogens are protected against the action of proteases. After binding its ligand conformational rearrangement of LBD of nuclear receptor and dissociation of complexes ER – heat shock proteins takes place. Except of the potential possibility to activate transcription, this rearrangement causes the change of topography of receptor regions, sensitive to proteolysis (**Ramsey & Klinge, 2001**). Phosphorylation of estrogen receptors is observed after their binding with hormone (**Kato et al., 1995**) that enhances the binding.

Transformed receptor forms dimers and in this form binds with DNA and may activate the transcription. Effective dimerization of ERα requires a weak constitutive activity of sequences in domain C (**Kumar & Chambon, 1988**). It is necessary to note, that AF1 and AF2 exhibit relatively weak activity, whereas the maximum of transcription induction is observed when they act together (**Tora et al., 1989; Pham et al., 1992**). From other side, in some cases the activation of AF-1 is enough to activate the transcription. Thus, 4-hydroxytamoxifen **4** is unable to induce AF-2 activity, but it is a strong agonist in cellular and promoter context where AF-1 is effective transcriptional activator (**Berry et al., 1990**).

| 4-hydroxytamoxifen | tamoxifen | raloxifene |
|:---:|:---:|:---:|
| **4** | **5** | **6** |

Transcriptional process is modulated by receptors' ligands and various co-regulators (**Cheskis et al., 1997; An et al., 1999; 2001; Tcherepanova et al., 2000; Wong et al., 2001; Liu, J. et al., 2003; Bai & Gugière, 2003; Xu & Li, 2003**). Conformation of ER changes upon interaction with coactivator proteins (**Tamrazi et al., 2005**), as result the activity of one ligand may change in depending on cell nature. Thus, tamoxifen **5** and raloxifene **6** are agonists of estradiol in cardiovascular system, whereas they show antagonistic properties in breast and endometrium (**Jordan, 2007**). Many others SERMs have similar properties.

Nowadays more 10 estrogen receptor-β isoforms are known, which have been identified starting from 2000 (**Lu et al., 2000**).

To study the roles of each receptor *in vivo*, a series of the mice were generated lacking either a functional ERα and ERβ or both (αERKO, βERKO, αβERKO) (**Emmel & Korach, 2001**).

ERβ may modulate the functions of ERα, if these receptors are in the same cells (**Matthews et al., 2006**). It became crucial during the diagnostics and the treatment of oncological diseases (**Leygue et al., 1998; Pujol et al., 1998; Hall & McDonnel, 1999; Lazennec et al., 2001; Monroe et al., 2005**). Compounds having the preferential binding to ERβ have great perspectives to be used for the treatment of autoimmune diseases, prostate disease, depression and ovulation disorders (**Gustafsson, 2005**). The noted above is the evidence for actuality of the search for modulators with preferable affinity to ERα or ERβ.

Obviously, determination of complexes structure of estrogen receptors with various ligands with known biological properties was supposed to contribute to the development of models for mechanisms of estrogens action and understanding of the connection between structure and hormonal activity of ligands and thus to solve the abovementioned problem.

X-rays data of ligand-binding domain of ERα with estradiol **1** and raloxifene **6** (**Brzozowski et al., 1997**), 4-hydroxytamoxifen **4** and diethylstilbestrole **7** (**Shiau et al., 1998**), and ligand-binding domain of ERβ with raloxifene **6** and genistein **8** (**Pike et al., 1999**) have been obtained. Estradiol **1** and diethylstilbestrol **7** are full agonists to ERα and ERβ, 4-hydroxytamoxifen **4**, raloxifene **6**, and genistein **8** are agonists/antagonists. Interestingly, synthetic compounds of type **9** bind with ERβ as effectively as genistein **8** (**Miller et al., 2003**). Removal of ligands **1, 4, 6, 7, 8** from its complexes in crystal with LBD of ERα and ERβ, docking of other potential ligands and the following optimization of its position in complex and binding energy by molecular modeling methods allow to evaluate the properties of new compounds independently from their belonging to steroid series. Some vagueness of evaluation of affinity to receptors is connected with the fact that the X-Ray data for complexes with different ligands are obtained only with LBD, but not with full-length receptors.

The last of utmost importance, because during the realization of transcriptional action the formation of complexes between the DNA binding domain of estrogen receptors and estrogen response element (ERE) of duplex DNA is necessary, which requires the exact disposition of these elements of structure. Earlier structure of the DNA-binding domain of the ERα has been investigated (**Schwabe et al., 1990**), however three-dimensional model of the DNA binding domain of ERα was proposed significantly later (**Deegan et al., 2010**). On account of the above mentioned the differences in RBA values of model compounds to full-length receptor and to its LBD could be significant. Thus, the affinity of (5S,11S)-5,11-diethyl-5,6,11,12-tetrahydrochrisene-2,8-diol **9** to full-length ERβ is in 10 times higher, than to its LBD (**Meyers et al., 1999**).

The results of quantum chemical calculations of ligand-receptor complexes allowed to synthesize a huge number of compounds having more then in 100-times higher effective binding to β-ER in comparison to α-ER (**Manas et al., 2004**).

There are other ways for evaluation of properties of new compounds. For example some of them are traditional QSAR methods (**Gantchev et al., 1994; Tong et. al., 1997; Wiese et. al, 1997; Azzaoui et al., 1998; Gao et al., 1999; Wurtz et al., 1998; Sippl, 2002; Klopman &**

**Chakravarti, 2003; Wolohan & Reichert, 2004; Pasha et al., 2005).** In spite of the fact that such approaches have moderate predicted force, they do not provide the deeper understanding of estrogen action mechanism. From our point of view, using the multimodal approach, based on the application of methods of comparative molecular field analysis and binding energy calculations is most perspective **(Wolohan & Reichert, 2004).**

The knowledge about conformational mobility of different groups of potential ligands of ERs has great importance **(Kym et al., 1993; Grese et al., 1998; Selivanov & Shavva, 2002).** These data have interest in connection with data about modeling of conformations of ligand-receptor complexes **(Kraichely et al., 2000; Egner et al., 2001)** and conformational dynamic of ERs **(Celic et al., 2007).**

Let's consider the examples of successful searching of modified estrogens which have selective binding affinity to hERα or hERβ **(Hillisch et al, 2004).**

Structure analysis of LBD of these receptors shows that the nearest surrounding of bound estradiol in these receptors differs from each other on two amino acid residues: Leu384 and Met421 in ERα are substituted by Met336 and Ile373 in ERβ. Volumes of side chains of these amino acid residues are 85.9 Å (Met), 82.6 Å (Leu) and 82.3 Å (Ile). It was predicted that the increased flexibility of the linear Met side chain would allow larger substituent to be accommodated. Met336 ERβ is situated closely to position 8β, and the introduction of small lipophilic substituent into this position must lead to the increasing of RBA of modified analogue to ERβ. Met421 of ERα is at region of D-ring, and analogue with substituent at positions 16α and/or 17α will have the increased affinity to ERα.

Experiments have proved the stated predictions. As reference compounds steroids **10** and **12** have been used. First one has selectivity hERα/hERβ is 20, and for second one this value hERβ/hERα is 22.5. Modified analogues **11** and **13** have the mentioned ratios as 70 and 180 correspondingly.

Unfortunately, there is no correlation between RBA values for hERα and hERβ with values obtained in the experiments with the corresponding receptors of animals.

In some cases the ratio between these values are opposite **(Hillisch et al., 2004).**

The investigation of RBA for 71 compounds (mainly, metabolites of estrogens) to hERα and hERβ have shown that the differences in experimental values are not more then one order **(Zhu et al., 2006).**

| 10 | 11 | 12 | 13 |

| 14 | 15 | 16 |

The introduction of relatively small linear substituents (4-5 carbon atoms) at position 11β of steroid skeleton may lead to the appearance of antagonistic activity to ERβ at agonistic properties to ERα (steroids **14** and **15**), whereas analogue **16** is agonist to both receptors (**Loosen, 1999**).

17          18          19

Steroids with small substituents at position 11β without aromatic ring possess significantly higher affinity and transcriptional activity of ERα (**Loosen et al., 2000**), for example, analogues **17-19** have been found.

ICI 182,780 (fulvestrant)          ICI 164,384

20          21

RU 58,668          RU 39,411

22          23

Finally, there are compounds, which fully block the binding of estradiol **1** with known ERs, for example steroids **20-23** (**Jordan, 2003**). A number of compounds with large substituents at C-7 (α) and C-11 (β) have been synthesized, such analogues are of great interest for the treatment of estrogen-dependent oncological diseases and hormones imbalance, caused by the increased formation of estrogens in the body.

## 3. Carcinogenicity causes of ER ligands

The establishment of at least major reasons of carcinogenicity of estrogens, their agonists/antagonists has significant importance, since this understandings lies in the fundament of the creation of medications with the improved properties.

At the present time two main types of carcinogenesis are known - promotive and genotoxic (mutagenic), action of them may add up. Existence of the fist one is confirmed by well-known facts of tumor formation under the estrogen action (**Russo et al., 2002**) and promotion of tumor induction under the action of various agents, for example, nitroso-butylurea (**Sumi et al., 1984**). The same results have been obtained in other models. For example, 17α-ethynylestradiol **24** enhances the tumor formation in rat males under the action of diethylnitrosamine (**Yoshida & Fukunishi, 1981**). Estradiol increased dysplasia of breast on androgenized rats, induced by 7,12-dimethylbenz[a]anthracene.

The explanation of this negative influence of estrogens is quite clear – when in active state the cells are vulnerable to attacks by reactive compounds.

24    25

Lately using 2-fluoroestradiol **25** as an example it was shown that there is no correlation between carcinogenicity and hormonal action of estrogens (**Liehr, 1983**). It is important that 17α-ethynylestradiol **24** possesses high hormonal activity and lowered carcinogenicity (**Li, J.J. et al., 1995**). These investigations (and earlier ones) became the basis for searching of other mechanisms of estrogens' carcinogenicity.

Specifically, it was established that estrogen metabolites may covalently bind with hamster microsomic proteins, and this process is inhibited by ascorbinic and cathehol-O-methytransferase action (**Haaf et al., 1987**). Therefore authors proposed that «active» metabolites are o-quinones, which possess heightened reactivity. In next 20 years it was clarified that the hydroxylation of estrogens in the body leads to the formation of 2- or 4-hydroxyestrogens of types **26** and **27**, which then converted to o-quinones of type **28** and **29** (**Liehr et al., 1995; 1996; Bolton et al., 1998; Bolton, 2002; Bolton & Thatcher, 2008; Zhang, F. et al., 1999; Liu, X. et al., 2002; Zhang, Q. et al., 2008**). Irreversible depuration of DNA that could not be regenerated by reparases may take place under the action of o-quinones. Compounds of types **31** and **32** are possible depuration products. Quinones of type **28** do not cause the damage of DNA. It is assumed that the reason of this is their heightened reactivity; therefore they may be deactivated before their migration into cell nucleus.

From our point of view one of possible variants for the decreasing of estrogens' carcinogenicity is the introduction of a substituent in the position 1, which blocks the interaction with DNA and thus prevents its depuration. In the case when compounds with substituent at position 1 will lead to decreasing of estrogenic activity, such modification (in dependence from the task) will be very perspective.

33                                  34                                  35

3                                    36

It is also known that metabolites with hydroxyl group at C-6 of types **33** and **34** may have carcinogenic properties (**Itoh et al., 1998**). Thus, compounds which can not be hydroxylated at position 6 are perspective potential candidates for synthesis and further investigations.

Another metabolite of estrogens - 16α-hydroxyestrone **35** is also considered as inductor of tumors' formation (**Lewis et al., 2001; Seeger et al., 2006**). Hydroxylation of estrone at position 16α is one of main directions of estrogen metabolism, which is elevated in women with high risk of breast cancer, as well with other oncological diseases. Estriol **3** content is informative as well: there is the correlation between breast tumors' development in mice (**Lewis et al., 2001**).

Products of hydroxylation of equilenin and equilin also possess carcinogenic properties (**Zhang, F. et al., 1999; Shen et al., 1997**). Corresponding quinones may damage DNA, and the investigation of this class of compounds with substituent at position 4 is of a great importance. Authors concluded that 4-fluoroequilenin derivatives **36** are promising alternatives to traditional estrogen replacement therapy due to their similar estrogenic properties with less overall toxicity (**Liu, X. et al., 2003**).

37                                    38

The hydroxylation of selective modulators of ERs and the following reaction products transformations may cause DNA depurination that leads to carcinogenicity of drugs. It was shown on the example of the formation of α-hydroxytamoxifen **37** and its possible transformation into compounds of type **38** (**Jordan, 2007**).

It is not surprising that during last years the efforts are directed to the methods of steroid estrogen level determination, because the exact value of their content in various tissues helps to diagnose differentially various hormone-sensitive diseases (**Arai et al., 2010; Blair et al., 2010**).

## 4. Inhibition of estrone formation in the body

It is known that about two thirds of all the breast cancers occur in postmenopausal women, when estrogen is no longer synthesized in ovaries. However the estradiol content in estrogen-dependent tumors is significantly higher than in blood plasma and in normal tissues on bourdes with tumors. Partly it can be explained by the ability of tumor to accept estradiol from the blood (Pasqualini et al., 1996), because estrogen synthesis may be enhanced in extragonadal organs. Furthermore, local synthesis of estrogens in tumor may be on high level (Pasqualini et al., 1997). In view of the aforesaid it is necessary to consider the ways of synthesis of these hormones and understand the influence on the formation of reactive estrogens in tumor (scheme).

Androst-4-en-3,17-dione
(Adione)
39

Estrone

Sulphate estrone (E1C)
40

Estradiol (E2)

It is well-known, that estrogens are formed in the body from testosterone or androst-4-en-3,17-dione 39. Aromatization is multistep process, proceeding under the action of enzymes of cytochrome P-450 system. The main steps of aromatization, key stage in estrogen formation are considered in many publications (Jordan & Brodie, 2007 and citations herein). It is reasonable that the great attention is directed to the search of irreversible inhibitors of aromatase.

Most often the initial investigations are carrying out on human placenta cells, the criterion for the evaluation of effectiveness of investigated compounds is value of $IC_{50}$ (concentration, at which the inhibition of enzyme activity is 50% from highest possible one under experimental conditions). Compounds having $IC_{50}$ in the range of nanomolar concentrations have perspectives to be further investigated. Next step for the evaluation of inhibitory activity of perspective compounds is the investigation on animal models, and very often the preliminary evaluation of effectiveness is in contrast with data obtained in second series.

Exemestane                    41                              42                              43

44                    45                    46

Steroid **41** and **42** properties investigation results could be used as an example (**diSalle & Robinson, 1990**). The $IC_{50}$ values in the experiments on human placenta cells are approximately equal - 42.5±4.3 and 20.3±2.2 nM correspondingly. However, in the experiments on rats the values of $ED_{50}$ (dose, at which the inhibition is 50% from highest possible one) are 3.7 and more 100 mg/kg under *per os* injection. Necessity of compounds investigation can be illustrated by huge number of examples in various animal models and by methods of steroids introduction into the body. In particular, compound **42** under subcutaneous introduction in doses 30 and 150 mg/kg blocks the growth of bearing DMBA-induced mammary tumors in female rats (**Nishino et al., 1989**) and after numerous investigations is clinically used with the trade name atamestane.

The main position for attack during demethylation of androst-4-en-3,17-dione is methyl group at C-19. Numerous derivatives at C-10 have been synthesized. Among them the most effective one is compound **43** with $K_i$ 3 nM to human placenta enzyme (**Cole & Robinson, 1990**). It comes as no surprise, that this compound is clinically used (**Numazava et al., 2005**). Compounds **44** (**Greway et al., 1990**) and **45** (**Peet et al., 1992**) demonstrated good properties.

Detailed search of aromatase inhibitors led to the creation of medications of steroid nature for the treatment of oncological diseases in clinic, from them, exemestane **41** and formestane **46** are also widely known. However clinical application of aromatase inhibitors revealed the presence of a number of non-specific toxic side effects: asthenia, nausea, headache etc. Certain endocrinological side effects in postmenopausal women are notable, namely hot flashes and vaginal dryness (**Goss, 1999**). Therefore the search of aromatase inhibitors in steroid series must be done in series that is not belonging to androgens.

**47** a) R=Cl, b) R=Br, c) R=CH₃          48                    49

25                    50

Because estrone **2** or estradiol **1** are formed as result of aromatization process it was possible to assume that these compounds will be reversible inhibitors of aromatase. Indeed, later it was found that even estradiol is anti-aromatase agent in human breast cancer cells (**Pasqualini & Chetrite, 2006**); the same was found for estrone sulfatase inhibition (**Pasqualini & Chetrite, 2001**). Simultaneously, reasoning from the same assumption, the synthesis of modified estrogens with substituents at C-2, C-4 or C-6 was carried out (**Numazava et al., 2005**).

These analogues are competitive inhibitors of aromatase. 2-Substituted steroids **47 a,b,c,** have the best properties, they are significantly active in comparison with estrone **2**, $K_i$ values are 0.130±0.017, 0.224±0.024, 0.360±0.019 and 2.50±0.22 µM correspondingly. Steroids **48** and **49** have similar activity - $K_i$ values are 0.10±0.006 and 0.21±0.009 µM, however their synthesis is more complicated. Inhibitory activity of estradiol derivatives is significantly lower. From our point of view, its worth to pay attention to 2-fluoroestradiol **25**, in spite of the value of $K_i$ 9.04±0.5 µM being higher in comparison to other compounds and the fact, that its synthesis is more complicated. It is more important that this analogue does not possess carcinogenic properties in the experiments on rats (**Liehr, 1983**). In the series of 4-substituted estrone derivatives – 4-fluoroanalogue **50** has the best properties ($K_i$ = 1.28±0.07). All presented investigations had extensive character and it was impossible to take into account many details of biological properties. X-Rays analysis of complex of aromatase from human placenta with androst-4-en-3,17-dione **39** has been obtained (**Ghosh et al., 2009**), that opened the perspectives for the targeted search of aromatase inhibitors. Using the data obtained resulted in the docking of new reversible inhibitors in aromatase structure that allowed to explain their activity (**Yadav et al., 2011**).

Aromatase inhibitors are widely used for the treatment of estrogen-dependent oncological diseases; however they have a number of side-effects. Thus, the decreasing of estrogen content in the body automatically results in the increasing of cholesterol level in blood, and hence to the increased risk of cardiovascular diseases. This is the main reason for the creation of inhibitors on the basis of steroids in comparison with non-steroid ones. For example, exemestane has minimal negative effects on bone and lipid metabolism in animal and clinical studies (**Carpenter & Miller, 2005**). There is an opinion that exemestane may improve lipid profile (**Bundred, 2005**).

Molecular bases of interactions of various groups of ligands with aromatase have been considered relatively not long ago, that may lead to the creation of inhibitors with improved properties (**Hong et. al., 2008**).

Aromatase inhibitors are important, but not sufficient for blocking of growth of hormone-sensitive tumors. Point is that there is at least one more way for estrogens' formation in tumors.

It is known that estrone sulphate concentration in blood plasma of postmenopausal women is in 5-10 times higher in comparison with free hormone concentration. Assumption was made that estrogen sulphates may play a role of "source" of free estrogens in various organs, because its «half-life time» is longer than life-time of free estrogens (**Reed & Potter, 1999**). Estrogen sulphates may migrate into hormone-depended tumor and then converted to free hormones under estrone sulfatase action. It was found that estrone sulfatase activity in tumors is in 130-200 times higher in comparison with aromatase activity (**Chetrite et al., 2000**). This was the basis for initiation of investigations for the search for irreversible estrone sulfatase inhibitors.

Estrone sulfatase from human placenta is suitable model object for searching for corresponding inhibitors. It is the transmembrane protein that consists of 583 amino acid residues (mainly it is hydrophobic amino acids).

On the basis of data about primary structure of this enzyme and taking into account its homology with human arylsulfatase A and human arylsulfatase B (X-Ray data of arylsulfatase were known), the structure of catalytic centre of estrone sulfatase was proposed (**Howard et al., 2002**). X-Ray data of estrone sulfatase has been obtained a little bit later and it was shown that its tertiary structure is formed by two domains – globular polar domain, containing the active center and transmembrane domain, formed by two antiparallel α-helixes. Polar domain consists of two sub-domains, one of them has the active centre of enzyme. Transmembrane domain opens the entrance into the active center of enzyme, which is situated deep under the "mashrooms hat", close to the membrane surface. Near the active center entrance a big amount of hydrophobic amino acids is concentrated, which are a part of TD (Phe178, 182, 187, 230, 233 and 237), and the polar domain (Phe104 and 557, Leu554). Side chains of these amino acids form a tunnel, which leads to the active center (**Hernandes-Guzman et al., 2003**). Catalytic area of active center of estrone sulfatase is highly homologous to active centers of arylsulfatase A and B. Nine from ten catalytically important amino acids Asp35, Asp36, FG75, Arg79, Lys134, His136, His290, Asp342 and Lys368 are in analogous positions to all three sulfatases. It is in quite correlation with the experimental data about the importance of hydrophobic interactions during the binding of enzyme with inhibitors of steroid series (**Ahmed S., 2001**).

Conceptions concerning estrogen sulfates hydrolysis mechanisms and ferment deactivation are presented in series of articles (**Reed et al., 2005**), where an important role is assigned to an unusual amino acid - formylglycine in 75 position.

Investigation of kinetic parameters of hydrolysis of estrone sulphate and dehydroepiandrosterone sulphate have shown that values of $V_{max}$ for these compounds are correspondingly 9.95 and 1.89 μM/min, values of $K_m$ are 72.75 and 9.59 μM (**Hernandez-Guzman et al., 2001**). These values could be used as standard for the evaluation of substrate specificity of estrone sulfatase of various natures.

In several investigations it was established that for the effective inhibition of estrone sulfatase molecules must have sulphamate group at position 3. Firstly the necessity of this group was demonstrated on the example of steroid **51a**, widely known as EMATE (**Purohit et al., 1995**). However this compound did not reach the clinical application as anti-tumor agent because its estrogenic activity under *per os* introduction is in 5 times higher in comparison with estrone (**Elger et al., 1995**).

| 51 | 52 | 53 |

The investigations of Professor M. Reed' group are examples of the successful creation of estrone sulfatase inhibitors with lowered hormonal activity (**Purohit et al., 1998**), authors have synthesized compounds **51a-j**. The selection of modifications in EMATE structure was done on the basis of experimental facts about significant fall of uterotropic activity of estrone derivatives when substituents like alkyl-, allyl- or nitro- groups were introduced at positions 2 and (or) 4 (**Purohit et al., 1999**). Some results on human placenta microsomes enzyme are presented in the Table 1.

| Steroid | $R^1$ | $R^2$ | $IC_{50}$, $\mu M$ | Steroid | $R^1$ | $R^2$ | $IC_{50}$, $\mu M$ |
|---------|-------|-------|--------|---------|-------|-------|--------|
| a | H | H | 0.004 | f | H | $CH_3(CH_2)_2$ | > 100 |
| b | OMe | H | 0.03 | g | $CH_3(CH_2)_2$ | $CH_3(CH_2)_2$ | > 100 |
| c | $NO_2$ | H | 0.07 | h | Allyl | H | 2.5 |
| d | H | $NO_2$ | 0.0008 | i | H | Allyl | 9 |
| e | $CH_3(CH_2)_2$ | H | 29 | j | Allyl | Allyl | > 100 |

Table 1.

Irreversible E-ST inactivation has been observed in all cases. Most active inhibitor from this series is – 4-nitro derivative **51d** – in 5 times stronger than EMATE *in vitro* and had comparable activity with EMATE activity *in vivo*. The investigation of uterotropic activity has shown that this steroid increases uterus weight of ovariectomized rats, although to lesser degree than EMATE (158% in comparison with control, and 414% - EMATE). Monoallylic analogues are weaker inhibitors estrone sulfatase, but they are more active in comparison with propyl- ones. The presence of large substituents at C-2 and/or C-4 leads to decreasing of inhibitory activity, which may be caused by shielding of oxygen atom at C-3.
Estrone formiate **52** (**Schreiner & Billich, 2004**) and boronic acids **53** (**Ahmed, V., 2006**) have shown irreversible inhibitory activity, however these investigations had no further progress.

54          55          56

57          58          59

60          61

Compounds of type **54** were chosen as an example and authors used another analogue (oxatiazine ring, condensed with A ring) instead of sulphamate group at C-3 **(Peters et al., 2003)**. In the experiments *in vitro* in an intact MCF-7 human breast cancer cells model steroids have shown high inhibitory activity. *In vivo*, agent **54** showed moderate antitumor activity against MCF-7 breast cancer xenografts in BALB/c athimic nude mice. 3,′4′-Oxathiazine analogues showed weak inhibitory activity.

Compounds **55-57** effectively inhibit estrone sulfatase **(Tanabe et al, 1999)**. It indicated specifically on the possibility for the creation of inhibitors in the series of D-homo analogues of estrogens that was confirmed using sulphamates **58** and **59** **(Reed & Potter, 1999)**.

The development of this direction led to the creation of strong inhibitors **60** and **61** with values of $IC_{50}$ - 1 nM **(Fischer et al., 2003)**.

One more group of perspective inhibitors of estrone sulfatase was found – sulphamates of estrogens with methoxy- group at C-2 **(Raobaikady et al., 2003)**. At the time of these investigations it was known that 2-methoxyestradiol **62** induces apoptosis in many various lines of tumor′ cells, including prostate cancer cells, exhibits antiproliferative activity and blocks angiogenesis processes, which became a basis for the selection of model compounds.

The fact that bis-sulphamates of 2-methoxyestradiol **63** and 2-ethylestradiol **66** inhibit the growth of breast cancer cells, which are resistant to the action of many medications, has a crucial importance **(Suzuki et al., 2003)**.

We have considered the ways for the search for modified estrogens for the inhibition of steroids metabolism enzymes which have been done in series of derivatives with natural rings junction. Obvious perspective direction is the investigation of analogues with unnatural rings junction since peculiarities of their structure have the number of important characteristics, comparable with ones in series of natural estrogens and comparable biological properties of both series.

It is known that high effectiveness of binding of estradiol **1** with ERα is a result of high hydrophobicity of steroid molecule and possibility to form hydrogen bonds of phenolic hydroxyl group at C-3 with Glu353, Arg394 and water molecule. Hydroxyl group at C-17 forms hydrogen bond with His524 **(Brzozowski et al, 1997)**. Modified 8α-analogues of steroid estrogens have relative high affinity to ERα, and model explaining the binding with

ERα has been proposed (**Shavva et al., 2002** and citation herein). Metabolism of steroids with unnatural rings junction may be quite different from metabolism of natural steroids, which will allow to find the alternative solutions of many medicinal-biological tasks.

The perspectives for the creation of new inhibitors of steroid metabolism have been demonstrated using 6-oxa-D-homo-8α-analogues of estrogens **67** as an example (**Gluzdikov et al., 2007**). Authors accomplished the docking of different compounds of this series into ligand-binding domain of ERα. And after the analysis the assumption was made that this compound must have weak binding affinity to ERα or must have none in total. Sulphamate **67a** has been synthesized and the analogue showed a quite good inhibitory activity to estrone sulfatase. Steroid **67b** - potential product of hydrolysis has no uterotropic activity. It became the basis for the improvement of synthesis scheme of 7β-methyl-D-homo-8α-analogues of steroid estrogens (**Morozkina et al., 2009**) and investigation of peculiarities of their spatial structure (**Shavva et al., 2008**). Steroids of such structure may be used for the solution of other tasks (for example, as vectors for the transport of other classes of compounds into estrogen target-tissues).

Finally, 17β-hydroxysteroid dehydrogenase type 1 plays the important role in the induction and development breast cancer (**Vihko et al, 2002**). In ER+ breast cancer cells under the action of this enzyme the dominate direction of the reaction is the transformation of estrone into more dangerous estradiol. In ER-positive breast cancer cells the reaction tends to proceed in the reverse direction. Another reason of tumor growth is inactivation of dehydroepiandrosterone **68**, which blocks tumor growth (**Aka et al., 2010**).

68        69 a) R=H, b) R= CH₃       70 a) R=H, b) R= CH₃

71            72              50

Substrate specificity of available enzyme from human placenta was investigated and it was found that steroids of unnatural series are also substrates for this enzyme (**Egorova et al., 1973**). High substrate specificity was observed only in the case of *trans*-junction of C and D rings. Values of $V_{max}$ of 8α-series steroids may be more than ones for compounds of natural series. For example, $V_{max}$ value of 8α-estradiol **69a** is 219% of $V_{max}$ value of estradiol. D-homo-8α-estradiol **70a** has value of $K_m$ in 5 times less than estradiol value, whereas values of $V_{max}$ are approximately equal. Methylation of phenolic group (analogue **69b**) leads to the decreasing of $K_m$ value in one order, steroid **70b** has value of $K_m$ in 2.5 times less than compound **70a**. It takes attention big values of $V_{max}$ of steroids **71** and **72**, correspondingly

635 and133% in comparison with estradiol (**Langer et al., 1959**). Values of $K_m$ and $V_{max}$ of 2-hydroxyestradiol **72** are comparable with these values for estradiol **1** (**Chernyaeva et al., 1972**), and such modification may be important during the search of inhibitors of 17β-hydroxysteroid dehydrogenase. Hence, the presence of free hydroxyl group at C-3 is not necessary for significant substrate specificity of such steroids. Modified androgens are also substrates for this enzyme, although they are notably less specific (**Chernyaeva et al., 1972**). The abovementioned fact gives a persuasion that the search of inhibitors of investigated enzyme is most perspective in the series of steroids with unnatural rings junction. As far as we know such investigations have not yet been done.

It is quite interesting, that 2F- and 4F-estradiols (correspondingly **25** and **50**) are not substrates for 17β-hydroxysteroid dehydrogenase (**Langer et al., 1959**), which may be important during the search of compounds with different spectrum of biological properties.

Primary structure of this enzyme was determinated after the analysis of corresponding cDNA (**Peltoketo et al., 1988**), lately X-rays analysis was obtained (**Ghosh et al., 1995**). The comparison of spatial structures of 17β-hydroxysteroid dehydrogenase and investigated earlier 3α,20β-hydroxysteroid dehydrogenase (**Ghosh et al., 1994**) led to the conclusion about participation of His in the binding of hydroxyl group at C-3 of steroid and structure of transition state with the participation of triad Tyr-Ser-Lys. Authors justly mention the importance of the data obtained for modeling of interactions of 17β-hydroxysteroid dehydrogenase with various ligands for the creation of effective inhibitors of the enzyme. Interesting developing of these investigations was the modeling of spatial structures of the enzymes of humans and rats, which are significantly different in primary structure and substrate specificity. Rat enzyme structure was modeled by the replacement of corresponding amino acids in the structure of human enzyme crystal (**Ghosh et al., 1995**) and following minimization of energy was done (**Putanen et al., 1997**). Results of calculations of rat enzyme are in good correlation with obtained experimental data. Clarification of mechanism of action of both enzymes was done using chimeric enzyme and site-directed substitution.

73          74

X-rays data of the complexes of 17β-hydroxysteroid dehydrogenase with estradiol **1** (**Azzi et al., 1996**), 5α-dihydrotestosterone **73** and 20α-hydroxy-analogue of progesterone **74** (**Lin et al., 1999**) have been obtained lately. Nevertheless the preliminary evaluation of characteristics for the searching the specific potential inhibitors is quite a difficult task because in human body types 1, 7 and 12 catalyze the transformation of estrone into estradiol (**Blanchard & Luu-The, 2007**). Substrate specificities of 17β-hydroxysteroid dehydrogenases type 1 and 2 are similar, but in the case of second enzyme the transformation reaction estradiol – estrone is mainly directed to estrone formation (**Miettinen et al., 1996**), therefore the inhibition of this enzyme during the treatment of hormone-sensitive breast cancer is quite undesirable. The search of specific inhibitors of

17β-hydroxysteroid dehydrogenases type 1 is complicated task, the attempts to solve this task by replacement oxygen-containing groups at position 17 and introduction of fluorine atoms into the same position of steroid skeleton were unsuccessful (**Deluca et al., 2006**).

Steroid **75** with big value of $IC_{50}$ (530±7 nM) to this enzyme was synthesized, and this analogue has no hormonal activity (**Fisher et al., 2005**). Authors also obtained X-Ray data for the complex of compound **76** with 17β-hydroxysteroid dehydrogenase type 1 that has importance for the solution of this task.

Investigation of inhibitory activity of estrogen analogues with large substituents at C-16 in β-position led to find steroids **77** and **78** with selective action (**Lawrence et al., 2005**). Analogue **77** has value of $IC_{50}$ 0.29 μM to 17β-hydroxysteroid dehydrogenase type 1 (**Purohit et al., 2006**).

Parallel investigations of properties of modified estrogens with substituents in β-position at C-16 led to obtain the compounds of type **79** (**Laplante et al., 2008**), this steroid has value of $IC_{50}$ 44±7 nM for the transformation estrone **2** into estradiol **1** in T-47D intact cells. Unfortunately, analogue **79** possesses estrogenic activity, although this activity is decreased.

Obviously, clinical application of specific inhibitors of all three discussed enzymes is an intermediate step in the search for medications for the treatment of estrogen-sensitive oncological diseases. The most perspective direction is the search for compounds with simultaneous/synchronous inhibition activity to aromatase, estrone sulfatase and 17β-hydroxysteroid dehydrogenase. The basis for this approach is the possibility for overexpression of aromatase in tumors, which was shown in experiments on MCF-7 cell lines (**Santen et al., 1999**). Aromatase may stimulate the growth of tumors through both autocrine and paracrine pathways (**Chen et al., 1999**). Moreover, long-term estrogen deprivation increases sensitivity to estradiol and enhances aromatase activity in MCF-7 cells (**Yue et al., 1999**).

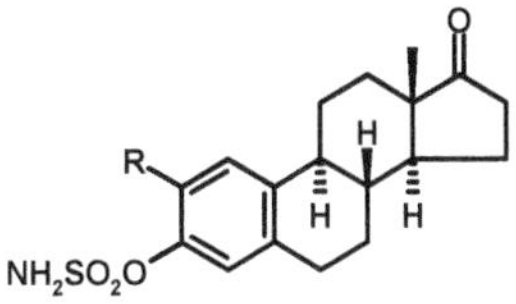

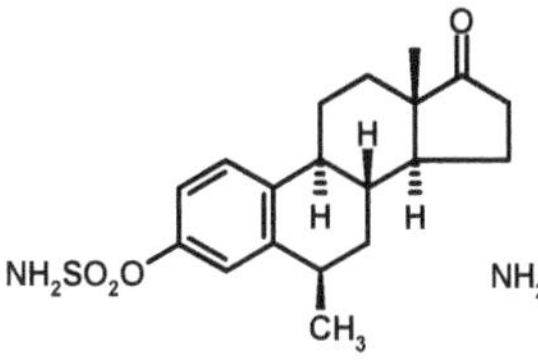

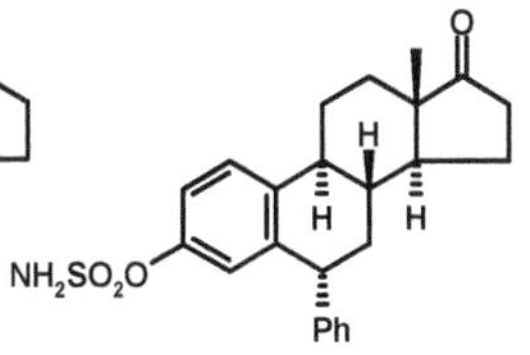

80 a) R=Cl, b) R=Br, c) R=CH₃          81          82

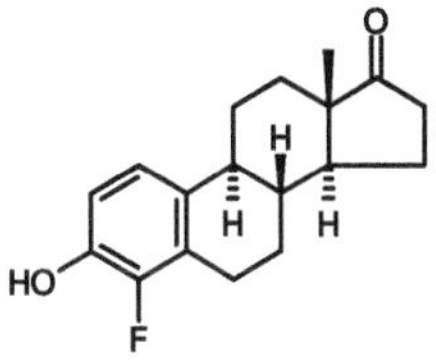

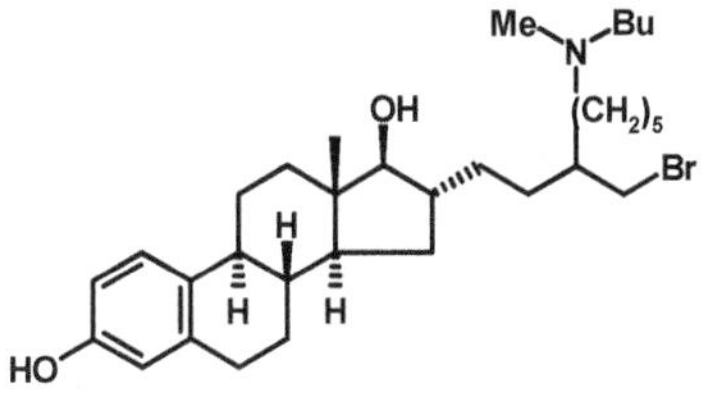

83          84

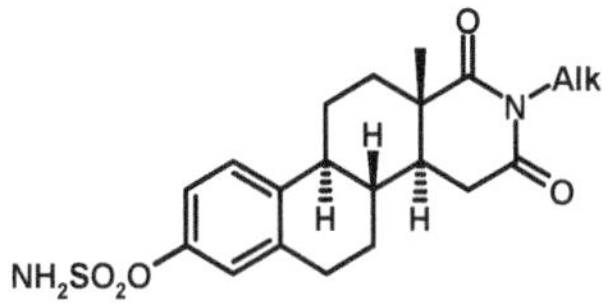

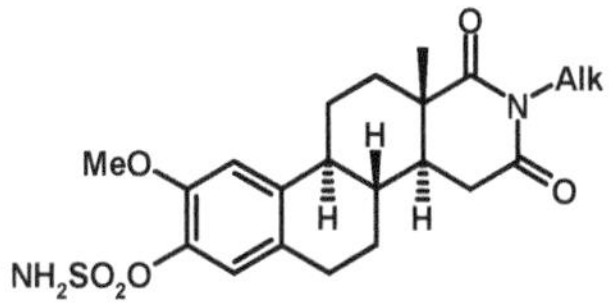

85          86

Both substrate specificity of enzymes and potential ways of inhibition metabolism must be taken into account during the search for steroid hormone synthesis inhibitors. The fine example of inhibitors which are able to inhibit the activity of aromatase and estrone sulfatase at the same time was demonstrated by Japanese authors (**Numazava et al., 2005; 2006**). In earlier investigation it was demonstrated that steroids **25, 47a,b,c** and **48-50** are good inhibitors of aromatase. Sulphamates **80a,b,c** and **81-83** having higher activity in comparison with EMATE have been synthesized. Authors justly think that these results may be useful for the development a new class of drugs having a dual function for the treatment of breast cancer. Additional benefits of the modifications at positions 2-, 4-, and 6 of steroid skeleton are perspective in respect of the fact that they may decrease the potential carcinogenicity of hydrolysis products (if they have) since the decreased possibility of formation of danger o-quinones of type **29** (**Liehr et al., 1995, 1996; Bolton et al., 1998; Bolton & Thatcher, 2008; Zhang, F. et al., 1999; Liu, X. et al, 2002; Zhang, Q. et al., 2008**) or 6-hydroxyestrogens (**Itoh et al., 1998**).

Search for non-steroidal inhibitors of aromatase and sulfatase is of interest as well. Such properties belong to heterocyclic sulphamates (**Reed & Potter, 2006**), however the perspectives for its using in clinic is not clear at the moment.

The attempts of synthesis of steroids with multifunctional action, in particular, inhibitors of ERs and 17β-hydroxysteroid dehydrogenase type 1 were done (**Tremblay & Poirier, 1996**).

Steroid **84** was selected as model compound by authors on the basis of previous data. Earlier it was established that in the series of 16-(bromoalkyl)estradiols for the realization of inhibitory action the presence of side chain (3-4 carbon atoms) at position 16α is optimal. Such substituents contribute to the appearance of antagonist activity to ERα. It is desirable to have the tertiary amide group with substituents on the amide nitrogen. Authors assumed that primary bromide will inactivate 17β-hydroxysteroid dehydrogenase. Thus, steroid was expected to be inhibitor of 17β-hydroxysteroid dehydrogenase and agonist-antagonist to nuclear estrogen receptor. These suppositions have been confirmed: model steroid caused 25% stimulation of cellular growth at concentration 0.1 μM, at the same concentration steroid inhibited by 45% the 0.1 nM estradiol-stimulated growth of ZR-75-1 cells. It means, that compound **84** is partial agonist of ER and inhibitor of 17β-hydroxysteroid dehydrogenase with moderate activity.

Sulphamates **85** and **86** are inhibitors of estrone sulfatase and 17β-hydroxysteroid dehydrogenase (**Potter & Reed, 2002; Messinger et al., 2006**).

The selection of ways for the treatment of oncological diseases mainly depends from individual peculiarities of patients, as result the methods of definition of aromatase, estrone sulphatase, 17β-hydroxysteroid dehydrogenase or mRNA (which realizes their synthesis), content have a crucial importance (**Irahara et al., 2006**).

## 5. Modified estrogens with antioxidant action as potential neuroprotective agents

Estradiol and its analogues have been known to have pro- and antioxidant features. These properties of estrogens are still subject of debate and depend on many factors, including animals or tissues, administration routes, concentrations, peroxidative model and so on. Antioxidant action of estrogens has been widely studied in vivo and in vitro. Aside from its effects on LDL-oxidation (**Badeau et al., 2005**), it has reported that estrogens decreased lipid peroxidation in brain homogenates and neuronal cultures (**Thibodeau et al., 2002**), reduced the superoxide anion production in different cells (**Florian et al., 2004**),

In vivo studies allow usage of different experimental models of neurological disease (**Azcoitia et al., 2002**). Among the steroid family, only estrogens have the capability to prevent neuronal cell death caused by oxidative stress. Estradiol has been reported to reduce mortality and cerebral damage in the models of brain ischemia including middle cerebral artery occlusion and common artery occlusion (**Perez et al., 2005**). The neuroprotective effect of estrogens have also been shown in animal model of Parkinson's disease induced by 1-methyl-4-phenyl-1,2,3,6-tetrahydropyridine and in experimental models with various toxicities including serum deprivation, amyloid β peptide, glutamate-induced excitotoxicity, kainic acid and so on (see **reviews Green & Simpkins, 2000; Amantea et al., 2005**). Estrogens may protect against injury via receptor-dependent and receptor-independent mechanisms and it has been suggested that antioxidant capacity is an important component of the complex neuroprotective effect (**Green & Simpkins, 2000; Prokai & Simpkins, 2007**).

Antioxidant activity of estrogens as well as other known antioxidants in vivo is determined by a lot of factors: concentrations, distribution, localization, fate of antioxidant-derived radical, interaction with other antioxidants, metabolism (**Niki & Noguchi, 2000**). Natural fluctuation of ovarian hormones during estrous cycle may influence the effect of exogenous hormones; therefore ovariectomized animals are often used. Another problem with this approach is that estrogens can be transformed in tissues into metabolites, for example to catecholestrogens, that have another antioxidant property and can produce prooxidants (**Picazo et al., 2003**). Most animal studied have utilized rodents (especially rats), that have a very high rate of estrogen degradation. Further, in case of brain the synthetic estrogens that are candidates for neuroprotective antioxidants in vivo should be able to cross the blood-brain barrier after their systemic administration. In vivo estrogens probably do not exert their own antioxidant action but interact synergistically with other antioxidants or reductants (**Hwang et al., 2000**). They can also affect the redox state of the cell through alteration of glutathione concentration and enhance the production of high energy compounds, stimulate antioxidant enzymes, such as SOD, catalase or glutathione transferase (**Perez et al., 2005; Akcay et al., 2006; Siow et al., 2007; Kumtepe et al., 2009**). Using in vivo methodology we can not understand molecular mechanisms of certain hormone antioxidant action, but it allows studying the manifestation of complex action of hormone treatment.

More than 12 different types of neuronal cells against the 14 different toxicities were used to investigate neuroprotective effect of estrogens, their analogues and derivatives (**Green & Simpkins, 2000; Wise et al., 2001**). The concentrations of estrogens that have produced protective action in these models vary from physiological (0.1 nM) to pharmacological (50 μM) and it is suggested that different neuronal types may have different sensitivities to estrogen-mediated protection. For example physiological concentrations of 17β-estradiol were neuroprotective in cultures that contain multiple cell types and maintain intact cellular architecture (**Dhandapani & Brann, 2007**). Several studies provide a positive correlation between in vitro neuroprotective potency and antioxidant activity of estrogens: they inhibited lipid peroxidation induced by glutamate, iodoacetic acid, amyloid β peptide (**Perez et al., 2005; Prokai-Tatrai et al., 2008**), reduced iron-induced lipid peroxidation (**Vedder, et al., 1999**), prevented intracellular peroxides accumulation induced by different toxicities (**Behl et al., 1997**). The neuroprotective antioxidant activity dependents on the presence of OH-group in the C-3 position on the A ring of the molecule. The formation of ether derivatives at C-2 position reduces effect because it abolishes the ability to donate a hydrogen atom (**Prokai et al., 2001; Perez et al., 2005**).

However, adjoin electron-donating methoxy groups to the phenolic ring may enhance antioxidant potency by weakening the phenolic O-H bond and provide stability of the formed phenoxyl radical (**Prokai & Simpkins, 2007**). Nevertheless generally higher concentrations of the hormones were required for antioxidant action than were needed for neuroprotection. This observation indicates that antioxidant effect is not a significant mechanism involved in the neuroprotective activity of estrogens in vivo (**Wise et al., 2001; Manthey & Behl, 2006**).

The simplest level of in vitro study of radical scavenging activity is investigation using cell-free models. Oxidation is induced by different systems of free radical generation and different types of prooxidants in order to gain a more precise view of the mechanism of inhibition. This methodology allows to investigate basic chemical properties (antioxidant or prooxidant) of natural estrogen molecules or synthetic analogues and compare compounds in each other.

There are multiple reactive oxygen and nitrogen species (ROS and NOS) and free radicals: superoxide radical ($O_2^{\bullet-}$), hydroxyl radical ($HO^{\bullet}$), hydrogen peroxide ($H_2O_2$), nitric oxide ($NO^{\bullet}$), peroxynitrite ($ONOO^-$), hypochlorous acid ($HOCl$), peroxyl radical ($ROO^{\bullet}$), lipoperoxy radical ($LOO^{\bullet}$). The reactivity toward various ROS or NOS can be measured by the inhibition methodology in which free radical species are generated in a special model system and the antioxidant effect is measured by inhibition of the reference reaction (Sanchez-Moreno C., 2002). For the superoxide anion radical generation a few model systems can be used: for example, hypoxanthine-xanthine oxidase system, autooxidation of riboflavine or non-enzymatic reaction of phenazine methosulphat in the presence of NADH and $O_2$. Then $O_2^{\cdot-}$ reduces nitro-blu tetrazolium into formazan at $25^0C$ and pH=7.4.

It is important to note that antioxidant action of estrogens is not necessarily depends on their receptors (Xia et al., 2002; Perez et al., 2005). This allows to search for modified analogues with lowered or depleted hormonal activity. It appeared that, for example, *ent*-estradiol 87 has antioxidant properties (Simpkins, 2004). The introduction of conjugated with aromatic ring double bond into steroid molecule leads to the increased antioxidant activity (steroids 88 and 89) (Römer, W.; Oettel, M.; Droescher, P.; Schwarz, S., 1997) and compound 90 (Römer et al., 1997) in comparison with estrogen without double bonds. Steroids of type 88 have significant hypothalamic action (Berliner, 1996), that allowed them to be recommended for the treatment of autoimmune diseases.

As we have noted earlier, presence of hydroxyl groups at C-3 and at C17 is important for effective binding of estrogens with estrogen receptors. As the first group is necessary for antioxidant activity of estrogen, synthesis of analogue with substituents at C-17 and/or aromatic ring, which would prevent receptor binding, would be an easy solution of the problem.

Thus, 17-methylensteroid **91** in the experiments on 23-day-old Sprague-Dowley rats exhibits only 1/70 of the uterotropic activity of estradiol. Moreover, this compound blocks the action of 7,12-dimethylbenzanthracene (**Jungblat et al., 1990**). Although in this work the investigation of antioxidant activity of compounds is not mentioned, it must be present in analogy with 17-difluoromethylene derivative **92** (**Bolhman & Rubanii, 1996**). In spite of that steroid has positive action on cardiovascular system; such compounds may have only restricted application because this steroid possesses contraceptive activity. We have to note that biological properties of 8α-analogue **93** are close to properties of steroid **92** (**Bolhman & Rubanii, 1996**). Analogues of type **93** decrease lipoprotein level.

The synthesis of steroid ethers in position 17 also could have lead to compounds having antioxidant activity coupled with lowered uterotropic action, as it was shown with compounds such as **96** (**Prokai et al., 2001; Prokai & Simpkins, 2007**). Thus, the presence of large substituents in ring D does not result in lowered antioxidant properties, hence synthesis of new compounds which would possess double bond at position 8(9) and large substituents at D-ring can be considered as the next step in the creation of new drugs. It is desirable that these substituents had free phenol hydroxyl group, which would automatically increase its antioxidant properties. In fact, steroids **94** and **95** do have desirable properties (**Römer et al, 1997**).

The introduction of large substituent at position 2 must lead to decrease of estrogenic properties of modifies analogue at the presence of antioxidant activity, that was demonstrated with compounds **97** (**Miller et al., 1996**) and **98** (**Simpkins et al., 2004**) as examples.

|  99  |  100  |  101  |

The high antioxidant activity of steroid **99** has been shown on different models (**Klinger et al., 2003**). Unfortunately this compound strongly inhibits monooxidaze activity of cytochrome P450 that is undesirable.

Hydroxyl group at C-17 in α-region of molecule does not prevent the appearance of antioxidant properties (compounds **100** and **101**), which opens additional possibilities for the obtaining compounds with the selective action (**W. Römer, M. Oettel, P. Droescher, S. Schwarz, 1997**).

Antioxidant properties of 6-oxa steroid estrogen analogues have undergone little investigation. Oxygen atom does obviously possess a big influence on electron density distribution in A ring, which can have an impact on antioxidant properties of such compounds. Difference in antioxidant action mechanisms between such compounds and those discussed earlier can be assumed (**Prokai-Tatrai et al., 2008**).

We carried out the search for modified steroid estrogen analogues in the series of steroids with unnatural rings junction having antioxidant properties and lowered/depressed uterotropic activity. Such properties belong to compounds **102** (**Pison et al., 2009**) and **103**. Some results of investigations of antioxidant properties of steroid **102** are presented in the Table 2.

102                                    103

| Experimental conditions | Schiff bases, conventional units / mg of phospholipids | Conjugated diene, nmol/mg of phospholipids | Triene conjugates, conventional units / mg of phospholipids | Klein coefficient | Malonic dialdehyde, nmol/mg of phospholipids |
|---|---|---|---|---|---|
| Control | 129±10 | 12.2±0.7 | 0.209±0.022 | 0.70±0.01 | 1.65±0.14 |
| Steroid **102** | 96±6 P<0.05 | 9.5±1.0 P<0.05 | 0.152±0.022 P < 0.05 | 0.71±0.05 P > 0.05 | 1.80±0.18 P > 0.05 |

P – Student' coefficient.

Table 2. Results of investigation of action of steroid **102** on lipid peroxidation in brain of rats

Steroid was given *per os* in olive oil in dose 5 mg per 100 g of weight of rats, for the day before the slaughter. Solutions of the steroids contain 5 mg in 0.3 ml. Control group of animals were treated by olive oil in equal volume.

Solely further investigations of such compounds may show the perspectives of this class of steroids. Depressed hormonal activity of investigated steroids may be a negative factor, inasmuch as during their using the capacity for the induction of the formation of enzymes with antioxidant properties will be decreased.

The presence of antioxidant activity leads to expect neuroprotective action of such modified estrogens, in spite of the fact that exact mechanisms of these properties have not yet been established. A huge amount of patents in this area is a proof of it. We shall cite some of those works (**Simpkins et al, 1994; Covey, 2002; Wuelfert et al, 2002; Peri et al., 2005; Pei, 2005**). Unfortunately clinical trials did not confirm neuroprotective action. Most probably it is connected with multifunctional activity of estrogens, and as a result their positive properties are "compensated" by negative action, but how and which ones are unknown. Further progress in this area must be connected with success in detailed investigation of mechanism of neuroprotective properties and synthesis of analogues with restricted action.

## 6. Osteoptotective action of estrogen receptors ligands

Several animal modes are used to test new compounds with osteoprotective properties. Ovariectomized mice are the ones most commonly used. Although aging in rats does not trigger osteoporosis development, ovariectomy-driven low estrogen concentration leads to changes in bone tissue, which mimic those occurring in aged women. At first phase of fast bone tissue loss triggered by accelerated bone remodeling occurs. Later on this process slows down. Trabecular tissue becomes depleted more so then cortical tissue. It should be noted that bone breaking is rarely observed in ovariectomized rats, thus is probably better to call this process osteopeny.

There are known several models for testing steroids on animals. When investigating the action of compounds in mature rats at the age of 3 months intensive growth of bones in longitudinal direction should be taken into account. 75 Days old (**Turner et al., 1994**) rats are more suitable for the investigation; rats model (6-12 months), which has very few skeletal changes, are much harder to work with. To test bone state several parameters are used, such as «bone mineral density» (g/cm$^3$) and «bone mineral content» (g/sm. length, g/sm$^2$). Last parameter has linear correlation with bone mass (r=0.999) (**Sato et al., 1995**) and calcium contain in ash after bone burning (r=0.90) (**Gaumet M., 1996**). By measuring dry weight of the bone (after drying at high temperature until the constant mass is obtained), ash weight after burning (**Bauss et al., 1996**), and also by investigating the ratio of this two parameters (**Broulik & Schreiber, 1994**) changes in mineral bone content can be measured. Results of dual-energy X-rays absorptiometry BMD correlate with fracture incidence and useful in evaluation progression of osteoporosis (**Sharp et al., 2000**). Yet, the final conclusion about steroid activity can only be given after the investigation of their influence on mechanical durability of the bone (**Turner et al., 1994; Sato et al., 1999**). All the works in this part were investigating naturally occurring steroids.

As we have already noted the significant structural similarity between natural steroids and their 8α-analogues, the osteoprotective and uterotropic action of these compounds were investigated. In experiments with ovariectomized Wistar rats parallel change in those effects was observed. It was suggested that osteoprotective activity is dependent on nuclear α-receptor of estrogens (**Morozkina et al., 2007**). Hence analogues were chosen as model compounds, despite the fact that presence of methoxyl group at C-3 was expected to trigger the lowering of activity. However in this case carcinogenicity was also expected to be lowered. In the experiments with Sprague-Dowley rats compounds **104** and **105** were shown to possess the same osteoprotective activity as ethynylestradiol, although they were administered in higher doses (**Morozkina et al., 2008**). The presence of substituents in positions 2 and 4 cancels the osteoprotective effect.

104                                    105

106

We assumed that steroid **106** may have osteoprotective action on the analogy with tibolone. It was confirmed experimentally; however compound **106** has embriotoxic action in experiments of contraceptive properties investigations which possibly decreases significantly the perspectives of such analogues.

| Droloxifene | Toremifene | GW5638 | LY353381 (arzoxifene) |
|:---:|:---:|:---:|:---:|
| **107** | **108** | **109** | **110** |

| CP335156 (Lasoxifen) | HMR3339 | Bazedoxifene |
|:---:|:---:|:---:|
| **111** | **112** | **113** |

As ER modulators are capable of displaying antagonistic properties in uterus and mammary gland while retaining agonistic features in bone, perspectives of using such compounds as osteoprotectors was investigated. Raloxifene has very effective osteoprotective properties. Clinical studies have shown that, aside from osteoprotective effects, the risk of breast cancer was also lowered (**Fontana & Delmas, 2001**). Interestingly that osteoprotective effect of raloxifene is not always mediated by ERs (**Miki et al., 2009**), and as the result the properties of its analogues may be quite interesting. However it was established that raloxifene in this case has some negative properties, peculiar to typical estrogens (high risk of hot flashes, leg crumps and venous thrombosis (**Deal & Draper, 2006**). In view of the aforesaid it is worth to remember about earlier synthesized compound LY357489 (**Grese et al., 1998**), whose osteoprotective action is significantly higher in comparison with raloxifene. This compound is the conformationally restricted raloxifene' analogue; its selective action was explained by specificity of interaction with ERs. Probably, it is necessary to investigate the mechanism of this compound' action.

Lately a huge number of SERMs with osteoprotective action have been synthesized, for example droloxifene **107** (**Ke et al., 1995; Chen, H.K. et al., 1995**), LY 353381 (arzoxifene **110**) (**Sato et al., 1998; Ma et al., 2002**), lasofoxifen (CP-336,156) **111** (**Ke et al., 1998; 2000, 2004**), GW5638 **109** (**Wilsson et al, 1997**) and many other compounds with interesting biological properties. For example, lasoxifen (CP-336,156) showed osteoprotective and cholesterol-lowering properties, decreased body weight in the experiments on ovariectomized rats. This compound had osteoprotective action in adult male orchideectomized rats, and has not influence on prostate (**Ke et al., 2000**).

Droloxifene showed interesting biological properties in the experiments with animals, such as osteoprotective action in aged female rats (**Chen, H.K. et al., 1995**). However it was shown to be less effective then tamoxifen in breast cancer treatment clinical studies, so its investigation was stopped (**Vogelvang et al., 2006**).

Lasoxifen showed osteoprotective and cholesterol-lowering action while lowering body weight of ovariectomized rats. This compound also displayed osteoprotective properties in adult male orchideectomized rats while having no effect on prostate (**Ke et al., 2000**). As far as we are aware, effectiveness of lasofoxifen have not undergone clinical studies.

Idoxifene was used in clinical trials on patients, whose tumors were resistant to tamoxifen, however third-generation aromatase inhibitors took its place, clinical data about its osteoprotective properties are conflicting (**Vogelvang et al., 2006**).

Preliminary studies of breast cancer treatment by HMR3339 and its osteoprotective properties provided results that may be considered positive (**Vogelvang et al., 2006**).

Bazedoxifen possesses promising properties. As a result of 5 years long clinical study on 4216 patients in postmenstrual period good osteoprotective properties were found (**Silverman et al., 2010**).

We have already mentioned the possibility of agents' synthesis in 8α-analogues of steroid estrogens series with osteoprotective properties. Preliminary results are presented in Table 3. 17α-ethynylestradiol was used as standard.

| Group of experimental rats (number of animals in the group) | Change of body weight, | Uterine weight, mg/100 g of body weight | Ash femur weight/wet femur weight | Bone mineral density, g/cm2 |
|---|---|---|---|---|
| Sham-operated (10) | 29±3* | 154 ± 4* | 0.432±0.007* | 0.258±0.005* |
| Ovariectomized (15) | 60±5 | 22.7 ± 0.5 | 0.398 ±0.005 | 0.231±0.003 |
| Ovariectomized, treated with EE (10) | 12±4* | 140± 6** | 0.433±0.005* | 0.255±0.006* |
| Ovariectomized, treated with steroid **69a** (10) | 7 ± 4* | 148± 6** | 0.425±0.006* | 0.258±0.007* |
| Ovariectomized, treated with raloxifen (10) | 33±5* | 46.5 ± 2.6* | 0.430±0.007 | 0.245±0.006* |
| Ovariectomized, reated with raloxifen and steroid **69a** (15) | 38±5* | 31.2 ± 1.2* | 0.425±0.005* | 0.248±0.006* |

Signs * and ** mean statistically significant difference between studied group and group of ovariectomized animals, $p<0.05$ and $p<0.01$ (Students t-criterion).

Table 3.

According to the data, this compound possesses osteoprotective properties. Also, in contrast to action of 17α-ethynylestradiol and steroid, combination of compound and raloxifene did not trigger hypertriglyceridonemy, yet cholesterol-lowering effect remained. There is no doubt that investigations regarding properties of 8α-series steroids are of great importance.

The new area in synthesis of compounds with osteoprotective properties should be noted – the creation of hybrid molecules having steroid and peptide fragments, for example compounds (**Wang et al., 2003**). Such compounds have stronger action in the experiments on rats in comparison with sum of action of these compounds.

| 114 | 115 |

Peptidylsteroid **114** has very interesting properties (**Yokogawa et al., 2006**). This hybrid compound during intranasal administration has a potent antiosteoporotic effect without side effects in experiments on female ddY mice.

In the treatment of estrogen-sensitive conditions aromatase inhibitors are to be used sometimes, which triggers estrogen concentration to drop, increasing osteoporosis and cardiovascular disease risk (**Ponzone et al., 2008; Reid, 2009; Gennari et al., 2011**). In each case the decision in using a drug depends on individual features of the patient. Usage combined drugs, which have calcitriol as a part of them, might prove useful to lower osteoporosis (**Krishnan et al., 2010**).

## 7. Steroid estrogens and cardiovascular system

Coronary heart diseases (CHD) is rare, and the incidence of CHD complications is much lower in premenopausal women then in man or postmenopausal women of similar age. After menopause the gender difference is lost and the incidence of CHD complications in women gradually approach that the men. In addition, menopause adversely affects several risk factors for CHD. It allows to assume the important role of estrogens in the protection of body from coronary heart diseases and expediency of their use as HRT medications.

Protective effect of estrogens has been shown in various animal models.

Rats have been used as a model system to study estrogenic effects on plasma lipid levels (**Lundeen et al., 1997**). On the whole this model has a lot of restrictions, first of all the main one is the predominant plasma cholesterol is HDL, not LDL, as it is in human. There are known: mouse models of atherosclerosis (**Hodgin & Maeda, 2002**) on rabbits (**Haarbo & Christiansen, 1996**) and primates (**Adams et al., 1990**). In all cases the main is the evaluation of influence of estrogens on the development of atherosclerotic plaque or lesion. In most cases it was shown the inhibitory activity of estrogens on atherosclerosis development.

Firstly it was postulated that main antiatherosclerotic action of estrogen is caused by the ability to decrease cholesterol level in serum; however in a number of investigations it was shown that this mechanism is not obligatory (**Shavva et al., 1987; Holm et al., 1997**).

At the present time it is postulated that atheroprotective effects of estrogen may be mediated by their nuclear receptors. ERα was found in endothelial cells (**Venkov et al., 1996**), in smooth-muscle cells (**Karas et al., 1994**) and in myocardial cells. A number of authors maintain the opinion about the importance for protective functions both ERα (**Gerard'es et al, 2006; Pare at al., 2002**), and ERβ (**Watanabe et al., 2003**). It is impossible to note the experimental data, showing the cardioprotective activity of estrogens, which is not mediated by nuclear receptors (**Shavva et al., 1987; Karas et al., 2001**).

Estrogens increase vasodilatation and inhibit the response of blood vessels to injury and the development of atherosclerosis, this action is referred to non genomic, this develops maximum after 20 min after estrogen introduction (**Mendelsohn & Karas, 1999**). Fast vasodilatation is possible due to the influence on both calcium-activated potassium ion-channel function (**Ghanam et al., 2000**), and on the synthesis of nitric oxide (the last relaxes vascular smooth muscle and inhibits platelet activation (**Holm et al., 1997; Node et al., 1997**). More detailed ways of non-genomic effects have been considered by **Mendelsohn & Karas (1999)**.

Of crucial importance is the influence of agents on hemodynamic functions (**Borissoff et al., 2011**).

One more factor of risk of arising of atherosclerosis and thrombosis is higher content of oxidized lipoproteins, possible mechanism of these diseases have been considered (**Steinberg et al., 1989; Holvoet & Collen, 1994**).

Antioxidant action of estrogens has been widely studied *in vivo* and *in vitro*. Besides its effects on LDL-oxidation (**Maziere et al., 1991; Markides et al., 1998; Ruiz-Larrea et al., 2000; Badeau et al., 2005**), it has reported that estrogens decreased lipid peroxidation in brain homogenates and neuronal cultures (**Vedder et al., 1999; Thibodeau P. et al., 2002**), reduced the superoxide anion production of different cells (**Bekesi et al., 2000; Florian et al., 2004**). All these effects may contribute to the beneficial consequences of estrogen replacement on the cardiac and vascular function, bone and mineral metabolism, brain function.

In the experiments on rabbits with hypercholesterinemic diet it was shown that 17α-dihydroequilin sulphate and 17α-ethynylestradiol significantly reduce atherosclerosis by 35% in the aortic arch and 75-80% in the thoracic and abdominal aorta, in spite of high level of LDL cholesterol (**Sulistiany at al., 1995**). High ration between HDL and LDL level is important but is not absolute parameter in prognosis of cardio-heart diseases risk. Clinical trials of estrone sulphate (at the same time 17α-ethynylestradiol has been investigated) in postmenopausal women have shown the significant improvement of this parameter. It is important that the action of estrone sulphate did not result in triglycerides level increasing in contrast to 17α-ethynylestradiol (**Colvin et al., 1990**).

Thus, numerous investigations on animal models (we described only few of them) give the evidence about the advisability of application of estrogens for HRT. First clinical trials for using of estrogens with this aim gave optimism, however wide-ranging investigations did not confirm the expectations. In older postmenopausal women with established coronary-artery atherosclerosis, 17β-estradiol had no significant effect on the progression of atherosclerosis (**Hodis et al., 2003**). Moreover, the combination: estrogen plus progestin may increase the risk of CHD (**Manson et al., 2003**). This is very important effect, because the content of triglycerides in blood is the independent factor of risk of cardio-vascular diseases (**Koren et al., 1996**).

This difference is very important because the increased level of triglycerides in blood is the independent factor of risk of cardiovascular diseases (**Koren et al., 1996**).

From other side, main and side effects of any medication depend on/from methods of the introduction into the body. Therefore the positive results obtained during transdermal introduction of estradiol takes attention (**Sumino et. al., 2006**). Oral estrogens raised triglycerides whilst transdermal estradiol lowered those (**Nerbrand et al., 2004**). The conclusion about propriety of such introduction of estrogens may be done only after wide-ranging long-term investigations.

The investigations of influence of estrogen receptors modulators, being already in clinical application, on coronary heart system have particular interest. First of them is raloxifen. Raloxifene blocks the sedimentation of redundant cholesterol in aorta in the experiments on rabbits **(Bjarnason et al., 1997; 2001)**.

One more new steroid has interesting properties **(Pelzer et al., 2005)**, this analogue in the experiments in estrogen-deficient spontaneously hypertensive rats has positive influence on hemodynamic function and inhibits cardiac hypertrophy.

## 8. Conclusion

From the data presented it became obviously the strategy for the searching of new medications on the basis of estrogen receptors ligands with the improved properties in comparison with clinically used. As far as the synthesis of such ligand is very complicated task, on the first stage the group with known structure peculiarities in the solution (including conformational dynamics) and determinate the possibilities for theoretical calculations of their spatial structure. The following docking of new possible agents into structures of macromolecule compounds (receptors, enzymes and other proteins) is used for the selection of most perspective compounds. And it is quite necessary to take into account the metabolic ways of new analogues.

## 9. References

Adams, M.R.; Kaplan, J.R.; Manuck, S.B.; Koritnik, D.R.; Parks, J.S.; Wolfe, M.S. & Clarkson, T.B. (1990). Inhibition of coronary artery atherosclerosis by 17beta estradiol in ovariectomized monkeys: lack of an effect of added progesterone. *Arteriosclerosis*, Vol.10, No.6, (November-December 1990), pp. 1051-1057, ISSN 0021-9150

Ahmed, S.; James, K.; Owen, C.P.; Patel, C.K. & Patel, M. (2001). Hydrophobicity, a Physicochemical Factor in the Inhibition of the Enzyme Estrone Sulfatase (ES). *Bioorg. Med. Chem. Letters*, Vol.11, No.11, (September 2001), pp. 2525-2528, ISSN 0960-894X

Ahmed, V.; Liu, Y.; Silvestro, C. & Taylor, S.D. (2006). Boronic acids as inhibitors of steroid sulfatase. *Bioorg. Med. Chem.*, Vol.14, No.24, (December 2006), pp. 8564-8573, ISSN 0968-0896

Aka, J.A.; Mazumdar, M.; Chen, C-Q.; Pourier, D. & Lin., S-X. (2010). 17β-Hydroxysteroid Dehydrogenase Type 1 Stimulates Breast Cancer by Dehydrotestosterone Inactivation in Addition to Estradiol Production. *Mol. Endocrinol.*, Vol.46, No.4, (April 2010), pp. 832-845, ISSN 0888-8809

Akcay, Y.D.; Sagin, F.G.; Sendag, F.; Oztekin, K. & Sozmen, E. (2006). Effects of estrogen-only therapy on LDL oxidation in women with hysterectomy: Does paraoxonase genotype play a role? *Maturitas*, Vol.53, No.3, (February 2006), pp. 325–332, ISSN 0378-512

Amantea, D.; Russo, R.; Bagetta, G. & Corasaniti, M. (2005). From clinical evidence to molecular mechanisms underlying neuroprotection afforded by estrogens. *Pharmacological Research*, Vol.52, No.2, (August 2005), pp. 119–132, ISSN 1043-6618

An, J.; Ribeiro, R.C.J.; Webb, P.; Gustaffson, J.-Å.; Kushner, P.J.; Baxter, J.D. & Leitman, D.C. (1999). Estradiol repression of tumor necrosis factor-α transcription requires estrogen receptor activation function-2 and is enhanced by coactivators. *Proc. Natl. Acad. Sci. USA*, Vol.96, No.26, (December 1999), pp. 15161-15166, ISSN 0027-8424

An, J.; Tzagarakis-Foaster, C.; Scharschmidt, T.C.; Lomri, N. & Leitman, D.C. (2001). Estrogen Receptor β-Selective Transcriptional Activity and Recruitment of Coregulators by Phytoestrogens. *J. Biol. Chem.*, Vol.276, No.21 (May 2001), pp. 17808-17814, ISSN 0021-9258

Arai, S.; Miyashiro, Y.; Shibata, Y.; Kashiwagi, B.; Tomaru, Y.; Kobayashi, M.; Watanabe, Y.; Honma, S. & Suzuki, K. (2010). New quantification method for estradiol in prostatic tissues of benign hyperplasia using liquid chromatography-tandem mass spectrometry. *Steroids*, Vol.75, No.1, (January 2010), pp. 13-19, ISSN 0039-128X

Azcoitia, I.; Doncarlos, L. & Garcia-Segura, L. (2002). Estrogen and Brain vulnerability. *Neurotoxicity Res.*, Vol.4, No.3, (January 2002), pp. 235-245, ISSN 1029-8428

Azzaoui, K.; Diaz-Perez, M.J.; Zannis-Hadjoupoulos, M.; Price, G.B. & Wainer, I.W. (1998). Effect of Steroids on DNA Synthesis in an in Vitro replication System: Initial Quantitative Structure-Activity Relationship Studies and Construction of Non-Estrogen Receptor Pharmacophore. *J. Med. Chem.*, Vol.41, No.9, (April 1998), pp. 1392-1398, ISSN 0022-2623

Azzi, A.; Rhese, P.H.; Zhu, D.-W.; Campbell, R.L.; Labrie, F. & Lin, S-X. (1996). Crystal structure of human estrogenic 17β-hydroxysteroid dehydrogenase complexed with 17β-estradiol. *Nature Struct. Biol.*, Vol.3, No.8, (August 1996), pp. 665-668, ISSN 1072-8368

Badeau, M.; Adlercreutz, H.; Kaihovaara, P. & Tikkanen, M. (2005). Estrogen A-ring structure and antioxidative effect on lipoproteins. *Journal of Steroid Biochemistry & Molecular Biology*, Vol.96, No.3-4, (August 2005), pp.271–278, ISSN 0960-0760

Bai, Y. & Gugière, V. (2003). Isoform-selective Interactions between Estrogen Receptors and Steroid Receptor Coactivators Promoted by Estradiol and ErbB-2 Signaling in Living Cells. *Mol. Endocrinol.*, Vol.17, No.4, (April 2003), pp. 589-599, ISSN 0888-8809

Bauss, F.; Esswein, A.; Reiff, K.; Sponer, G. & Müller-Beckmann, B. (1996). Effect of 17β-Estradiol-Bisphosphonate Conjugate, Potential Bone-Seeking Estrogen Pro-Drugs, on 17β-Estradiol Serum Kinetics and Bone Mass in Rats. *Calcif. Tissue Int.*, Vol.59, No.3, (September 1996), pp. 168-173, ISSN 0171-967X

Behl, C.; Skutella, T.; Lezoualch, F.; Post, A.; Widmann, M.; Newton, C. & Holsboer, F. (1997). Neuroprotection against Oxidative Stress by Estrogens: Structure-Activity Relationship. *Molecular Pharmacology*, Vol.51, No.4, (April 1997), pp. 535–541, ISSN 0026-895X

Bekesi, G.; Kakucs, R.; Varbıro, S.; Racz, K.; Sprintz, D.; Feher, J. & Szekacs, B. (2000). In vitro effects of different steroid hormones on superoxide anion production of human neutrophil granulocytes. *Steroids*, Vol.65, No.12, (December 2000), pp. 889–894, ISSN 0039-128X

Beral, V. & Million Women Study Collaborators. (2003). Breast cancer and hormone-replacement therapy in the Million Women Study. *Lancet*, V.362, No.9382, (August 2003), pp. 419-427, ISSN 0140-6736

Beral, V.; Bull, D. & Reeves G. &Million Women Study Collaborators. (2005). Endometrial Cancer and hormone-replacement therapy in Million Women Study. *Lancet,* Vol.365, No.9469, (April 2005), pp. 1543-1551, ISSN 0140-6736

Berliner, D.L.; Adams, N.W. & Jennings-White, C.L. (1996). Novel estrenes for inducing hypothalamic effects. *PCT Int. Appl. WO 96 10032,* filed 29 September 1994, issued 4 April 1996

Berry, M.; Metzger, D. & Chambon, P. (1990). Role of the two activating domains of the estrogen receptor in the cell-type and promoter-context dependent agonistic activity of the anti-oestrogen 4-hydroxytamoxifen. *EMBO J.,* Vol.9, No.9, (September 1990), pp. 2811-2818, ISSN 0261-4189

Blair, J.A. (2010). Analysis of estrogen in serum and plasma for postmenopausal women: Past present, and future. *Steroids,* V.75, No.4-5, (April 2010), pp. 298-306. ISSN 0039-128X

Blanchard, P-G. & Luu-The, V. (2007). Differential androgen and estrogen substrates specificity in the mouse and primate type 12 17β-hydroxysteroid dehydrogenase. *J. Endocrinol.,* Vol.194, No.2, (August 2007), pp. 449-455, ISSN 0022-0795

Bjarnason, N.H.; Haarbo, J.; Byrjalsen, I.; Kaufman, R.F. & Christiansen, C. (1997). Raloxifene Inhibits Aortic Accumulation of Cholesterol in Ovariectomized, Cholesterol-Fed Rabbits. *Circulation,* Vol.96, No.6, (September 1997), pp. 1964-1969, ISSN 0009-7322

Bjarnason, N.H.; Haarbo, J.; Kaufman, R.F.; Alexandersen, P. & Christiansen, C. (2001). Raloxifene and estrogen reduce progression of advanced atherosclerosis- a study in ovariectomized, cholesterol-fed rabbits. *Atherosclerosis* (Irel, Channon), Vol.154, No.1, (February 15, 2001), pp. 97-102, ISSN 0021-9150.

Bolhman, R. & Rubanii, G.M. (1996). 17-Difluoromethylenestratrienes with antioxidant and vasodilating activity. *Ger. Offen DE 19509729,* filed 13 March 1995, issued 19 September 1996

Bolton, J.L.; Pisha, E.; Zhang, F. & Qui, S. (1998). Role of Quinoids in Estrogen Carcinogenesis. *Chem. Res. Toxicol.,* Vol.11, No.10, (October 1998), pp. 1113-1127, ISSN 0893-228SX

Bolton, J.L. (2002). Quinoids, quinoid radicals, and phenoxyl radicals formed from estrogens and antiestrogens. *Toxicology,* Vol.177, No.1, (January 2002) pp. 55-65, ISSN 0893-228SX

Bolton, J. & Thatcher, G.R.J. (2008). Potential Mechanisms of Estrogen Quinone Carcinogenesis. *Chem. Res. Toxicol.,* Vol.21, No.1, (January 2008), pp. 93-101, ISSN 0893-228SX

Borissoff, J.I.; Spronk, H.M.H. & ter Cate, H. (2011). The Haemostatic System as Modulator of atherosclerosis. *New Engl. J. Med.,* Vol.364, No.18, (May 2011), pp. 1746-1760, ISSN 0028-4793

Broulik, P.D. & Schreiber, V. (1994). Methylene Blue Inhibits the Stimulation of Bone Mass by High Dose of Estradiol in Male Rats. *Endocrine Regulation,* Vol.28, No.3, (September 1994), pp. 141-144, ISSN 1210-0668

Brzozowski, A.M.; Pike, A.C.; Dauter, Z.; Hubbard. B.E.; Bonn, T.; Engstrom, O.; Ohman, L.; Green, G.L.; Gustafsson, J.A. & Carlquist, M. (1997). Molecular basis of antagonism and antagonism in the estrogen receptor. *Nature,* Vol.389, No.6652, (October 1997), pp. 753-758, ISSN 0028-0836

Bundred, N.J. (2005). The effects of aromatase inhibitors on lipids and thrombosis. *British J. Cancer*, Vol.93, No.12, Suppl.1, (August 2005), S23-S27, ISSN 0007-0920

Bushnell, C.D. (2005). Oestrogen and stroke in women: assessment of risk. *Lancet Neurology*, Vol.4, No.11, (November 2005), pp. 743-752, ISSN 1474-4422

Carpenter, R. & Miller, W.R. (2005). Role of aromatase inhibitors in breast cancer. *British J. Cancer*, Vol.93, No.12, Suppl.1, (August 2005), S1-S5, ISSN 0007-0920

Celic, L.; Lund, J.D.D. & Schiøtte, B. (2007). Conformational Dynamics of the Estrogen Receptor α: Molecular Dynamics Simulation of the Influence of Binding Site Structure on Protein Dynamics. *Biochemistry*, Vol.46, No.7, (February 2007), pp. 1743-1758, ISSN 0006-2960

Chen, H.K.; Ke, H.Z.; Jee, W.S.S.; Ma, Y.F.; Pirie, C.M.; Simmons, H.A.; Thompson, D.D. (1995). Droloxifene Prevents Ovariectomy-Induced Bone Loss in Tibia and Femora of Aged Female Rats: a Dual-Energy X-Rays Absorptiometric and Histomorphometric Study. *J. Bone Miner. Res.*, Vol.10, No.8, (July 1995), pp. 1256-1262, ISSN 0884-0431

Chen, S.; Okubo, B.; Kao, Y-C. & Yang, C. (1999). Breast tumor aromatase and transcriptional regulation. *Endocrine-Related Cancer*, Vol.6, No.2, (June 1999), pp. 149-156, ISSN 1351-0088

Chernyaeva, M.E.; Segal, G.M. & Torgov, I.V. (1972). Interaction peculiarities of 17β-hydroxysteroid dehydrogenase from the human placenta with some steroid compounds. *Russian Chem. Bull.*, No.4, (July-August 1972), pp. 588-596, ISSN 0002-3329

Cheskis, B.J.; Karanthanasis, S. & Lyttle, C.R. (1997). Estrogen Receptor Ligands Modulate Its Interaction with DNA. *J. Biol. Chem.*, Vol.272, No.17, (April 1997), pp. 11384-11391, ISSN 0021-9258

Chetrite, G.S.; Cortes-Prieto, J.; Philippe, J.C.; Wright, F. & Pasqualini, J.R. (2000). Comparison of estrogen concentrations, estrone sulfatase and aromatase activities in normal, and in cancerous, human breast tissues. *J. Steroid Biochem. Mol. Biol.*, Vol.72, No.1, (January 2000), pp. 23-27, ISSN 0960-0760

Cole, P.A. & Robinson, C.H. (1990). Mechanism and Inhibition of Cytochrome P-450 Aromatase. *J. Med. Chem.*, Vol.33, No.11, (November 1990), pp. 2933-2942, ISSN 0022-2623

Colvin, P.L.; Auerbach, B.J.; Koritnik, D.R.; Hazzard, W.R. & Appelbaum-Bowden, D. (1990). Differential Effects of Oral Estrone Versus 17β-Estradiol on Lipoprotein in Postmenopausal Women. *J. Clin. Endocrinol. Metab.*, Vol.70, No.6, (June 1990), pp. 1568-1573, ISSN 0021-972X

Covey, D.F. (2002). Preparation of enantiomeric estrogen derivatives containing unsaturated bonds in conjugation with the terminal or A ring as potential cytoprotective and neuropretective agents. *PCT Int. Appl. WO 02 40032*, filed 17 November 2000, issued 23 May 2002.

Davison, S. & Davis, S.R. (2003). Hormone replacement therapy: current controversies. *Clin. Endocrinol.*, Vol.58, No.1, (January 2003), pp. 249-261, ISSN 0300-0664

Deal, C.L. & Draper, M.W. (2006). Raloxifene: a selective estrogen-receptor modulators for postmenopausal osteoporosis - a clinical update on efficacy and safety. *Women's Health*. Vol.2, No.2, (March 2006), pp. 199-210, ISSN 1745-5057

Deegan, B.J.; Seldeen, K.L.; McDonald, C.B.; Bhat, V. & Farooq, A. (2010). Binding of the ERα Nuclear Receptor to DNA Is Coupled to Proton Uptake. *Biochemistry*, Vol.49, No.29 (July 27, 2010), pp. 5978-5988, ISSN 0006-2960.

Deluca, D.; Möller, G.; Rosinus, A.; Elger, W.; Hillish, A. & Adamski, J. (2006). Inhibitory effects of fluorine-substituted estrogens on the activity of 17β-hydroxysteroid dehydrogenases. *Mol. Cell. Endocrinol.*, Vol.248, No.1-2, (March 2006), p. 218-224, ISSN 0303-7207

Dhandapani, K. & Brann, D. (2007). Role of astrocytes in estrogen-mediated neuroprotection. *Experimental Gerontology*, Vol.42, No.1-2, (January-February 2007), pp. 70-75, ISSN 0531-5565

Egner, U.; Heunrich, N.; Ruff, M.; Gangloff, M.; Mueller-Fahrnow, A. & Wurtz, J.M. (2001). Different ligands-different receptor conformation: Modeling of the hER LBD in complex with agonists and antagonists. *Med. Res. Rev.*, Vol.21, No.6, (November 2001), pp. 523-539. ISSN 0198-6325

Egorova, V.V.; Zakharychev, A.V. & Ananchenko, S.N. (1973). Structure and Reactivity of steroids. VI. Long range effects in a series of 1,3,5(10)-estratriene compounds. *Tetrahedron*, Vol.29, No.2, (January 1973), pp. 301-307

Elger, W.; Schwarz, A.; Hedden, A.; Reddersen, G. & Schneider, B. (1995). Sulfamates of various estrogens are prodrugs with increased systemic and reduced hepatic estrogenicity at oral application. *J. Steroid Biochem. Mol. Biol.*, Vol.55, No.3-4, (December 1995), pp. 395-403, ISSN 0960-0760

Emmel, J.M.A. & Korach, K.S. (2001). Developing Animal Models for analyzing SERM Activity . *Ann. N-Y. Acad. Sci.*, Vol.949, (December 2001), pp. 36-43, ISBN 1-57331-359-9

Fischer, D.S.; Woo, L.W.L.; Mahon, M.F.; Purohit, A.; Reed, M.J. & Potter B.V.L. (2003). Novel D-ring Modified Estrone Derivatives as Novel Potent Inhibitors of Steroid Sulfatase. *Bioorg. Med. Chem.*, Vol.11, No.2-3, (February 2003), pp. 1685-1700, ISSN 0968-0896

Fischer, D.S.; Allan, G.M.; Bubert, C.; Vicker, N.; Smith, A.; Tutill, H.J.; Purohit, A.; Wood, L.; Packham, G.; Mahon, M.F.; Reed, M.J. & Potter, B.V.L. (2005). E-Ring Modified Steroids as Novel Potent Inhibitors of 17β-Hydroxysteroid Dehydrogenase Type 1. *J. Med. Chem.*, Vol.48, No.18, (September 2005), pp. 5749-5770, ISSN 0022-2623

Florian, M.; Freiman, A. & Magder, S. (2004). Treatment with 17-β-estradiol reduces superoxide production in aorta of ovariectomized rats. *Steroids*, Vol.69, No.13-14, (December 2004), pp. 779–787, ISSN 0039-128X

Fontana, A. & Delmas, P.D. (2001). Clinical use of selective estrogen receptor modulators. *Current Opinion in Rheumatology*, Vol.13, No.4, (July 2001), pp. 333-339, ISSN 1040-8711

Gantchev, T.G.; Ali, H. & van Lier, J.E. (1994). Quantitative Structure-Activity Relationships /Comparative Molecular Field Analysis (QSAR/CoMFA for Receptor-Binding Properties of Halogenated Estradiol Derivatives. *J. Med. Chem.*, Vol.37, No.24, (November 1994), pp. 4164-4176, ISSN 0022-2623

Gao, H.; Williams, C.; Labute, P. & Bajorath, J. (1999). Binary Quantative-Activity Relationship (QSAR) Analysis of Estrogen Receptor Ligands. *J. Chem. Inf. Comput. Sci.* Vol.39, No.1, (January-February 1999), pp. 164-168, ISSN 0095-2338

Gaumet, N.; Seibel, M.J.; Braillon, P.; Giry, J.; Lebecque, P.; Davicco, M.J.; Coxam, V.; Rouffet, J.; Delmas, P.D. & Barlet, J.P. (1996). Influence of Ovariectomy on Bone Metabolism in Very Old Rats. *Calcif. Tissue Int.* Vol.58, No.4, (April 1996), pp. 256-262, ISSN 0008-0594

Gennari, L.; Merlotti, D.; Nuti, R. (2011). Aromatase activity and bone loss. *In Advanced in clinical chemistry,* Vol.54, (2011), pp. 129-164, ISSN 0065-2423. Elsevier, ed. by Makovsky, G.S.

Gerardes, P.; Gagnon, S.; Hajadj S.; Merhi, Y.; Sirois, M.G.; Cloutier, I. & Tagguay, J.-F. (2006). Estradiol blocks the induction of CD40 and CD40L expression on endothelial cells and prevents neutrophil adhesion: an ERα-mediated pathway. *Cardiovasc. Res.,* Vol.71, No.3, (August 2006), pp. 566-573, ISSN 0008-6363.

Ghanam, K.; Ea-Kim, L.; Javellaud, J. & Oudart, N. (2000). Involvement of potassium channels in the protection effect of 17β-estradiol on hypercholesterolemic rabbit carotid artery. *Atherosclerosis (Shannon, Irel),* Vol.152, No.1, (September 2000), pp. 59-67, ISSN 0021-9150

Ghosh D.; Wawzak, X.; Week, C.M.; Duex, W.L. & Erman, M. (1994). The refined three-dimensional structure of 3α,20β-hydroxysteroid dehydrogenase and possible roles of the residues conserved in short-chain dehydrogenase. *Structure,* Vol.2, No.7, (July 1994), pp. 629-640, ISSN 0969-2126

Ghosh, D.; Pletnev, V.Z.; Zhu, D.-W.; Wawrzak, Z.; Duax, W.L.; Pangborn, W.; Labrie, F. & Lix, S.-X. (1995). Structure of human estrogenic 17β-hydroxysteroid dehydrogenase at 2.2 Å resolution. *Structure,* Vol.3, No.5, (May 1995), pp. 503-513, ISSN 0969-2126

Ghosh, D.; Griswold, J.; Erman, M. & Pangborn, W. (2009). Structural basis for androgen specificity and oestrogen synthesis in human aromatase. *Nature,* Vol.457, No.7226, (January 2009), pp. 219-223, ISSN 0028-0836

Gluzdikov, I.A.; Purohit A.; Reed, M.J. & Shavva A.G. (2007). Novel estrone sulphatase inhibitors. *XVIII Mendeleev congress on general and applied chemistry.* Moscow, September 23-28, 2007. Abstract Book, 2056.

Goss, P.E. (1999). Risk versus benefits in the clinical application of aromatase inhibitors. *Endocrine-Related Cancer,* Vol.6, No.2, (June 1999), pp. 325-332, ISSN 1351-0088

Green, G.L.; Gilna, P.; Waterfield, M.; Baker, A.; Hort, Y. & Shine, J. (1986). Sequence and expression of human estrogen receptor complementary DNA. *Science,* Vol.231, (March 1986), pp. 1150-1154, ISSN 0036-8075

Green, P. & Simpkins, J. (2000). Neuroprotective effects of estrogens: potential mechanisms of action. *Int. Journal of Devl. Neuroscience,* Vol.18, No.4-5, (July 2000), pp. 347-358, ISSN 0736-5748

Grese, T.A.; Pennington, L.D.; Sluka, J.P.; Adrean, M.D.; Cole, H.W.; Fuson, T.R.; Magee, D.E.; Phyllips, D.L.; Rowley, E.R.; Shetler, P.K.; Short, L.L.; Venugopalan, M.; Yang, Na, N.; Sato, M.; Glasebrook, A.L. & Bryant, H.U. (1998). Synthesis and Pharmacology of Conformationally Restricted Raloxifene Analogues: Highly Potent Selective Estrogen Receptor Modulators. *J. Med. Chem.,* Vol.41, No.8, (April 1998), pp. 1272-1283, ISSN 0022-2623

Greway, A.T.; Mentzer, M. & Levy, M.A. (1990). Enzyme interactions of 2,10-ethanoandrostene-3,17-dione with aromatase and 17β-dehydrogenase. *Biochem. Int.,* Vol.20, No.3, (1990), pp. 591-597, ISSN 1039-9712

Gruber, D.M. & Huber, J.C. (1999). Conjugated estrogens–the natural SERMs. *Gynecol. Endocrinol.*, Vol.13, Suppl.6, (December 1999), pp. 9-12, ISSN 0951-3590

Gustafsson, J-Å. (2003). What pharmacologists can learn from recent advances in estrogen signaling. *Trends Pharmacol. Sci.*, Vol.24, No.9, (September 2003), pp. 479-485, ISSN 0165-8147

Gustafsson, J-Å. (2005). Steroids and Scientist. *Mol. Endocrinol.*, Vol.19, No.6, (June 2005), pp. 1412-1417, ISSN 0888-8809

Haaf, H.; Li, S.A.; Li, J.J. (1987). Covalent binding of estrogen metabolites to hamster liver microsomal proteins: inhibition by ascorbic acid and catechol-O-methyl transferase. *Carcinogenesis*, Vol.8, No.2, (January 1987), pp. 209-215, ISSN 0143-3334

Haarbo, J. & Christiansen, C. (1996). The impact of female sex hormones on secondary prevention of atherosclerosis in ovariectomized cholesterol-fed rabbits. *Atherosclerosis (Shannon, Irel)*, Vol.123, No.1-2, (June 1996), pp. 139-144, ISSN 0021-9150

Hall, J.M. & McDonnel, D.P. (1999). The estrogen-receptor β-isoform (ERβ) of the human estrogen receptor modulates ERα transcriptional activity and is a key regulator of the cellular response to estrogens and antiestrogens. *Endocrinology*, Vol.140, No.12, (December 1999), pp. 5566-5578, ISSN 0013-7227

Hernandez-Guzman, F.G.; Higashiyama, T.; Osawa, Y. & Ghosh D. (2001). Purification, characterization and crystallization of human placental estrone/ dehydroepiandrosterone sulfatase, a membrane-bound enzyme of the endoplasmic reticulum. *J. Steroid Biochem. Mol. Biol.*, Vol.78, No.5, (November 2001), pp. 441-450, ISSN 0960-0760

Hernandez-Guzman, F.G.; Higashiyama, N.; Pangborn, W.; Osawa, Y. & Ghosh D. (2003). Structure of Human Estrone Sulfatase Suggests Functional Roles of Membrane Association. *J. Biol. Chem.*, Vol.78, No.25, (June 2003), pp. 22989-22997, ISSN 0021-9258

Hillisch, A.; Peters, O.; Kosemund, D.; Müller, G.; Walter, A.; Schneider, B.; Reddersen, G.; Elger, W. & Fritzemeier, K-H. (2004). Dissecting Physiological Roles of Estrogen Receptor α and β with Potent Selective Ligands from Structure-Based Design. *Molecular Endocrinology*, Vol.18, No.7, (July 2004), pp. 1599-1609, ISSN 0888-8809

Hodgin, J.B. & Maeda, N. (2002). Minireview: Estrogen and Mouse Models of Atherosclerosis. *Endocrinology*, Vol.143, No.12, (December 2002), pp. 4495-4501, ISSN 0013-7227

Hodis, H.N.; Mack, W.J.; Azen, S.P.; Lobo, R.A.; Shoupe, D.; Mahrer, P.R.; Faxon, D.P.; Cashin-Hemphill, L.; Sanmareo, M.E.; French, W.J.; Shook, T.L.; Gaarder, T.D.; Mehra, A.O.; Rabbani, R.; Sevanian, A.; Shil, A.B.; Torres, M.; Vogelbach, K.N.; Selzer, R.H. (2003). For the Women's Estrogen-Progestine Lipid-Lowering Hormone Atherosclerosis Regression Trial Research Group. Hormone Therapy and Progression of Coronary-Artery Atherosclerosis in Postmenopausal Women. *New Engl. J. Med.*, Vol.349, No.6, (August 2003), pp. 535-545, ISSN 0028-4793

Holm, P.; Korsgaard, N.; Shalmi, M.; Andersen, H.L.; Hougaard, P.; Skouby, S.O. & Stender, S. (1997). Significant Reduction of the Antiatherogenic Effect of Estradiol by Long-term Inhibition of Nitric Oxide Synthesis in Cholesterol-clamped Rabbits. *J. Clin. Invest.*, Vol.100, No.4, (August 1997), pp. 821-828, ISSN 0021-9738

Holvoet, P. & Collen, D. (1994). Oxidized lipoproteins in atherosclerosis and thrombosis. *FASEB J*, Vol.8, No.15, (December 1994), pp. 1279-1284, ISSN 0892-6638

Hong, Y.; Cho, M.; Yuan, Y.-C. & Chen, S. (2008). Molecular basis for the interaction of four different classes of substrates and inhibitors with human aromatase. *Biochem. Pharmacol.*, Vol.75, No.5, (March 2008), pp. 1161-1169, ISSN 0960-0760

Howard, N.M.; Purohit A.; Robinson, J.J.; Vicker, N.; Reed M.J. & Potter B.V.L. (2002). Estrone 3-sulfate mimics, inhibitors of estrone sulfatase activity: homology model construction and docking studies. *Biochemistry*, Vol.41, No.50, (December 2002), pp. 14801-14814, ISSN 0006-2960

Hwang, J.; Peterson, H.; Hodis, H.; Choi, B. & Sevanian A. (2000). Ascorbic acid enhances 17β-estradiol-mediated inhibition of oxidized low density lipoprotein formation. *Atherosclerosis*, Vol.150, No.2, (June 2000), pp. 275-284, ISSN 0021-9150

Irahara, N.; Miyoshi, Y.; Tagushi, T.; Tamaki, Y. & Noguchi, S. (2006). Quantitative analysis of aromatase, sulfatase and 17β-HSD$_1$ mRNA expression in soft tissue metastases of breast cancer. *Cancer Letters*, Vol.243, No.1, (November 2006), pp. 23-31, ISSN 0008-5472

Itoh, S.; Hirai, T.; Totsuka, Y.; Takagi, H.; Tashiro, Y.; Wada, K.; Wakabayashi, K.; Shibutani, S. & Yoshizawa, I. (1998). Identification of Estrogen-Modified Nucleosides from Calf Thymus DNA Reacted with 6-hydroxiestrogen 6-Sulfates. *Chem. Res. Toxicol.*, Vol.11, No.11, (November 1998), pp. 1312-1318, ISSN 0893-228X

Jordan, V.C. (2003). Antiestrogens and Selective Estrogen Receptor Modulators as Multifunctional Medicines. 2. Clinical Considerations and New Agents. *J. Med. Chem.*, Vol.46, No.7, (March 2003), pp. 1081-1111, ISSN 0022-2623

Jordan, V.C. (2007). New insights into the metabolism of tamoxifen and its role in the treatment and prevention of breast cancer. *Steroids*, Vol.72, No.13, (November 2007), pp. 829-842, ISSN 0039-128X

Jordan, V.C. & Brodie, A.M.H. (2007). Development and evolution of therapies targeted to the estrogen receptor for the treatment and prevention of breast cancer. *Steroids*, Vol.72, No.1, (January 2007), pp. 7-25, ISSN 0039-128X

Jungblat, P; Wiechert, R. & Bittler, D. (1990). 17-Methylene- and 17-ethylidene-estratrienes. 1990. *US Pat. 4977147*, filed 7 December 1988, issued 11 December 1990

Karas, R.H.; Patterson, B.L. & Mendelsohn, M.E. (1994). Human vascular smooth muscle cells contain functional estrogen receptor. *Circulation*, Vol.89, No.5, (May 1994), pp. 1943-1950, ISSN 0009-7322

Karas, R.H.; Schulton, H.; Pare, G.; Aronovitz, M.; Ohlsson, C.; Gustafsson, J-A. & Mendelsohn, M.E. (2001). Effects of Estrogen on the Vascular Injury Response in ER α,β (double) knockout mice. *Circulation Res.*, Vol.89, No.6, (September 2001), pp. 534-539, ISSN 0009-7330

Kato, S.; Endoh, H.; Masuhiro, Y.; Kitamoto, T.; Uchiyama, S.; Sasaki, H.; Masushige, S.; Gotoh, Y.; Nishida, E.; Kawashima, H.; Metzger, D. & Chambon P. (1995). Activation of the estrogen receptor through phosphorylation by mitogen-activated protein kinase. *Science*, Vol.270, (December 1995), pp. 1491-1494, ISSN 0036-8975

Kauser, K. & Rubanyi, G. (1998). A method using 17-difluoromethylene-estratrienes for lowering plasma level of lipoprotein(a). *PCT Int. App. WO 98 18429*, filed 3 June 1996 and issued 11 December 1997.

Kauser, K. & Rubanyi, G. (1998). Use of raloxifene and related compounds for the manufacturing of a medicament for lowering plasma level of lipoprotein(a). *PCT Int. App. WO 98 18428*, filed 30 October 1996 and issued 7 May 1997

Ke, H.Z.; Simmons, H.A.; Pirie, C.M.; Crawford, D.T. & Tompson, D.D. (1995). Droloxifene, a New Estrogen Antagonist/Agonist, Prevent Bone Loss in Ovariectomised Rats. *Endocrinology*, Vol.136, No.6, (June 1995), pp. 2435-2441, ISSN 0013-7227

Ke, H.Z.; Paralkar, V.M.; Grasser, W.A.; Crawford, D.T.; Qi, H.; Simmons, H.A.; Pirie, C.M.; Chidsey-Frink, K.L.; Owen, T.A.; Smock, S.L.; Chen, H.K.; Jee, W.S.S.; Cameron, K.O.; Rosati, R.L.; Brown, T.A.; DaSilva-Jardine, P. & Thompson, D.D. (1998). Effects of CP-336,156, a new, nonsteroidal estrogen agonist/antagonist, on bone, serum cholesterol, uterus, and body composition in rat models. *Endocrinology*, Vol.139, No.4, (April 1998), pp. 2068-2076, ISSN 0013-7227

Ke, H.Z.; Qi, H.; Crawford, D.T.; Chidsey-Frink, K.L.; Simmons, H.A. & Thompson, D.D. (2000). Lasofoxifene (CP-336,156), a Selective Estrogen Receptor Modulator, Prevents Bone Loss Induced by Aging and Orchidectomy in the Adult Rat. *Endocrinology*, Vol.141, No.4, (April 2000), pp. 1338-1344, ISSN 0013-7227

Ke, H.Z.; Simmons, H.A.; Shen, V. & Thompson, D.D. (2004). Long-term treatment of lasofoxifene preserves bone mass and bone strength and does not adversely affect the uterus in ovariectomized rats. *Endocrinology*, Vol.145, No.4, (April 2004), pp. 1996-2005, ISSN 0013-7227

Kelly, M.J.; Qiu, J. & Rønnekleiv, O.K. (2003). Estrogen Modulation of G-Protein-Coupled Receptor activation of Potassium Channels in the Central Nervous System. *Ann. N.-Y. Acad. Sci.*, Vol.1007, (December 2003), pp. 6-16, ISBN 1-57331-487-0

Klinger, W.; Lupp, A.; Karge, E.; Baumbach, H.; Eichhorn, F.; Feix, A.; Fuldner, F.; Gernhardt, S.; Knels, L.; Kost, B.; Mertens, G.; Werner, F.; Oettel, M.; Romer, W.; Schwarz, S.; Elger, W.; Schneider, B. (2002). Estradiol, testosterone, dehydroepiandrosterone and androsteronedione: novel derivatives and enantiomers. Interactions with rat liver microsomal cytochrome P450 and antioxidant radical scavenger activities *in vitro*. *Toxicol. Lett.*, Vol.128, No.1-3, (March 2002) p. 129-144.

Klopman, G. & Chakravarti, S.K. (2003). Structure-activity relationship study of a diverse set of estrogen receptor ligands (I) using MultiCASE expert system. *Chemosphere*, Vol.51, No.6, (May 2003), pp. 445-459. ISSN 0045-6535

Koike, S.; Sakai, M. & Maramatsu, M. (1987). Molecular cloning and characterization of rat estrogen receptor DNA. *Nucleic Acid Res.*, Vol.15, No.6, (March 1987), pp. 2499-2513, ISSN 0305-1048

Koren, E.; Corder, C.; Mueller, G.; Centurion, H.; Hallum, G.; Fesmire, J.; McDonathy, W. & Alapovic, P. (1996). Triglycerides enriched lipoprotein particles correlate with the severity of coronary artery disease. *Atherosclerosis (Shannon, Irel)*, Vol.122, No.1, (April 1996), pp. 105-115, ISSN 0021-9150

Kraichely, D.M.; Sun, J.; Katzenellenbogen, J.A. & Katzenellenbogen, B.S. (2000). Conformational Changes and Coactivator Recruitment by Novel Ligands for Estrogen Receptor α and Estrogen Receptor β: Correlations with Biological Character and Distinct Differences among SRC Coactivator Family Members. *Endocrinology*, Vol.141, No.10, (October 2000), pp. 3534-3545, ISSN 0013-7227

Krishnan, A.V.; Swami, S.; Peng, L.; Wang, J.; Moreno, J. & Feldman, D. (2010). Tissue-selective regulation of aromatase expression by calcitriol: implication for breast cancer therapy. *Endocinology*, Vol.151, No.1, (January 2010), pp. 32-42, ISSN 0013-7227.

Kuipper, G.G.; Enmark, E.; Pelto-Huikko, M.; Nilsson, S. & Gustafsson, J.A. (1996). Cloning of a novel receptor expressed in rat prostate and ovary. *Proc. Natl. Acad. Sci. USA*, Vol.93, No.12, (June 1996), pp. 5925-5930, ISSN 0027-8424

Kumar, V. & Chambon, P. (1988). The estrogen receptor binds tightly to its responsible element as a ligand-induced homodimer. *Cell*, Vol.55, No.1, (October 1988), pp. 145-156, ISSN 0092-8674

Kumtepe, Y.; Borekci, B.; Karaca, M.; Salman, S.; Alp, H. & Suleyman, H. (2009). Effect of acute and chronic administration of progesterone, estrogen, FSH and LH on oxidant and antioxidant parameters in rat gastric tissue. *Chemico-Biological Interactions*, Vol.182, No.1, (November 2009), pp. 1–6, ISSN 0009-2797

Kym, P.R.; Anstead, G.M.; Pinney, K.G.; Wilson, S.R. & Katzenellenbogen, J.A. (1993). Molecular Structure, Conformational Analysis, and Preferential Modes of Binding of 3-Aroyl-2-arylbenzo[b]thiophene Estrogen Receptor Ligands: LY117018 and Aryl Photoaffinity Labelling Analogs. *J. Med. Chem.*, Vol.36, No.24, (November 1993), pp. 3910-3922, ISSN 0022-2623

Langer, L.J.; Alexander, J.A. & Engel, L.L. (1959). Human Placental Estradiol-17β Dehydrogenase. II. Kinetics and substrate specificities. *J. Biol. Chem.*, Vol.234, No.10, (October 1959), pp. 2609-2614

Laplante, Y.; Cadot, C.; Fournier, M.-A. & Poirier, D. (2008). Estradiol and estrone C-16 derivatives as inhibitors of type 1 17β-hydroxysteroid dehydrogenase: Blocking of ER+ breast cancer cell proliferation induced by estrone. *Bioorg. Med. Chem.*, Vol.16, No.4, (February 2008), pp. 1849-1860, ISSN 0968-0896

Lawrence, H.R.; Vicker, N.; Allan, G.M.; Smith, A.; Mahon, M.F.; Tutill, H.J.; Purohit, A.; Reed, M.J. & Potter, B.V.L. (2005). Novel and potent 17β-hydroxysteroid dehydrogenase type 1 inhibitors. *J. Med. Chem.*, Vol.48, No.8, (April 21, 2005), pp. 2759-2762, ISSN 0022-2623

Lazennec, G.; Bresson, D.; Lucas, A., Chauveau, C. & Vignon, F. (2001). ERβ Inhibits Proliferation and Invasion of Breast Cancer Cells. *Endocrinology*, Vol.142, No.9, (September 2001), pp. 4120-4130, ISSN 0013-7227

Levin, E.L. (2002). Cellular function of plasma membrane estrogen receptors. *Steroids*, Vol.7, No.6, (May 2002), pp. 471-475, ISSN 0039-128X

Lewis, J.P.; Thomas, T.J.; Kling, C.M.; Gallo, M.A. & Thomas, T. (2001). Regulation of cell cycle and cyclins by 16α-hydroxyestrone in MCF-7 breast cancer cells. *J. Mol. Endocrinol.*, Vol.27, No.3, (December 2001), pp. 293-307, ISSN 0952-5041

Leygue, E.; Dotzlaw, H.; Watson, P.H. & Murphy, L.C. (1998). Altered estrogen receptor α and β messenger RNA expression during human breast tumorogenesis. *Cancer Res.*, Vol.58, No.15, (August 1998), pp. 3197-3201, ISSN 0008-5472

Li, J.J.; Li, S.A.; Oberley, T.D. & Parsons, J.A. (1995). Carcinogenic Activities of Various Steroidal and Nonsteroidal Estrogens in the Hamster Kidney: Relation to Hormonal Activity and Cell Proliferation. *Cancer Res.*, Vol.55, No.19, (October 1995), pp. 4347-4351, ISSN 0008-5472

Liehr J.G. (1983). 2-Fluoroestradiol. Separation of estrogenicity from carcinogenicity. *Molec. Pharmacol.*, Vol.23, No.2, (March 1983), pp. 278-281, ISSN 0002-895X

Liehr, J.G.; Ricchi, M.J.; Jefcoat, C.R.; Hannigan, E.V.; Hokanson, J.A. & Zhu, B.T. (1995). 4-Hydroxilation of estradiol by human uterine myometrium and myoma microsomes: implication for the mechanism of uterine tumorogenesis. *PNAS*, Vol.92, No.20, (September 1995), pp. 9220-9224, ISSN 0027-8424

Liehr, J.G. & Ricchi, M.J. (1996). 4-Hydroxylation of estrogens as marker of human mammary tumors. *PNAS*, Vol.93, No.8, (April 1996), pp. 3294-3296, ISSN 0027-8424

Lin, S.X.; Han, Q.; Azzi, A.; Zhu, D-W.; Gongloff, A. & Campbell, R.L. (1999). 3D-Structure of human estrogenic 17β-HSD1: binding with various steroids. *J. Steroid Biochem. Mol. Biol.*, Vol.69, No.1-6, (April-June 1999), pp. 425-429, ISSN 0960-0760

Liu, J.; Knappenberger, K.S.; Kack, H.; Andersson, G.; Nilsson, E.; Dartsh, C. & Scott, C.W. (2003). A Homogenous in Vitro Functional Assay for Estrogen Receptor: Coactivator Recruitment. *Mol. Endocriol.*, Vol.17, No.3, (March 2003), pp. 346-355, ISSN 0888-8809

Liu, X.; Yao, J.; Pisha, E.; Yang, Y.; Hua, Y.; van Breeman, R.B. & Bolton, J.L. (2002). Oxidative DNA damage induced by equine estrogen metabolites: role of estrogen receptor alpha. *Chem. Res. Toxicol.*, Vol.15, No.4, (April 2002), pp. 512-519, ISSN 0893-228X

Liu, X.; Zhang, F.; Liu, H.; Burdette, J.; Li, Yan, O.; Cassia, R.; Pisha, E.; Yao, J.; van Breemen, R.B.; Swanson, S.M; Bolton, J.L. (2003). Effect of halogenated substituents on the metabolism and estrogenic effects of the equine estrogen, equilenin. *Chem. Res. Toxicol.* Vol.16, No.6, (June 2003), pp. 741-749, ISSN 0893-228X

Loosen, H.J.J. (1999). Estrogenic estra-1,3,5(10)-trienes with differential effects on the alpha and beta estrogen receptors, having a linear hydrocarbon chain of from 5-9 carbon atoms in position 11. *PCT Int. Appl. WO 00/31112*, filed 20 November, 1998, and issued 18 November, 1999

Loosen, H.J.J.; Veeneman, G.H.; Schoonen, W.G.E.J. (2000). Non-aromatic estrogenic steroids with a hydrocarbon substituent in position 11. *PCT Int. Appl. WO 01/18027*, filed 6 September, 1999, and issued 28 August 2000

Lu, B.; Leugue, E.; Dotzlaw, H.; Murphy, L.G. & Murphy, L.C. (2000). Functional characteristics of a novel murine estrogen receptor-β isoform, estrogen receptor-β 2. *J. Mol. Endocrinol.*, Vol.25, No.2, (October 2000), pp. 229-242, ISSN 0952-5041

Lundeen, S.G.; Carver, J.M.; McKean, M-L. & Winneker R.C. (1997). Characterization of the Ovariectomized Rat Model for the Evaluation of Estrogen Effects on Plasma Cholesterol Levels. *Endocrinology*, Vol.138, No.4, (April 1997), pp. 1552-1558, ISSN 0013-7227

Ma, Y.L.; Bryant, H.U.; Zeng, Q.; Palkowitz, A.; Jee, W.S.S.; Turner, C.H. & Sato, M. (2002). Long-Term Dosing of Arzoxifene Lowers Cholesterol, Reduces Bone Turnover, and Preserves Bone Quality in Ovariectomized Rats. *J. Bone Miner. Res.*, Vol.17, No.12, (December 2002), p. 2256-2264, ISSN 0884-0431

Manas, E.S.; Unwalla, R.J.; Xu, Z.B.; Malamas, M.S.; Miller, C.P.; Harris, H.A.; Hsiao, C.; Akopian, T.; Hum, W-T.; Malakian, K.; Wolfrom, S.; Bapat, A.; Bhat, R.A.; Stahl, M.L.; Somers, W.S. & Alvarez, J.C. (2004). Structure-based design of estrogen-receptor-beta selective ligands. *J. Am. Chem. Soc.*, Vol.126, No.46, (November 2004), pp. 15106-15119, ISSN 0002-7853

Manson, J.E.; Hsia, J.; Jonhson, K.C.; Rossouw, J.E.; Assaf, A.R.; Lasser, L.N.; Travisan, M.; Black, H.R.; Heckbert, S.R.; Detrano, R.; Strickland, O.L.; Wong, N.D.; Crouse, J.R.; Dtein, E. & Cushman, M. (2003). Estrogen plus Progestin and the risk of Coronary Heart Disease. *New Engl. J. Med.*, Vol.349, No.6, (August 2003), pp. 523-534, ISSN 0028-4793

Manthey, D. & Behl C. (2006). From structural biochemistry to expression profiling: neuroprotective activities of estrogen. *Neuroscience*, Vol.138, No.3, (March 2006), pp. 845-850, ISSN 0306-4522

Markides, C.; Roy, D. & Liehr, J. (1998). Concentration dependence of prooxidant and antioxidant properties of catecholestrogenes. *Arch. Biochem. Biophys.*, Vol.360, No.1, (December 1998), pp. 105-112, ISSN 0003-9861

Matthews, J.; Wihlén, B.; Tujague, M.; Wan, J.; Ström, A. & Gustafsson, J.-Å. (2006). Estrogen receptor (ER) Modulates ERα-Mediated Transcriptional Activation by Altering the Recruitment of c-Fos and c-Jun to Estrogen-Responsible Promoters. *Mol. Endocrinol.*, Vol.20, No.3, (March 2006), pp. 534-543, ISSN 0888-8809.

Maziere, C.; Auclair, M.; Ronveaux, M.; Salmon, S.; Santus, R. & Maziere, J-C. (1991). Estrogens inhibit copper and cell-mediated modification of low density lipoprotein. *Atherosclerosis*, Vol.89, No.2-3, (August 1991), pp. 175-182, ISSN 0021-9150

Mendelsohn, M.E. & Karas, R.H. (1999). The Protective Effects of Estrogens on Cardiovascular System. *New Engl. J. Med.*, Vol.340, No.23, (June 1999), pp. 1801-1811, ISSN 0028-4793

Messinger, J.; Thole, H-H.; Husen, B.; Koskimies, P.; Pirkkala, L. & Weske, M. (2006). Preparation of estratrienes as 17β-hydroxysteroid dehydrogenase type 1 and steroid sulfatase inhibitors. *PCT Int. Appl. WO 2006 125800*, filed May 26, 2005, and issued 30 November, 2006

Meyers, M.J.; Sun, J.; Carlson, K.E.; Katzenellenbogen, B.S. & Katzenellenbogen, J.A. (1999). Estrogen Receptor Subtype-Selective Ligands: Asymmetric Synthesis and Biological Evaluation of cis- and trans-5,11-Dialkyl-5,6,11,12-tetrahydrochrysenes. *J. Med. Chem.*, Vol.42, No.13, (July 1999), pp. 2456-2468, ISSN 0022-2623

Miettinen, M.; Mustonen, M.V.; Poutanen, M.H.; Isomaa, V.V. & Vihko, R.K. (1996). Human placental 17β-hydroxysteroid dehydrogenase type 1 and type 2 isoenzyme have opposite activities in culturated cells and characteristic cell- and tissue-specific expression. *Biochem. J.*, Vol.314, No.3, (March 1996), pp. 839-845, ISSN 0013-7227

Miki, Y.; Suzuki, T.; Nagasaki, S.; Hata, S.; Akahira, J. & Sasano, H. (2009). Comparative effects of raloxifene, tamoxifen and estradiol on human osteoblasts *in vitro*: Estrogen receptor dependent or independent pathways of raloxifene. *J. Steroid Biochem. Mol. Biol.*, Vol.113, No.3-5, (February 2009), pp. 281-289, ISSN 0960-0760

Miller, C.P.; Jirkovski, I.; Hayhurst, D.A. & Adelman, S.A. (1996). In vitro antioxidant effects of estrogens with a hindered-3-hydroxy function on the copper-induced oxidation of low density lipoproteins. *Steroids*, Vol.61, No.5, (May 1996), pp. 305-308, ISSN 0039-128X

Miller, C.P.; Collini, M.D. & Harris, H.A. (2003). Constrained Phytoestrogens and Analogues as ERβ Selective Ligands. *Bioorg. Med. Chem. Lett.*, Vol.13, No.14, (July 2003), pp. 2399-2403, ISSN 0960-894X

Monroe, D.G.; Secreto, F.J.; Subramaniam, M.; Getz, B.J.; Khosla, S. & Spelberg, T.C. (2005). Estrogen receptor α and β heterodimers exert unique effects on estrogen- and tamoxifen-dependent gene expression in human U2OS osteosarcoma cells. *Mol. Endocrinol.*, Vol.19, No.6, (June 2005), pp. 1555-1568, ISSN 0888-8809

Morozkina, S.N. & Shavva, A.G. (2007). Synthesis, investigation of molecular structures, and biological properties of 8α-steroid estrogen analogues. Screening and MedChemEurope. 20-21 February, 2007. Palau De Congressor De Catalunia. Barcelona, Spain. Presentation.

Morozkina, S.N.; Egorov, M.S.; Eliseev, I.I.; Selivanov, S.I.; Eschenko, N.D.; Putilina, F.E.; Vilkova, V.A.; Zakharova, L.I. & Shavva, A.G. (2008). Synthesis and investigation of osteoprotective action of some 8α-analogues of steroid estrogens. *Vestnik Sankt-Peterburgskogo Universiteta*, Seriya 4: Fizika, Khimiya, Ser.4, No.3, (September 2008), pp. 104-108, ISSN 1024-8579 (Rus. Ed.)

Morozkina, S.N.; Chentsova, A.S.; Khasan, T.; Selivanov, S.I.; Shavarda, A.L. & Shavva, A.G. (2009). New variant of synthesis of D-homo-6-oxa-8α steroid estrogen analogues with 7β-methyl group. *Chem. Heterocycl. Comp.*, No.9, (September 2009), pp. 1427-1429, ISSN 0132-6244 (Rus. Ed.)

Mosselman, S.; Polman, J.; Dijkema, R. (1996). ER beta: identification and characterization of a novel human estrogen receptor. *FEBS Lett.*, Vol.392, No.1, (August 1996), pp. 49-53, ISSN 0014-5793

Nerbrand, C.; Lidfeldt, J.; Niberg, P.; Scherstén, P. & Samsioe, G. (2004). Serum lipids and lipoproteins in relation to endogenous and exogenous female sex steroids and age. The Women's Health in the Lund Area (WHILA) study. *Maturitas*, Vol.48, No.2, (June 2004), pp. 161-169, ISSN 0378-5122

Niki, E. & Noguchi, N. (2000). Evaluation of Antioxidant Capacity. What Capacity is being Measured by Which Method? *IUBMB Life*, Vol.50, No.4-5, (October 2000), pp. 323-329, ISSN 1521-6543

Nishino, Y.; Schneider, M.R.; Michna, H. & El Etreby, M.F. (1989). Antitumor effect of a specific aromatase inhibitor, 1-methyl-androsta-1,4-diene-3,17-dion (Atamestane), in female rat bearing DMBA-induced mammary tumors. *J. Steroid Biochem.*, Vol.34, No.1-6, (1989), pp. 435-437, ISSN 0022-4731

Node, K.; Kitakaze, M.; Kosaka, H.; Minamino, T.; Funaya, H. & Hori, M. (1997). Amelioration of Ischemia- and Reperfusion –induced Myocardium Injury by 17β-Estradiol Role of Nitric Oxide and Calcium-activated Potassium Channels. *Circulation*, Vol.96, No.6, (September 1997), pp. 1953-1963, ISSN 0009-7322

Numazava, M.; Ando, M.; Watari, Y.; Tominaga, T.; Hayata, Y. & Yoshimura, A. (2005). Structure-activity relationship of 2-, 4-, or 6-substituted estrogens as aromatase inhibitors. *J. Steroid Biochem. Mol. Biol.*, Vol.96, No.1, (June 2005), pp. 51-57, ISSN 0960-0760

Numazava, M.; Tominaga, T.; Watari, Y. & Tada, Y. (2006). Inhibition of estrone sulfatase by aromatase inhibitor-based estrogen 3-sulfamates. *Steroids*, Vol.71, No.5, (May 2006), pp. 371-379, ISSN 0960-0760

Ogawa, S.; Inoue, S.; Watanabe, T.; Hiroi, H.; Hosoi, T.; Oushi, Y. & Muramatsu, M. (1998). The complete primary structure of human estrogen receptor β (hERβ) and its heterodimerization with ERα in vivo and in vitro. *Biochem. Biophys. Res. Commun.*, Vol.243, No.1, (February 1998), pp. 122-126, ISSN 0006-291X

Pare, G.; Krust, A.; Karas, R.H.; Dupont, S.; Aronovitz, M.; Chambon, P. & Mendelsohn, M.E. (2002). ERα mediate the protective effect of estrogen against vascular injury. *Circulation Res.*, Vol.90, No.10, (May 2002), pp. 1087-1092, ISSN 0009-7330

Pasha, F.A.; Srinivasta, H.K. & Singh, P.P. (2005). Semiempirical QSAR study and ligand receptor interactions of estrogens. *Molecular Diversity*, Vol.9, No.1-3, (January 2005), pp. 215-220. ISSN 1381-1991

Pasqualini, J.R.; Chetrite, G.; Blacker, C.; Feinstein, M.-C.; Delalonde, L.; Talbi, M. & Maloch, C. (1996). Concentrations of estrone, estradiol and estrone sulfate and evaluation of sulfatase and aromatase activities in pre- and postmenopausal breast cancer. *J. Clin. Endocrinol. Metab.*, Vol.81, No.4, (April 1996), pp. 1460-1464, ISSN 0021-972X

Pasqualini, J.R.; Cortes-Prieto, J.; Chetrite, G. & Ruis, A. (1997). Concentrations of estrone, estradiol, and their sulfates and evaluation of sulfatase and aromatase activities in patient with breast fibroadenoma. *Int. J. Cancer*, Vol.70, No.6, (March 1997), pp. 639-643, ISSN 0020-7136

Pasqualini, J.R. & Chetrite, G. (2001). Paradoxical effect of estradiol: it can block its own bioformation in human breast cancer cells. *J. Steroid Biochem. Mol. Biol.*, Vol.78, No.1, (July 2001), pp. 21-24, ISSN 0960-0760

Pasqualini, J.R. & Chetrite, G.S. (2006). Estradiol as an anti-aromatase agent in human breast cancer cells. *J. Steroid Biochem. Mol. Biol.*, Vol.98, No.1, (January 2006), pp. 12-17, ISSN 0960-0760

Pedram, A; Razandi, M. & Levin, E.R. (2009). Nature of Functional Estrogen Receptors at the Plasma Membrane. *Molec. Endocrinol.*, Vol.20, No.9, (September 2009), pp. 1996-2009, ISSN 0888-8809

Peet, N.P.; Burkhard, J.P.; Wright, C.L. & Jonhston, J. & O'Neil. (1992). Time-dependent inhibition of human placental aromatase with 2,19-methylenoxy-bridget androstenedione. *J. Med. Chem.*, Vol.35, No.17, (August 1992), pp. 3303-3306, ISSN 0022-2623

Pei, Y. (2005). Preparation of estrone derivatives as cytoprotective agents for use in pharmaceutical compositions for the treatment of degenerative diseases. *U.S. Pat. Appl. Publ.* US 2005 267085, filed 27 May 2004 and issued 1 December 2005.

Peltoketo, H.; Isomaa, V.; Mäentausta, O. & Vihko, R. (1988). Complete amino acid sequence of human placental 17β-Hydroxysteroid dehydrogenase deduced from cDNA. *FEBS Letters*, Vol.239, No.1, (October 1988), pp. 73-77, ISSN 0014-5793

Pelzer, T.; Jazbutyte, V.; Hu, K.; Segerer, S.; Nahrendorf, M.; Nordbeck, P.; Bonz, A.W.; Muck, J.; Fritzemeier, K.-H.; Hedele-Hurtung, C.; Ertl, G. & Neyses, L. (2005). The estrogen receptor-α agonist 16α-LE2 inhibits cardiac hypertrophy and improve hemodynamic function in estrogen-deficient spontaneously hypertensive rats. *Cardiovasc. Res.*, Vol.67, No.4, (September 2005), pp. 604-612, ISSN 0008-6363

Perez, E.; Liua, R.; Yang, S.-H.; Cai, Z.; Covey, D. & Simpkins J. (2005). Neuroprotective effects of an estratriene analog are estrogen receptor independent in vitro and in vivo. *Brain Research*, Vol.1038, No.2, (March 2005), pp. 216–222, ISSN 0006-8993

Peri, A.; Benvenuti, S.; Luciani, P. & Serio, M. (2005). Pharmaceutical compositions containing selective estrogen receptor modulators for the treatment of Alzheimer's disease. *PCT Int. Appl.* WO 2005 105063, filed 3 May 2004 and issued 10 November 2005.

Peters, R.H.; Chao, W-Ru; Sato, B.; Shigeno, K.; Zaveri, N.T. & Tanabe, M. (2003). Steroidal oxathiazine inhibitors of estrone sulfatase. *Steroids*, Vol.68, No.1, (January 2003), pp. 97-110, ISSN 0039-128X

Pham, T.A.; Hwung, Y.P.; Santiso-Mere, D.; Mc.Donnel, D.P. & O'Malley, D.P. (1992). Ligand-dependent and -independent function of the transactivation regions of the human receptor in yeast. *Mol. Endocrinol.*, Vol.6, No.7, (July 1992), pp. 1043-1050, ISSN 0888-8809

Picazo, O.; Azcoitia, I. & Garcia-Segura, L. (2003). Neuroprotective and neurotoxic effects of estrogens. *Brain Research*, Vol.990, No.1-2, (November 2003), pp. 20-27, ISSN 0006-8993

Pike, A.C.W.; Brzozowski, A.M.; Hubbard, R.E.; Bonn, T.; Thorsell, A-G.; Engström, O.; Ljunggren, J.; Gustafsson, J-Å. & Carlquist, M. (1999). Structure of the ligand-binding domain of estrogen receptor beta in the presence of a partial agonist and a full antagonist. *EMBO J.*, Vol.18, No.17, (September 1999), pp. 4608-4618, ISSN 0261-4189.

Pison, U.; Shavva, A.G. & Morozkina, S.N. (2009). Preparation of 6-oxa-8α-steroid estrogen analogues - a group of unnatural estrogens and their use in medicine. *PCT Int. Appl. WO 2008 009619*, filed 10 November 2008 and issued 14 May 2009.

Ponzone, R.; Mininanni, P.; Cassina, E.; Pastorino, F. & Sismondi, P. (2008). Aromatase inhibitors for breast cancer: different structure, same effects? *Endocrine Relat. Cancer*, Vol.15, No.1, (March 2008), pp. 27-36, ISSN 1351-0088

Potter, B.V.L. & Reed, M.J. (2002). Preparation of estrone derivatives for treatment use as steroid sulfatase and steroid dehydrogenase inhibitors for treatment of breast cancer. *PCT Int. Appl. WO 02 32409*, filed 20 October, 2000, and issued 25 April, 2002.

Prokai, L.; Oon, S.-M.; Prokai-Tatrai, K.; Abboud, K. & Simpkins, J. (2001). Synthesis and Biological Evaluation of 17β-Alkoxyestra-1,3,5(10)-trienes as Potential Neuroprotectants Against Oxidative Stress. *J. Med. Chem.*, Vol.44, No.1, (January 2001), pp. 110-114, ISSN 0022-2623

Prokai, L. & Simpkins, J. (2007). Structure–nongenomic neuroprotection relationship of estrogens and estrogen-derived compounds. *Pharmacology & Therapeutics*, Vol.114, No.1, (April 2007), pp. 1–12, ISSN 0163-7258

Prokai-Tatrai, K.; Perjesi, P.; Rivera-Portalatinc, N.; Simpkins, J. & Prokai, L. (2008). Mechanistic investigation on the antioxidant action of neuroprotective estrogen derivative. *Steroids*, Vol.73, No.3, (March 2008), pp. 280-288, ISSN 0039-128X

Pujol, P.; Rey, J.M.; Nirde, P.; Roger, P.; Gastaldi, M.; Laffargue, F.; Rochefort, H. & Maudelonde, T. (1998). Differential expression of estrogen receptors α and β messengers RNAs as potential marker of ovarian carcinogenesis. *Cancer Res.*, Vol.58, No.3, (December 1998), pp. 5367-5373, ISSN 0008-5472

Purohit, A.; Williams, G.A.; Howarth, N.M.; Potter, B.V.L. & Reed, M.J. (1995). Inactivation of steroid sulfatase by an active site-directed inhibitor, estrone-3-O-sulfamate. *Biochemistry*, Vol.34, No.36, (September 1995), pp. 11508-11514, ISSN 0006-2960

Purohit, A.; Vernon, K.A.; Hummelinck, A.E.W.; Woo, L.W.L.; Hejaz, H.A.M.; Potter, B.V.L. & Reed, M.J. (1998). The development of A-ring modified analogues of oestrone 3-O-sulphamate as potent steroid sulphatase inhibitors with reduced oestrogenicity.

*J. Steroid Biochem. Mol. Biol.*, Vol.64, No.5-6, (March 01, 1998), pp. 269-275, ISSN 0960-0760

Purohit, A.; Hejaz, H.A.M.; Woo, L.W.L.; van Strien, A.E.; Potter, B.V.L. & Reed, M.J. (1999). Recent advances in the development of steroid sulphatase inhibitors. *J. Steroid Biochem. Mol. Biol.*, Vol.69, No.1-6, (April-June 1999), pp. 227-238, ISSN 0960-0760

Purohit, A.; Tutill, H.J.; Day, J.M.; Chander, S.K.; Lawrence, H.R.; Allan, G.M.; Fisher, D.S.; Vicker, M.; Newman, S.P.; Potter, B.V.L. & Reed, M.J. (2006). The regulation and inhibition of 17β-hydroxysteroid dehydrogenase in breast cancer. *Mol. Cell. Endocrinol.*, Vol.248, No.1-2, (March 2006), pp. 199-203, ISSN 0303-7207

Putanen, T.; Poutanen, M.; Ghosh, D.; Vihko, R. & Vihko, P. (1997). Origin of Substrate Specificity of Human and Rat 17β-Hydroxysteroid Dehydrogenase Type 1, Using Chimeric Enzyme and Site-Directed Substitutions. *Endocrinology*, Vol.138, No.8, (August 1997), pp. 3532-3539, ISSN 0013-7227

Ramsey, Y.L. & Klinge, C.M. (2001). Estrogen response element binding alteration in estrogen receptor-α conformation as revealed by susceptibility to partial proteolysis. *J. Molec. Endocrinol.*, Vol.27, No.3, (December 2001), pp. 275-292, ISSN 0952-5041

Raobaikady, B.; Purohit, A.; Chander, S.K.; Woo, L.W.L.; Leese, M.P.; Potter, B.V.L. & Reed, M.J. (2003). Inhibition of MCF-7 breast cancer cell proliferation and in vivo steroid sulphatase activity by 2-methoxyestradiol-bis-sulfamate. *J. Steroid Biochem. Mol. Biol.*, Vol.84, No.2-3, (February 2003), p. 351-358, ISSN 0960-0760

Reed, M.J. & Potter, B.V.L. (1999). Steroid 3-sulphamate derivatives as inhibitors of oestrone sulphatase. *PCT Int. Appl. WO 99 27935*, filed December 4, 1997, and issued December 3, 1999.

Reed, M.J.; Purohit, A.; Woo, L.V.L.; Newman, S.P. & Potter, B.V.L. (2005). Steroid Sulfatase: Molecular Biology, Regulation, and Inhibition. *Endocrine Rev.*, Vol.26, No.2, (April 2005), pp. 171-202, ISSN 0163-769X

Reed, M.J. & Potter, B.V.L. (2006). Preparation of heterocyclic sulfamate compounds as inhibitors of oestrone sulfatase and aromatase for treating of cancer. *U.S. Pat. Appl. Publ. US 2006 241173*, filed 17 November 2004, 1997, and issued 26 October, 2006.

Reid, D.M. (2009). Prevention of osteoporosis after breast cancer. *Maturitas*, Vol.64, No.1, (September 2009), pp. 1-3, ISSN 0378-5122

Römer, W.; Oettel, M.; Droescher, P. & Schwarz, S. (1997). Novel «scavestrogens» and their radical scavenging effects, iron-chelating, and total antioxidative activities: Δ8(9)-dehydro derivatives of 17α-estradiol and 17β-estradiol. *Steroids*, Vol.63, No.2, (March 1997), pp. 304-310, ISSN 00390128X

Römer, W.; Oettel, M.; Menzenbach, B.; Droescher, P. & Schwarz, S. (1997). Novel estrogens and their radical scavenging effects, iron-chelating, and total antioxidative activities: 17α-substituted analogs of Δ9(11)-dehydro-17β-estradiol. *Steroids*, Vol.62, No.10, (November 1997), pp. 689-694, ISSN 0039-128X

diSalle, E. & Robinson, C.H. (1990). Novel Irreversible Aromatase Inhibitors. *Ann. N-Y Acad. Sci.*, Vol.595, (June 1990), pp. 357-367, ISBN 0-89766-566-X

Ruiz-Larrea, M.; Martin, C.; Martınez, R.; Navarro, R.; Lacort, M. & Miller, N. (2000). Antioxidant activities of estrogens against aqueous and lipophilic radicals; differences between phenol and catechol estrogens. *Chemistry and Physics of Lipids*, Vol.105, No.2, (April 2000), pp. 179–188, ISSN 0009-3084

Russo, J.; Lareef, M.H.; Tahin, Q.; Hu, Y.-Fu; Slater, C.; Ao, X. & Russo, I.H. (2002). 17β-Estradiol is carcinogenic in human breast epithelial cells. *J. Steroid Biochem. Mol. Biol.*, Vol.80, No.2, (February 2002), pp. 149-162, ISSN 0960-0760

Sak, K.; Evaraus, H. (2004). Nongenomic effects of 17β-estradiol-diversity of membrane binding sites. *J. Steroid Biochem. Mol. Biol.*, Vol.88, No.4-5, (April 2004), pp. 323-335, ISSN 0960-0760

Sanchez-Moreno, C. (2002). Methods used to evaluate the free radical scavenging activity in foods and biological systems. *Food Sci. Tech. Int.*, Vol.8, No.3, (June 2002), pp. 121-137, ISSN 1082-0132

Santen, R.J.; Yue, W.; Naftolin, E.; Mor, G. & Berstein, L. (1999). The potential of aromatase inhibitors in breast cancer prevention. *Endocrine-Related Cancer*, Vol.6, No.2, (June 1999), pp. 235-243, ISSN 1351-0088

Sato, M.; Kim, J.; Short, L.L.; Slemend, C.W. & Bryant, H.U. (1995). Longitudinal and Cross-Sectional Analysis of Raloxifene Effects on Tibiae from Ovariectomized Aged Rats. *J. Pharmacol. Exp. Ther.*, Vol.272, No.3, (March 1995), pp. 1252-1259, ISSN 0022-3565

Sato, M.; Turner, C.H.; Wang, T.; Agrian, M.D.; Rowley, E. & Bryant, H.U. (1998). LY353381.HCl: a novel raloxifene analog with improved SERM potency and efficacy in vivo. *J. Pharmacol. Exp. Ther.*, Vol.287, No.1, (January 1998), pp. 1-7, ISSN 0022-3565.

Sato, M.; Crese, T.A.; Dodge, J.A.; Bryant, H.U. & Turner, C.H. (1999). Emerging Therapy for the Prevention or Treatment of Postmenopausal Osteoporosis. *J. Med. Chem.*, Vol.42, No.1, (January 1999), pp. 1-24, ISSN 0022-2623.

Schreiner, E.P. & Billich, A. (2004). Estrone formiate: a novel type of irreversible inhibitors of human steroid sulfatase. *Bioorg. Med. Chem. Letters*, Vol.14, No.19, (October 2004), pp. 4999-5002, ISSN 0968-0896

Schwabe, J.W.R.; Neuhaus, D. & Rhodes, D. (1990). Solution structure of the DNA-binding domain of the oestrogen receptor. *Nature*, Vol.348, No.6300, (November 1990), pp. 458-461, ISSN 0028-0836

Seeger, H.; Wallwiener, D.; Kraemer, E. & Mueck, A.O. (2006). Comparison of possible carcinogenic estradiol metabolites: Effect on proliferation, apoptosis and metastasis of human breast cancer cells. *Maturitas*, Vol.54, No.1, (April 2006), pp. 72-77, ISSN 0378-5122

Selivanov, S.I. & Shavva, A.G. (2002). An NMR Study of the Spatial Structure and Intramolecular Dynamics of Modified Analogues of Steroid Hormones. *Russ. J. Bioorg. Chem.*, Vol.28, No.3 (May-June 2002), pp. 194-208, ISSN 1068-1620

Sharp, J.C.; Copps, J.C.; Liu, Q.; Ryner, L.N.; Sebastian, R.A.; Zeng, G.Q.; Smith, S.; Niere, J.O.; Tomanek, B. & Sato, M. (2000). Analysis of Ovariectomy and Estrogen Effects on Body Composition in Rats by X-Rays and Magnetic Resonance Imaging Techniques. *J. Bone Miner. Res.*, Vol.15, No.1, (January 2000), p. 138-136, ISSN 0884-0431

Shavva, A.G.; Zlobina, I.V.; Nersisyan, G.G.; Matevosyan, I.N.; Ryzhenkov, V.E. & Prokop'ev, A.A. (1987). Racemic B-nor-18,D-bishomo-9-isoestrone with hypocholesterolemic activity. *U.S.S.R. SU 1371962*, filed 20 February 1981, and issued 8 October 1987.

Shavva, A.G.; Vlasova, K.V.; Tsogoeva, S.B.; Egorov, M.S. & Yakutseni, P.P. (2002). A Study of the Binding of Estradiol and 8-Isoestraiol to the Estrogen α-Receptor by

Molecular Modeling. *Russ. J. Bioorg. Chem.*, Vol.28, No.3, (May-June 2002), pp. 209-214, ISSN 0132-3423

Shavva, A.G.; Starova, G.L.; Selivanov, S.I. & Morozkina, S.N. (2008). Molecular structures of some D-homo-6-oxa-8α steroid estrogen analogues. *Chem. Heterocycl. Comp.*, No.2, (February 2008), pp. 202-207, ISSN 0132-6244 (Rus. Ed.)

Shen, Li; Qui, S.; van Breeman, R.B.; Zhang, F.; Chen, Y. & Bolton, J.L. (1997). Reaction of Premarin Metabolite 4-Hydroxyequilenine Semiquinone Radical with 2'-Deoxyguanosine: Formation of Unusual Cyclic Adducts. *J. Am. Chem. Soc.*, Vol.119, No.45, (November 1997), pp. 11126-11127, ISSN 0002-7863

Shiau, A.K.; Barstad, D.; Loria, P.M.; Cheng, L.; Kushner, P.J.; Agard, D.A. & Green, G.L. (1998). The structure based of estrogen receptor/coactivator recognition and the antagonism of this interaction by tamoxifen. *Cell*, Vol.95, No.7, (December 1998), pp. 927-937. ISSN 0092-8674

Silverman, S.; Chines, A.; Zanchetta, J.; Genant, H.; Kendler, D.; de la Losa, F.R.; Kung, A.; Constantine, G. & Adachi, J. (2010). Sustained Efficacy of Bazedoxifen in preventing Fracture in Postmenopausal Women with Osteoporosis: Results of a 5-year, Randomized, Placebo-controlled Study. *Bone*, Vol.46, Suppl.1, (March 2010), S-63, ISSN 8756-3282

Simpkins, J.A.; Yang, S-H.; Liu, R.; Perez, E.; Cai, Zu Y., Covey, D.F. & Green, P.S. (2004). Estrogen-Like Compounds for Ischemic Neuroprotection. *Stroke*, Vol.35, No.11, Suppl.1, (November 2004), pp. 2648-2651, ISSN 0039-2499

Simpkins, J.W.; Singh, M. & Bishop, J. (1994). Methods for neuroprotection. *US Pat. 5554601*, filed 4 October 1994, and issued 10 September 1994.

Siow, R.; Li, F.; Rowlands, D.; de Winter, P. & Mann, G. (2007). Cardiovascular targets for estrogens and phytoestrogens: Transcriptional regulation of nitric oxide synthase and antioxidant defense genes. *Free Radical Biology & Medicine*, Vol.42, No.1, (April 2007), pp. 909–925, ISSN 0891-5849

Sippl, W. (2002). Binding Affinity Prediction of Novel Estrogen Receptor Ligands Using Receptor-Based 3D QSAR Methods. *Bioorg. Med. Chem.*, Vol.10, No.12, (December 2002), pp. 3741-3755, ISSN 0968-0896

Steinberg, D.; Parthasarathy, S.; Carev, T. E.; Khoo, J.C. & Witztum, J.L. (1989). Beyong Cholesterol. Modifications of Low-Density Lipoprotein That Increase Its Atherogenicity. *New Engl. J. Med.*, Vol.320, No.14, (April 1989), pp. 915-924, ISSN 0028-4793

Sulistiany, S.J.; Adelman, A.C.; Jayo, J. & St. Clair, R.W. (1995). Effects of 17α-Dihydroequilin Sulfate, a Conjugate Equine Estrogene, and Ethynylestradiol on Atherosclerosis in Cholesterol-Fed Rabbits. *Atherosclerosis, Thrombosis, and Vascular Biology*, Vol.15, No.6, (June 1995), pp. 837-846, ISSN 1079-5642

Sumi, C.; Yokoro, K. & Matsushima, R. (1984). Preventive effects of antiestrogen on mammary and pituitary tumorogenesis in rats. *Br. J. Cancer*, Vol.50, No.6, (December 1984), pp. 779-784, ISSN 0007-0920

Sumino, H.; Ichikawa, S.; Kasama, S.; Takahashi, T.; Kumakura, H.; Takayama, Y.; Kanda, T. & Kurabayashi, M. (2006). Different effects of oral conjugated estrogen and transdermal estradiol on arterial stiffness and vascular inflammatory markers in postmenopausal women. *Atherosclerosis* (Amsterdam, Neth.), Vol.189, No.2, (December 2006), pp. 436-442, ISSN 1809-2942.

Suzuki, R.N.; Newman, S.P.; Purohit, A.; Leese, M.P.; Potter, B.V.L. & Reed, M.J. (2003). Growth inhibition of multi-drug-resistant breast cells by 2-methoxyoestradiol-bis-sulphamate and 2-ethyloestradiol-bis-sulphamate. *J. Steroid Biochem. Mol. Biol.*, Vol.84, No.2-3, (February 2003), pp. 269-278, ISSN 0960-0760

Tamrazi, A.; Carlson, K.E.; Rodrigues, A.L. & Katzenellenbogen, J.A. (2005). Coactivator Proteins as Determinants of Estrogen Receptor Structure and Function: Spectroscopic Evidence for a novel Coactivator-Stabilized Receptor Conformation. *Mol. Endocrinol.*, Vol.19, No.6, (June 2005), pp. 1516-1528, ISSN 0888-8809

Tanabe, M.; Peters, R.; Chao, W-R. & Shigeno, K. (1999). Estrone sulfamate inhibitors of estrone sulfatase, and associated pharmaceutical compounds and methods of use. *PCT Int. Appl. WO 99/33858*, filed 24 December 1997 and issued 21 December 1999.

Tcherepanova, I.; Puigserver, P., Norris, J.D.; Spiegelman, B.M. & McDonnel, D.P. (2000). Modulation of Estrogen Receptor-α Transcriptional Activity by the Coactivator PGC-1. *J. Biol. Chem.*, Vol.275, No.21, (May 2000), pp. 16302-16308, ISSN 0021-9258

Thibodeau, P.; Kachadourian, R.; Lemay, R.; Bisson, M.; Day, B. & Paquette, B. (2002). In vitro pro- and antioxidant properties of estrogens. *Journal of Steroid Biochemistry & Molecular Biology*, Vol.81, No.3, (July 2002), pp. 227–236, ISSN 0960-0760

Tong, W.; Perkins, R.; Xing, Li; Welsh, W.J. & Sheehan, D.M. (1997). QSAR Models for Binding of Estrogenic Compounds to Estrogen Receptor α and β Subtype. *Endocrinology*, Vol.138, No.9, (September 1997), pp. 4022-4025, ISSN 0013-7227

Tora, L.; White, J.; Brou, C.; Tasset, D.; Webeter, V.; Scheer, E. & Shambon, P. (1989). The human estrogen receptor has two independent nonacidic transcriptional activation functions. *Cell*, Vol.59, No.3, (November 1989), pp. 477-487, ISSN 0092-8674

Tremblay, G.B.; Tremblay, A.; Copeland, N. G.; Gilbert, D. J.; Jenkins, N. A.; Labrie, F.; Giguere, V. (1997). Cloning, chromosomal localization, and functional analysis of the murine estrogen receptor beta. *Mol. Endocrinol.*, Vol.11, No.3, (March 1997), pp. 353-365, ISSN 0888-8809

Tremblay, M.R.; Auger, S. & Poirier, D. (1995). Synthesis of 16-(bromoalkyl)-estradiols having inhibitory effects on human placental estradiol 17β-hydroxysteroid dehydrogenase (17-beta-HSD type 1). *Bioorg. Med. Chem.*, Vol.3, No.5, (May 1995), pp. 505-523, ISSN 0968-0896

Tremblay, M.R. & Poirier, D. (1996). Synthesis of 16-[carbamoyl(bromomethyl)-alkyl]estradiol: a potential dual-action inhibitor designed to blockade estrogen action and biosynthesis. *J. Chem. Soc., Perkin Trans. 1*, No.22, (November 1996), pp. 2765-2771, ISSN 0300-922X

Turner, C.H.; Sato, M. & Bryant, H. (1994). Raloxifene Preserves Bone Strength and Bone Mass in Ovariectomized Rats. *Endocrinology*, Vol.135, No.5, (May 1994), pp. 2001-2005, ISSN 0013-7227

Tzukerman, M.T.; Esty, A.; Santiso-Mere, D.; Danielian, P.; Parker, M.G.; Stein, R.B.; Pike, J.W. & McDonnell, D.P. (1994). Human estrogen receptor transcriptional capacity is determined by both cellular and promoter context and mediated by functionally distinct intramolecular regions. *Mol. Endocrinol.*, Vol.8, No.1, (January 1994), pp. 21-30, ISSN 0888-8809

Vedder, H.; Anthes, N.; Stumm G.; Wurz C.; Behl C. & Krieg J. (1999). Estrogen hormones reduce lipid peroxidation in cell and tissues of central nervous system. *J. of Neurochemistry*, Vol.72, No.6, (December 1999), pp. 2531-38, ISSN 1471-4159

Venkov, C.D.; Rankin, A.B. & Vaughan, D.E. (1996). Identification of authentic estrogen receptor in cultured endothelial cells: a potential mechanism for steroid hormone regulation of endothelial function. *Circulation*, Vol.94, No.4, (August 1996), pp. 727-733, ISSN 0009-7322

Vihko, P.; Härkönen, P.; Oduwole, O.; Törn, S.; Kurkela, R.; Porvari, K.; Pulkka, A. & Isomaa, V. (2002). 17β-Hydroxysteroid dehydrogenases and cancers. *J. Steroid Biochem. Mol. Biol.*, Vol.83, No.1-5, (December 2002), pp. 119-122, ISSN 0960-0760

Vogelvang, T.E.; van der Mooren, M.J.; Mijatovic, V. & Kenemas, P. (2006). Emerging Selective Estrogen Receptor Modulators Special Focus on Effects on Coronary Heart Disease in Postmenopausal Women. *Drugs*, Vol.66, No.2, (2006), pp. 191-221, ISSN 0012-6667

Green, S.; Walter, P.; Kumar, V.; Krust, A.; Bornert, J-M.; Argos, P. & Chambon, P. (1986). Human estrogen receptor cDNA: sequence, expression and homology to v-erb-A. *Nature*, Vol.320, No.6058, (March 1986), pp. 134-139, ISSN 0028-0836

Wang, C.; Cui, W.; Zhao, M.; Yang, J.; Peng, S. (2003). Studies on the synthesis and anti-osteoporosis of estrogen-GHRPs linkers. *Bioorg. Med. Chem. Letters*, Vol.13, No.1, (January 2003), pp. 143-146, ISSN 0960-984X

Warner, M. & Gustafsson, J-A. (2006). Nongenomic effect of estrogen: Why all the uncertainty? *Steroids*, Vol.71, No.1, (January 2006), pp. 91-95, ISSN 0039-128X

Watanabe, T.; Akishita, M.; Nakaoka, T.; Kozaki, K.; Miyahara, Y.; He, H.; Ogita, T.; Inoue, S.; Marumatsu, M.; Yamashita, M. & Ouchi, Y. (2003). Estrogen receptor β mediate the inhibitory effect of estradiol on vascular smooth muscle cell proliferation. *Cardiovasc. Res.*, Vol.59, No.3, (September 2003), pp. 734-744, ISSN 0008-6363

Wiese, T.E.; Polin, L.A.; Palomino, E. & Books, S.C. (1997). Induction of the Estrogen Specific Mitogenic Response of MCF-7 Cells by Selected Analogues of Estradiol-17β: A 3D QSAR Study. *J. Med. Chem.*, Vol.40, No.22, (October 1997), pp. 3659-3669, ISSN 0022-2623

Willson, T.M.; Norris, J.D.; Wagner, B.L.; Asplin, I.; Baer, P.; Brown, H.R.; Jones, S.A.; Henke, B.; Sauls, H.; Wolfe, S.; Morris, D.C. & McDonnel, D.P. (1997). Dissection of the molecular mechanism of action of GW5638, a novel estrogen receptor ligand, provides insights into the role of estrogen receptor in bone. *Endocrinology*, Vol.138, No.9, (September 1997), pp. 3901-3911, ISSN 0013-7227

Wise, P.; Dubal, D.; Wilson, M.; Rau, S. & Bottner, M. (2001). Neuroprotective effects of estrogens – new insights into mechanisms of action. *Endocrinology*, Vol.142, No.3, (March 2001), pp. 969-973, ISSN 0013-7227

Wolohan, P. & Reichert, D.E. (2004). Use of binding energy in comparative molecular field analysis of isoform selective estrogen receptor ligands. *J. Mol. Graphics Modeling*, Vol.23, No.1, (September 2004), pp. 23-38, ISSN 1093-3263

Wong, C.W.; Komm, B. & Cheskis, B.J. (2001). Structure–Function Evaluation of ER α and β Interplay with SRC Family Coactivators. ER Selective Ligands. *Biochemistry*, Vol.40, No.23, (June 2001), pp. 6756-6765, ISSN 0006-2960

Wuelfert, E.; Pringle, A.K. & Sundstrom, L.E. (2002). Preparation of neuroprotective 7-beta-hydroxy-steroids. *PCT Int. Appl. WO 02 00224*, filed 29 June 2000 and issued 3 January 2002.

Wurtz, J.-M.; Egner, U.; Heinrich, N.; Moras, D. & Mueller-Fahrnow, A. (1998). Three-Dimensional Models of Estrogen Receptor Ligand Binding Domain Complexes,

Based on Related Crystal Structure and Mutational and Structure-Activity Relationship Data. *J. Med. Chem.*, Vol.41, No.11, (May 1998), pp. 1803-1814, ISSN 0022-2623

Xia S., Coi, Z-Y., Thio, L.L., Kim-Han, S.S., Dugan, L.L., Covey D.F., Rothman, S.M. (2002). The estrogen receptor is not essential for all estrogen neuroprotection: new evidence from a new analog. *Neurobiology of Disease*, Vol.9, No.3, (April 2002), pp. 282-293, ISSN 0969-9961

Xu, J. & Li, Q. (2003). Review of the in Vitro Functions of the p160 Steroid Receptor Coactivators Family. *Mol. Endocrinol.*, Vol.17, No.9, (September 2003), pp. 1681-1692, ISSN 0888-8809

Yadav, M.R.; Sabale, P.M.; Giridhar, R.; Zimmer, C. & Haupenthal, J. (2011). Synthesis of some novel androstanes as potential aromatase inhibitors. *Steroids*, Vol.76, No.5, (May 2011), pp. 464-470, ISSN 0039-128X

Yokogawa, K.; Toshima, K.; Yamoto, K.; Nishioka, T.; Sakura, N.; Sakura, N. & Miyamoto, K. (2006). Pharmacokinetic Advantage of an Intranasal Preparation of a Novel Anti-osteoporosis Drug, L-Asp-Hexapeptide-Congugated Estradiol. *Biol. Pharm. Bull.*, Vol.29, No.6, (June 2006), pp. 1229-1233, ISSN 0928-6158

Yoshida, H. &, Fukunishi, R. (1981). Effect of sex steroids on the development of 1,2-dimethyl-benz[a]antracene-induced mammary dysplasia in neonatally and androgenized rats. *Gann*, Vol.72, No.2, (April 1981), pp. 315-317, ISSN 0016-450X

Yue, W.; Santen, R.J.; Wang, J.P.; Hamilton, C.J. & Demers, L.M. (1999). Aromatase within the breast. *Endocrine-Related Cancer*, Vol.6, No.2, (June 1999), pp. 157-164, ISSN 1351-0088

Zhang, F.; Chen, Y.; Pisha, E.; Shen, Li; Xiong, Y.; van Breeman, R.B. & Bolton, J.L. (1999). The major metabolite of equilenine, 4-hydroxyequilenine, autooxidized to an o-quinone which isomerizes to potent cytotoxin 4-hydroxyequilenine-o-quinone. *Chem. Res. Toxicol.*, Vol.12, No.2, (February 1999), pp. 204-213, ISSN 0893-228X

Zhang, Q.; Aft, R.L. & Gross, M.L. (2008). Estrogen Carcinogenesis: Specific Identification of Estrogen-Modified Nucleobase in Breast Tissue from Women. *Chem. Res. Toxicol.*, Vol.21, No.8, (August 2008), pp. 1509-1513, ISSN 0893-228X

Zhu, B.T.; Han, G-Z.; Shim, J-Y.; Wen, Y. & Jiang, X-R. (2006). Quantitative Structure-Activity Relationship of Various Endogenous Estrogen Metabolites for Human Estrogen Receptor $\alpha$ and $\beta$ Subtypes: Insights into the Structural Determinants Favoring a Differential Subtype Binding. *Endocrinology*, Vol.147, No.3, (September 2006), pp. 4132-4150, ISSN 0013-7227

# Permissions

The contributors of this book come from diverse backgrounds, making this book a truly international effort. This book will bring forth new frontiers with its revolutionizing research information and detailed analysis of the nascent developments around the world.

We would like to thank Hassan Abduljabbar, for lending his expertise to make the book truly unique. He has played a crucial role in the development of this book. Without his invaluable contribution this book wouldn't have been possible. He has made vital efforts to compile up to date information on the varied aspects of this subject to make this book a valuable addition to the collection of many professionals and students.

This book was conceptualized with the vision of imparting up-to-date information and advanced data in this field. To ensure the same, a matchless editorial board was set up. Every individual on the board went through rigorous rounds of assessment to prove their worth. After which they invested a large part of their time researching and compiling the most relevant data for our readers. Conferences and sessions were held from time to time between the editorial board and the contributing authors to present the data in the most comprehensible form. The editorial team has worked tirelessly to provide valuable and valid information to help people across the globe.

Every chapter published in this book has been scrutinized by our experts. Their significance has been extensively debated. The topics covered herein carry significant findings which will fuel the growth of the discipline. They may even be implemented as practical applications or may be referred to as a beginning point for another development. Chapters in this book were first published by InTech; hereby published with permission under the Creative Commons Attribution License or equivalent.

The editorial board has been involved in producing this book since its inception. They have spent rigorous hours researching and exploring the diverse topics which have resulted in the successful publishing of this book. They have passed on their knowledge of decades through this book. To expedite this challenging task, the publisher supported the team at every step. A small team of assistant editors was also appointed to further simplify the editing procedure and attain best results for the readers.

Our editorial team has been hand-picked from every corner of the world. Their multi-ethnicity adds dynamic inputs to the discussions which result in innovative outcomes. These outcomes are then further discussed with the researchers and contributors who give their valuable feedback and opinion regarding the same. The feedback is then collaborated with the researches and they are edited in a comprehensive manner to aid the understanding of the subject.

Apart from the editorial board, the designing team has also invested a significant amount of their time in understanding the subject and creating the most relevant covers. They scrutinized every image to scout for the most suitable representation of the subject and create an appropriate cover for the book.

The publishing team has been involved in this book since its early stages. They were actively engaged in every process, be it collecting the data, connecting with the contributors or procuring relevant information. The team has been an ardent support to the editorial, designing and production team. Their endless efforts to recruit the best for this project, has resulted in the accomplishment of this book. They are a veteran in the field of academics and their pool of knowledge is as vast as their experience in printing. Their expertise and guidance has proved useful at every step. Their uncompromising quality standards have made this book an exceptional effort. Their encouragement from time to time has been an inspiration for everyone.

The publisher and the editorial board hope that this book will prove to be a valuable piece of knowledge for researchers, students, practitioners and scholars across the globe.

# List of Contributors

**Roberto Domínguez and Angélica Flores**
Facultad de Estudios Superiores Zaragoza, Universidad Nacional Autónoma de México, México

**Sara E. Cruz-Morales**
Facultad de Estudios Superiores Iztacala, Universidad Nacional Autónoma de México, México

**Raghava Varman Thampan**
MIMS Research Foundation, A Division of Malabar Institute of Medical Sciences, Ltd. (MIMS), Calicut, Kerala, India

**Karin Tamm, Marina Suhorutshenko, Miia Rõõm, Jaak Simm and Madis Metsis**
Centre for Biology of Integrated Systems, Tallinn University of Technology, Tallinn, Estonia

**Karin Tamm and Madis Metsis**
Competence Centre on Reproductive Medicine and Biology, Tartu, Estonia

**Karin Tamm**
Nova Vita Clinic, Tallinn, Estonia

**Marzena Kamieniczna and Maciej Kurpisz**
Institute of Human Genetics Polish Academy of Sciences, Poland

**Anna Havrylyuk**
Danylo Halytsky Lviv National Medical University, Department of Clinical Immunology and Allergology, Ukraine

**Hajime Ueshiba**
Department of Internal Medicine, Toho University School of Medicine, Tokyo, Japan

**Maria Felicia Faienza and Luciano Cavallo**
Department of Biomedicine of Developmental Age, University of Bari, Italy

**Kyoko Sakai, Tomoyuki Ohno, Kazuyuki Kanemasa and Yoshio Sumida**
Center for Digestive and Liver Diseases, Nara City Hospital, Japan

**Yutaka Inada, Naohisa Yoshida, Kohichiroh Yasui, Yoshito Itoh, Yuji Naito and Toshikazu Yoshikawa**
Department of Gastroenterology and Hepatology, Kyoto Prefectural University of Medicine, Kyoto, Japan

**Leonie Quinn, Nicola Cranna, Jue Er Amanda Lee and Naomi Mitchell**
Department of Anatomy and Cell Biology, University of Melbourne, Australia

**Jane Lin and Ross Hannan**
Peter MacCallum Cancer Centre, St Andrews Place, East Melbourne, Australia

**Ross Hannan**
Department of Biochemistry and Molecular Biology, University of Melbourne, Australia
Department of Biochemistry and Cell Biology, Monash University, Australia

**Scott J. Lusher and Jacob de Vlieg**
Departments of Molecular Design & Informatics, The Netherlands
Netherlands eScience Center, The Netherlands

**Paolo Conti and Pedro H. Hermkens**
Departments of Medicinal Chemistry, The Netherlands

**Wim Dokter**
Departments of Immune Therapeutics, MSD, Oss, The Netherlands

**Pedro H. Hermkens**
Institute of Molecules & Materials, The Netherlands

**Jacob de Vlieg**
Computational Drug Discovery Group, Radboud University, Nijmegen, The Netherlands

**Alexander Shavva, Svetlana Morozkina and Olga Galkina**
Saint-Petersburg State University, Chemistry Faculty, Department of Natural Products Chemistry, Russia

Printed in the USA
CPSIA information can be obtained
at www.ICGtesting.com
JSHW011429221024
72173JS00004B/729